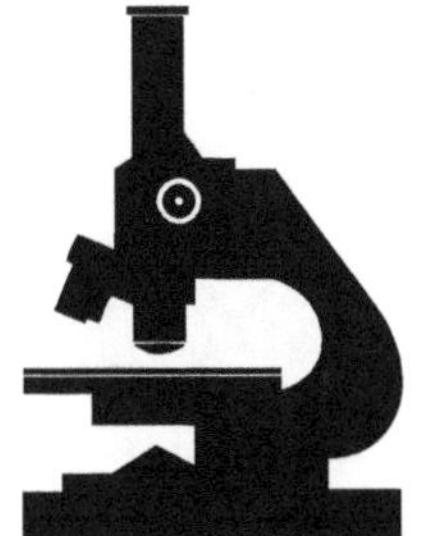

HOW HIV / AIDS SET THE STAGE FOR THE COVID CRISIS

NEVILLE HODGKINSON

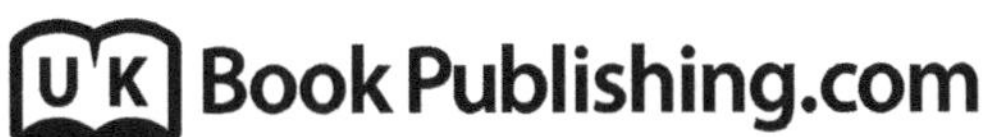

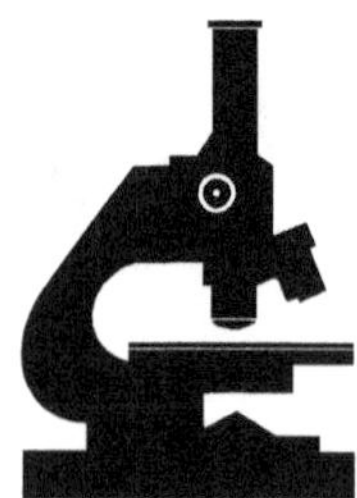

Editing, design, typesetting and publishing by UK Book Publishing

www.ukbookpublishing.com

ISBN: 978-1-915338-50-1

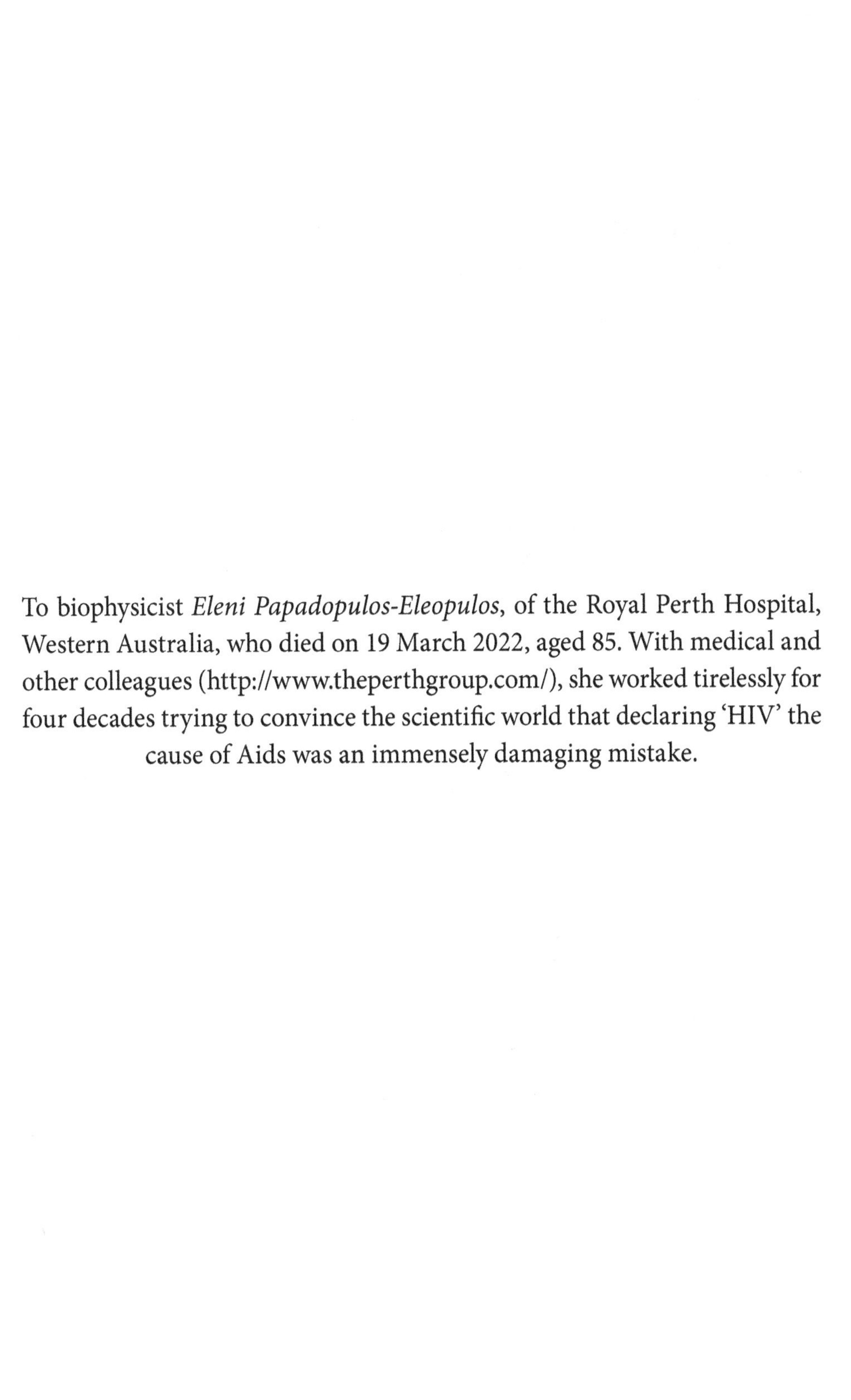

To biophysicist *Eleni Papadopulos-Eleopulos*, of the Royal Perth Hospital, Western Australia, who died on 19 March 2022, aged 85. With medical and other colleagues (http://www.theperthgroup.com/), she worked tirelessly for four decades trying to convince the scientific world that declaring 'HIV' the cause of Aids was an immensely damaging mistake.

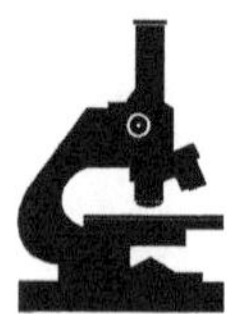

AUTHOR BIOGRAPHY

Neville Hodgkinson is an author and journalist who specialised for much of his career in writing about health and medicine. His posts included social policy correspondent of *The Times*, health editor of the *Sunday Express*, and medical and science correspondent of the *Daily Mail* and *Sunday Times*. After a break of several years concentrating on spiritual study and the emerging science of consciousness, he returned to medical journalism in 2021 with a series of more than 60 articles challenging Covid orthodoxy. His books include *Will To Be Well - the Real Alternative Medicine* and *I Know How to Live, I Know How to Die – the Teachings of Dadi Janki.*

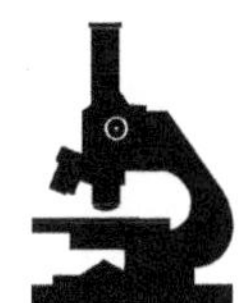

CONTENTS

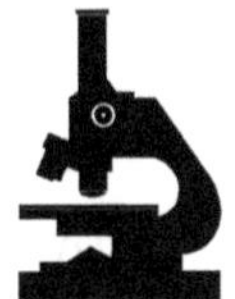

FOREWORD

Oxford, July 2022

When Covid-19 started to shake the world in early 2020, I felt a disturbing sense of *déjà vu* – not primarily because of the damage caused by the virus, but because of the response to it.

In an instant, powerful, state-funded bureaucracies, supported by anxious politicians, were mishandling the emergency in such a way as to devastate millions of lives. Most of the parties involved may have meant well, but between them, Big Brother, Big Pharma, Big Tech, mass media and academia came together in an alliance that caused a far-reaching betrayal of individual, social, and national interests.

As a former medical and science correspondent with UK newspapers, I was starkly reminded of the arrival in the 1980s of Aids, the immune system failure seen initially in a small subset of gay men and subsequently said to be caused by HIV, a killer virus putting everyone on the planet at risk.

In enormously expensive public health campaigns, we were told: 'Aids does not discriminate'. That turned out to be just as untrue as the pretence that all of us were equally at risk from SARS-COV-2.

I do not believe that in either case, the individuals centrally involved started out with a deliberate attempt to cause harm. That is despite indications to the contrary with Covid, including a trail of patents for genetic sequences subsequently found in SARS-COV-2.* These were, however, a sign that gene technology was advancing in ways that could wreak havoc on humanity. On the basis that 'If we don't do it, someone else will', preparations were being made in anticipation of a public health disaster, whether it should come about

---

* Painstakingly documented by the author and financial advisor Dr David Martin.

through accident or design.

With both HIV/Aids and Covid, a combination of immediate, urgent needs and pressures brought into being illusory ideas and policies that then took on a life of their own, as powerful commercial, political and social forces came into play.

This book reproduces a work first published in 1996 called *Aids: The Failure of Contemporary Science – How a Virus That Never Was Deceived the World*. It tells of my own gradual and reluctant awakening to the weakness of the 'deadly new virus' beliefs about Aids, and to the strengths of a completely different scientific account of what was going on. It describes massive resistance met by *The Sunday Times*, my newspaper at the time, when we put multiple aspects of the case against HIV before the public.

Damaging illusions about Aids persist to this day. My hope is that re-publishing the account of how these arose may accelerate their demise, and also help illuminate aspects of the dynamics behind the Covid catastrophe. Socially and politically, Covid-19 is HIV/Aids *writ large*.

With Aids, sympathy for early gay victims made the virus theory far more acceptable than linking the syndrome to specific lifestyle risks, as had first been proposed. Hundreds of billions of dollars subsequently flowed into research and treatment, a bonanza continuing to this day. The main beneficiaries have been drug companies, health bureaucrats, science journals, researchers, media groups, and countless non-governmental organisations.

With Covid, embarrassment surrounding the genetically engineered origins of SARS-COV-2 led to organised deception of the public over what was going on, and to exaggerated fears about the risks involved. An unholy alliance between public health bureaucrats and commercial interests led to the betrayal of long-established principles for pandemic management as well as vaccine safety.

Scientific *hubris* and institutional corruption contributed to both disasters.

Anthony Fauci, who as head of the US National Institute of Allergy and Infectious Diseases became America's Aids 'tsar' in the 1980s, played the same role with Covid nearly 40 years on. He set a lead in creating the global panic, dismissing medical pleas that protection should be focused on the most vulnerable rather than through generalised lockdowns. Fauci, along with Jeremy Farrar of the UK's Wellcome Trust, was at the heart of the scientific establishment's efforts to hide SARS-COV-2's origins, as resulting from genetic modification of a bat virus by US and Chinese researchers.

Health agencies in the UK and many other countries quickly fell into step. They recklessly promoted the mass administration of experimental vaccines, which brought billions in profits but were far from 'safe and effective', as widely touted. It is already clear, for those willing to see, that by stimulating the body into producing the toxic 'spike protein' characteristic of the virus, the jabs are capable of doing immeasurable harm. Apart from immediate death and injury suffered by many, long-term risks include a threat to fertility arising from a concentration of vaccine contents in the ovaries.

Cheap, off-patent drugs such as Ivermectin, used by some doctors to good effect as early treatment for Covid, were marginalised or banned, while US regulators fast-tracked vastly more expensive products such as Remdesivir ($3,000 per course), without proof of effectiveness and with serious safety concerns.

Likewise, in the first years of Aids, Fauci and other government scientists promoted to the hilt the idea that a deadly new virus was the cause, suppressing all other theories about how the syndrome came about. On the basis of fraudulent studies, they drove widespread administration of an immensely toxic and expensive drug, AZT. This earned hundreds of millions for the American company Burroughs-Wellcome and its UK parent, the Wellcome Foundation (now subsumed in the British pharmaceutical giant GSK). The drug was later recognised to have killed thousands of people.

The US Government's National Institutes of Health, the largest biomedical research agency in the world, dispenses billions of taxpayer dollars globally and many of its own scientists receive millions in royalties, mostly from drug companies. Supposedly philanthropic organisations such as the Gates Foundation, and the Wellcome Trust, also wield massive influence on biomedical research that in many instances benefits their own investment arms, distorting spending priorities.

This concentration of power, much of it also reflected in the financing, outlook and activity of the World Health Organization (WHO), meant that with both Aids and Covid, panic and profiteering ruled while genuine science flew out of the window.

In the case of Aids, it took nearly three decades for the WHO to admit there was no general heterosexual Aids epidemic. Even then, many die-hard HIV advocates refused to accept the verdict and in 2018 the WHO was still claiming the existence of a hidden epidemic, with one in four people unaware that they are victims of the purported virus. 'HIV=Aids=Death' was a horrible curse bestowed on those who tested positive when the panic was at its height and it is still a 'hex' blighting the lives of many, especially in Africa.

Wall of silence protecting virus theory

Aids: The Failure of Contemporary Science takes the reader gently, step by step, towards the 'impossible' conclusion that the entire HIV construct is an illusion.

At the time of writing it, I was still reeling from the intensity of the attacks on my newspaper work as well as from the challenge I was experiencing to my own faith in science, which I had long regarded as humanity's best hope for a better future.

But by the time the book was completed I knew for sure that the test for 'HIV' is not just inaccurate, but that it had never been shown to specify the presence of a unique disease agent. I discovered during my researches that this was implicitly understood by regulators from the very beginning, even while the tests were being rolled out internationally. One hundred experts from 34 countries were told at a WHO meeting in Geneva in 1986 that the test kits could only be used as a broad screen for possible abnormalities in blood, and not to diagnose HIV infection. Despite that cautionary warning, a representative from the US Food and Drug Administration told the meeting that public health needs had caused usage to expand and 'it was simply not practical' to stop this.

The falsehoods and errors are such a huge potential embarrassment to leaders within the worlds of science and medicine, and their followers in government and the media, that there have been decades of stony silence around the issue, largely kept from public view until now. The late Tom Bethell, a British-born author and journalist, put *Aids: The Failure of*

Contemporary Science top of his list of 'Books You're Not Supposed to Read' on the subject in his 2005 work *The Politically Incorrect Guide to Science**.

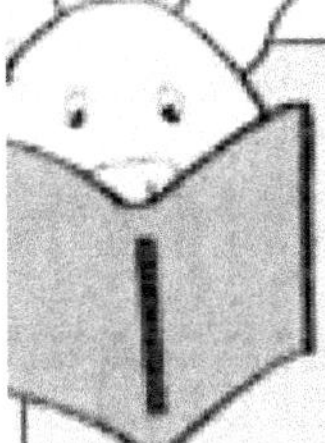

Books You're Not Supposed to Read

AIDS: The Failure of Contemporary Science by Neville Hodgkinson; London: The Fourth Estate, 1996.

Inventing the AIDS Virus by Peter H. Duesberg; Washington, D.C.: Regnery Publishing, 1996.

Oncogenes, Aneuploidy and AIDS: A Scientific Life and Times of Peter H. Duesberg by Harvey Bialy; Berkeley: North Atlantic Books, 2004.

The mishandling of Covid, however, has led to a reopening of the case against 'HIV', with critics arguing that unless the scientific community examine and own up to the failures surrounding Aids science, we will be at risk of similar public health disasters in the future.

* Regnery Publishing, Washington, D.C., 2005

A crucial point of departure between Aids and Covid is that whereas 'HIV' is mythological in character, SARS-COV-2 is a genuine disease entity.*

In both crises, however, positive results with rushed and inappropriately applied tests were misinterpreted as 'cases'. This misuse promoted the false idea that well people, without symptoms, were infecting others, further inflating the fears.

With Aids, a generation was taught to equate sex with death because of a supposedly lethal, new, sexually transmitted virus. To drive home this message, public health officials internationally promoted 'safer sex' measures including the use of condoms, already instituted within the gay community as a general precaution against disease transmission.

With Covid, interference in our lives was even more dramatic. Millions were forced into unnecessary isolation. Enforced mask-wearing and restrictions on movement and social engagement wrought massive harm. Children's development was interrupted. Elderly people died alone, prisoners of their care homes, not even allowed to experience healing sunshine. Millions more were impoverished as governments printed hundreds of billions in extra currency to pay for the loss of economic activity.

Perhaps the biggest commonality between Covid and Aids is the way both outbreaks triggered a response more religious than scientific in nature. Wildly inaccurate statistics that supported the official, fear-inducing dogma, earned immediate acceptance.

Questioning the orthodoxy was portrayed as heresy, and punished by ridicule, marginalisation, censorship, and defunding. With both Covid and Aids, doctors who stepped outside officially approved clinical guidelines became scapegoats for vicious media attacks, supported by academic and medical institutions dependent for their finances on toeing the line.

In the Aids years, for example, molecular biologist Professor Peter Duesberg lost a $300,000 'outstanding investigator' US Government award

* Some leading scientists have claimed persuasively that genes attributed to HIV were inserted into the coronavirus to facilitate its entry into human cells, but these are short, biologically active sequences that in no way demonstrate the existence of HIV as such. Rather, they are a sign of cell disorder. Similar sequences have been documented in breast and ovarian cancer tissues.

after challenging the HIV theory. Security of tenure meant his university couldn't fire him, but they stripped him of students and, laughably, reduced his role to chairman of the annual picnic committee.

With Covid, Dr Peter McCullough, one of America's most distinguished cardiologists, has been 'cancelled' by university colleagues and threatened by his professional associations for condemning drug and vaccine policies that he sees as harmful. Censorship has been widespread, and not only within social media. *The Conservative Woman*, a UK-based newsletter and website which fearlessly champions scientific challenges to Covid orthodoxy, and who published nearly 60 of my own articles on Covid, faced a prolonged internet blackout.

Perhaps it is not surprising that most doctors and scientists prefer discretion to valour, and are not prepared to question the official line when a pandemic mind-set has taken grip. Money and job security are important factors.

Seductive appeal of crusading spirit

Corruption in medical science is not by any means the whole story, however. I know from personal experience how seductive the desire to fall in with a 'crusading' spirit can be when a public health emergency has been declared.

In 1984, when US Government researcher Robert Gallo claimed to have found the virus causing Aids, my first reaction was sceptical. In the 1970s, as social policy correspondent at *The Times* and later as medical correspondent of the *Daily Mail*, I had learned of modernity's strong bias in favour of finding technical, product-oriented solutions for health care issues.

Just three years later, however, in 1987, now working as medical correspondent of *The Sunday Times*, I returned from an international Aids conference in Washington, USA, convinced that HIV was set to put millions of lives at risk. The threat was said to arise because of a long time-lag between infection, when a person would be capable of passing on the virus, and development of actual illness. There were no data to support this claim, but that did not matter; it was the *zeitgeist* of the time. Also swept off my feet by a personal visit to the White House, I became a convert to the cause of sounding a global alert over the virus's spread.

'Convert' is an appropriate word. Despite the very real emergency of Aids, an infectious joy flowed among many of those present at the Washington event, and similar huge international conferences that followed over many years. It was as though the delegates, who included drug company representatives as well as gay campaigners, became brothers-in-arms against this new, common peril. Reporters felt that for once, our work in this area meant more than simply selling newspapers – it might 'save lives'.

The same impulse has been in play throughout the Covid crisis. It is very dangerous, because it distorts judgment and stops reason dead in its tracks. I believe it tends to arise when we become separated from our real nature – our human kindness. When this happens, we risk filling the gap with compulsive 'do-gooding' in order to feel better about ourselves. We dress up our compulsion as a noble cause, such as 'Save our National Health Service', when the actual result, in the case of Covid, was to do the opposite. Billions in public funds were siphoned into private hands, NHS waiting times went through the roof, staff morale was (further) weakened and trust in doctors was damaged, perhaps irreparably.

The late Kary Mullis, who won the 1993 Nobel prize for chemistry for inventing the PCR (polymerase chain reaction) test used widely in both Aids and Covid work, and who was one of the HIV theory's sternest and most authoritative critics, did not suffer from this complaint.

Told that his stand was 'encouraging people to risk their lives', he replied: 'So what? I'm not a lifeguard, I'm a scientist. And I get up and say exactly what I think. I'm not going to change the facts around because I believe in something and feel like manipulating somebody's behaviour by stretching what I really know.'

The English poet and artist William Blake also understood the problem, famously writing that 'He who would do good to another must do it in minute particulars. General good is the plea of the scoundrel, hypocrite, and flatterer'.

Lack of kindness, of course, is no better than bogus kindness, and when Aids was first reported there was a period of heartless neglect under a right-wing administration in the US, who dismissed it as a 'gay plague'. Gay rights campaigners, fighting for years to end discrimination over sexual orientation, saw a threat to the future of the movement and grew increasingly angry and vociferous, demanding that government researchers provide an answer to the syndrome.

That was the atmosphere in which Gallo, a buccaneering virologist, claimed he had found a new virus to be circulating surreptitiously among us such that eventually almost all sexually active people would risk infection, disease, and death. A test to detect the virus was available, he said, and a protective vaccine would follow within two years. His claims were accepted unquestioningly by the global scientific community, with a huge sigh of relief, and the fight against what came to be called the Human Immunodeficiency Virus was set in motion.

I first learned that the purported cause of Aids was not all it seemed in 1991, when Joan Shenton, a medical documentary maker in London, told me of the challenge from Duesberg. He was renowned for his work on retroviruses, tiny slugs of genetic information, of which HIV was supposed to be one. A pioneer in the field, Duesberg did not regard them as causing disease and when Gallo claimed to have found one producing as devastating an illness as Aids, he was openly disbelieving.

He set out his case against the virus theory in a 21-page paper published in the journal *Cancer Research* in March 1987, entitled 'Retroviruses as Carcinogens and Pathogens: Expectations and Reality'. The journal's editor, Peter McGee, was astonished that the challenge produced zero response.

Suppression of its message came from the very top, as this leaked memo from the office of the Secretary of Health and Human Services, sent among others to the Surgeon General and the White House, revealed:

> This obviously has the potential to raise a lot of controversy (If this isn't the virus, how do we know the blood supply is safe? How do we know anything about transmission? How could you all be so stupid and why should we ever believe you again?) and we need to be prepared to respond.

Duesberg discovered that when HIV protagonists were asked to comment on the paper, most refused to reply on the record. Instead, they told reporters how terrible it was to question the hypothesis, because of the public health implications. Fauci told the *New York Times* that 'the evidence that HIV causes Aids is so overwhelming that it almost doesn't deserve discussion any more'.

So the critique was buried, despite the persistent efforts of a handful of US journalists – notably Celia Farber, who wrote a series of passionate articles on the topic for the rock magazine *Spin;* the late John Lauritsen, author of *Poison By Prescription* and *The AIDS War*; and Jon Rappoport, whose 1988 book *AIDS INC. – Scandal of the Century* long preceded my own efforts to have the topic aired.

Sunday Times challenges Aids orthodoxy

I heard nothing of the issue at the 1987 Washington conference, but four years later, now working as the *Sunday Times*'s science correspondent, I was persuaded by Shenton to examine Duesberg's case.

Sunday Times news executives recommended not wasting time on such a story, predicting – rightly, as it turned out – that it would bring a storm of criticism on our heads. The editor at the time, however, was Andrew Neil, a feisty Scot unafraid of disturbing established ideas just because they were supported by powerful interests.

In a long memo, I explained that a scientific challenge to HIV as the cause of Aids was about to be mounted at an 'alternative' Aids conference in Amsterdam. As well as Duesberg, speakers were to include Luc Montagnier, later to receive the Nobel prize for work that Gallo had in effect hijacked within his own laboratory and 'marketed' as the cause of Aids. Montagnier (who died, aged 89, in February 2022) was always conflicted between on the one hand knowing that Gallo oversold the virus theory, while on the other not wanting to let go of the money and fame that came to him for his discovery of 'HIV'.

On 26 April 1992, Neil ran my memo as a report across the top of the front page headlined 'Experts Mount Startling Challenge to Aids Orthodoxy'. A two-page spread inside, under the heading 'Aids: Can We Be Positive?' set out the detail of the challenge.

Outrage greeted this report, not least from among fellow medical and science correspondents, and for months I was unable to get another story on the subject into the paper. Then a new news editor, Mark Skipworth, arrived who urged me to return to the issue.

Over a two-year period I went on to examine the critique from a multitude of angles, eventually arriving at the conclusion that a small but brave group of researchers based in Perth, Western Australia – 2,000 miles from the nearest city – had probably come closest to the truth on Aids, challenging every pillar of the virus theory.

Their work indicated that in the rush to find a specific cause for the syndrome, biochemical changes in the bodies of people at risk of Aids became misinterpreted as meaning the presence of a unique viral entity. The real cause of the syndrome was heavy and prolonged exposure to several chemically different agents, including semen, nitrite inhalants, recreational drugs, multiple infectious microbes and the drugs used to treat them, and Factor VIII treatment for haemophilia (obtained at that time from pooled blood donations). These had the common property of injuring cells, including those of the immune system, through a process known as oxidative stress.*

A distinguished supporter of the newspaper's challenging investigation was the late Professor Gordon Stewart, an early WHO adviser on Aids, who had a lifetime's work in public health. He recognised that the diseases registrable as Aids were occurring in people suffering various types of toxic assault, regardless of 'HIV'. Predictions of spread based on this multi-factorial understanding proved highly accurate. That was not the case with forecasts made in an influential 150-page report based on the virus model, published in September 1989 by the Royal Society, the national academy of science for the UK.

A year later, as one of the society's most eminent and experienced members, Stewart submitted an 8,000-word analysis highlighting the discrepancy. The society gave him a heart-breaking, four-year run-around (described in chapter five, 'A Conspiracy of Humbug'), before finally refusing to publish. They never relented, nor apologised for the false predictions.

'Coming from the top scientific body in the country, this is a pretty disgraceful state of affairs,' Stewart told me before his death in 2016. 'It was

* Our bodies exist in a delicate state between levels of reactive oxygen species produced during metabolism, and the antioxidant defence system that scavenges them. When this gets out of balance, the resulting oxidative stress can lead to far-reaching cell and tissue damage.

the Royal Society that convened the meeting that made the wrong predictions. They are honour bound to put it right.' A demonstrable error had been made that in other walks of life 'would have been washed out years ago'. His findings and recommendations also remained unpublished by the WHO.

One of the consequences, as with Covid, was a huge misallocation of money to the detriment of genuine medical need. A 1993 report from the University of Northumbria Business School, to which Stewart contributed, found that for each Aids death, health authorities were spending an average of £290,000 on HIV prevention and research, compared with £50 for each death from heart disease. Many UK health regions had considerably more Aids workers than patients.

Africa's suffering

Tragically, the HIV theory brought a far more damaging and persistent distortion of health spending in Africa, where long-established illnesses accompanying extreme poverty were the real killers, as I discovered during a six-week investigation there in late 1993 (chronicled in detail in Chapter 10).

My reports provoked a chorus of condemnation back in the UK, led by the prestigious science journal *Nature*, whose editor was so upset that he contemplated picketing the *Sunday Times* offices.

Occasionally a truly authoritative voice was raised in support of the newspaper's work. *New African* magazine interviewed Professor P.A.K. Addy, editor-in-chief of the *African Journal on Sexually Transmitted Diseases*, about an explosive report I had filed after meeting two medical missionaries running a large charity for Aids orphans in Tanzania. They had been there for several years, only gradually to discover that their belief in an 'HIV' epidemic was completely ill-founded.

Addy, head of clinical microbiology at the University of Science and Technology in Kumasi, Ghana, was asked if he took their confession seriously.

> ADDY: Why not, I am really impressed that the very people who first blew the alarm bells that Africans were dying of Aids in fantastic numbers now say they got it all wrong.

NEW AFRICAN: Have you been to Uganda, Kenya and Tanzania where the medical world claims is the epicentre of AIDS?

ADDY: I have been to Uganda. And I've worked as a WHO personnel at the East African Virus Research Institute. I've known for a long time that Aids is not a crisis in Africa as the world is being made to understand. But in Africa it is very difficult to stick your neck out and say certain things.

NEW AFRICAN: Why?

ADDY: Some of us get funding for our research projects from some institutions in the West. So it is suicidal for us to stand up and challenge the advanced parts of the world on certain issues.

In answer to other questions, Addy said: 'These Europeans and Americans came to Africa with prejudiced minds and so they are seeing what they always wanted to see...The diagnosis itself, merely being told you have Aids, is enough to kill, and is killing people. The moment you tell somebody you are HIV-positive, the person loses his or her psychological capacity to fight diseases.'

In mid-1994 Andrew Neil was moved by Rupert Murdoch, the *Sunday Times* owner, to New York and his successor as editor made it plain that he did not want me to continue with the critique. I put in my notice immediately. David Godwin, a London literary agent, had suggested I should write a book on the controversy, and it took shape over the following year, being published by Fourth Estate in 1996.

With Neil gone from *The Sunday Times*, the book found few friends. The late Beverley Griffin, professor of virology at the Royal Postgraduate Medical School in London, was alone among senior scientists in the UK in issuing a supportive statement.

The Observer newspaper, under the guise of reviewing the book, ran a story ridiculing me headlined 'Sunday Times Science Editor Awaits Flat Earth'. It contained quotes fabricated by editorial staff, for which the paper later published an apology and correction, but hidden away where hardly anyone would see it.

Following fiercely hostile reaction from some gay activist leaders – including Larry Kramer, who urged delegates at a UK Aids conference to tear the pages of my book and spit in it if they came across it in a bookshop – 'that will soon stop it from being stocked' – Fourth Estate effectively 'cancelled' it, disposing of remaining copies without telling me.

In the year 2000, it looked as though the issue might resurface when President Thabo Mbeki of South Africa became a rarity among world leaders in using his high office to challenge Aids orthodoxy. He could not be ignored – but he paid a heavy price.

With the 13th International Aids Conference due to take place in Durban, South Africa, that July, he instigated two international AIDS Advisory Panel meetings to provide a platform for scientists with varying views (including two representatives from the Perth group). I attended the second of these meetings, in Johannesburg, at which the declared aim was to try to 'gain a full knowledge' on the subject.

This was seen as dangerous heresy by the high priests of the HIV faith, and those benefiting from the Aids belief system. The virus theory had brought a huge and unexpected bonanza in the form of funds for research, treatment, and health promotion. Much of this wealth came from taxpayer-funded government bodies in the US and elsewhere, as well as from tax-deductible contributions to supposedly philanthropic foundations, and from sales of drugs and test kits to already impoverished countries.

In the weeks before the conference, *Nature* facilitated a pre-emptive strike against Mbeki, helping to organise an international round-robin condemnation of any questioning of the faith. The move was initiated by retrovirologist Simon Wain-Hobson*, of the Pasteur Institute in Paris, who recruited signatures to a 'Durban Declaration' asserting that the evidence for HIV as the cause of Aids was 'clear-cut, exhaustive and unambiguous, meeting the highest standards of science'. Published by *Nature* to coincide with the conference, it was signed by more than 5,000 scientists and doctors from 43 countries, including many of those attending the event.

* Wain-Hobson chairs the US-based Foundation for Vaccine Research, whose website trumpets the safety and effectiveness of the Covid jabs, and 'resounding validation' of the experimental RNA technology for future vaccines.

In his welcome address to the delegates, Mbeki highlighted the fact that in the African context, Aids appeared wherever there was extreme poverty, suffering, social disadvantage and inequity. He pointed out that more than 12 million children under five were dying every year in the developing world, mostly from causes that could be prevented for just a few US cents per child.

He was polite and non-combative, but not enough to appease the critics. 'Mbeki is expected to dispense drugs like sweets and make himself the darling of the drug companies,' *New African* magazine noted. 'He will not. So he must be given a bad name, and hanged...And unfortunately, in our midst, are the Judases of South Africa (and Africa) who will betray a presidency for 30 pieces of silver.'

Mbeki was not just hanged but drawn and quartered. He suffered a coordinated international campaign of denigration. President Clinton formally designated Aids a threat to US national security because of alleged fears that it could topple foreign governments, the rand (South Africa's currency) plummeted, and a rash of scurrilous headlines appeared in newspapers around the world. Examples from the UK included 'Mbeki "lets Aids babies die in pain",' (*Observer*, 20 August); 'Thabo Mbeki: Enemy of the People' (*Sunday Times*, 27 August); and 'A second Black Death looms in South Africa: President Mbeki should face the fact that Aids could be a modern Holocaust' (*The Times*, 29 August). This was just as imaginary a prediction as the scenarios produced by Covid scare-mongers. South Africa's population continued to rise steadily, from 45 million in 2000 to 61 million in 2022.

In response to the Durban Declaration, the Perth Group coolly wrote: 'We wish it to be understood that the claim...cannot be substantiated'. Theirs was a voice in the wilderness, but they never stopped trying to reason their way past the wall of silence protecting the virus theory.

Journal editor fired

In 2010 a breakthrough appeared imminent when the respected journal *Medical Hypotheses* accepted a paper from the Perth scientists, reviewing the evidence for sexual transmission of Aids and HIV.

The abstract stated:

> It is claimed that tens of millions of people have acquired AIDS as a result of sexual transmission of HIV. Sexually transmitted diseases or infections are invariably spread from active to passive partners and *vice versa*. We have critically analysed the published data on AIDS acquisition. These data indicate that AIDS is certainly sexually acquired but not sexually transmitted. Conceptually the difference is subtle indeed but nonetheless pivotal in the understanding of AIDS pathogenesis.

The paper was accompanied by a second manuscript, 'Would Montagnier please clarify what method he used to prove the existence of HIV?' Both papers, with their every assertion supported by detailed references, were put in the pipeline for publication.

A prolonged silence followed, in the wake of which Professor Bruce Charlton, the journal's editor, explained that Elsevier, a giant, Netherlands-based publisher specializing in scientific and medical content, had intervened. He wrote:

> Unfortunately, I have already been deprived of editorial control of *Medical Hypotheses*. After I accepted your submitted paper for publication, and without my knowledge, it was 'intercepted' by the Elsevier management who are apparently holding it for some kind of evaluation. Presumably you have not had an acknowledgement of the paper so far? This is why. However, since I as editor accepted the paper for publication, and there is no process in the journal's official organization which allows for managers to counter this decision – your paper counts as 'in press'.

That was not to be. The group's work was too threatening to an entire industry, of which Elsevier is a major part, to be allowed to surface, even in a science journal specialising in radical ideas. On 11 May 2010, Charlton wrote in his blog:

> Just to note that I was sacked from the editorship of *Medical Hypotheses* today.

> *Medical Hypotheses* was very much a 'one man band' as a journal – its content being selected by the editor (occasionally after seeking advice from a member of the editorial advisory board) over a period of some 35 years. The journal's essence was that it was editorially reviewed (not peer reviewed), and favoured revolutionary science over normal science; that is, it favoured ideas on the basis that they were (for example) radical, interesting, dissenting, or sometimes amusing in a way likely to stimulate thought.
>
> The journal had just two editors during its lifespan: the founder David Horrobin from 1975 to his death in 2003, and his chosen successor, myself, from 2003-2010. As a consequence of mergers, *Medical Hypotheses* fell into the hands of Elsevier in 2002. Aside from a few issues still in the pipeline, the real *Medical Hypotheses* is now dead: killed by Elsevier 11 May 2010. RIP.

Charlton's successor as editor rejected both of the Perth group's new papers.

A few years earlier, the Perth scientists experienced an equally frustrating setback after engaging in a protracted online debate with Brian Foley, custodian of the Los Alamos HIV database, over whether an HIV genome actually exists. It took place between February 2003 and April 2005 through a 'Rapid Responses' feature of the *British Medical Journal* website, featuring electronic rather than print letters.

Even this online exposure to contrary perspectives and data was too much for the HIV/Aids mainstream.

Nature, self-appointed chief defender of the HIV faith, put the BMJ under pressure to stop the correspondence in an article published in November 2003 headed 'Medical journal under attack as dissenters seize Aids platform'. In it, Foley, Wain-Hobson and John P. Moore, a particularly belligerent HIV/Aids protagonist, complained of the misuse of a respectable scientific journal to contribute to the dissemination of 'disinformation' – the same blanket term used in the Covid era to suppress valid criticism of disastrous lockdown and vaccine policies. 'I do not think responding to BMJ posts is a worthwhile use of my time,' Foley told *Nature*.

Richard Smith, the BMJ's editor, responded vigorously in a reply published by *Nature* the following January. Quoting a famous 17th century pamphlet in which John Milton, the English poet, wrote: 'Whoever knew Truth put to the worse, in a free and open encounter?', he commented: 'I find it disturbing to see scientists arguing for restrictions on free speech. Surely open communication and argument is a fundamental value of science?'

Perhaps discomfited by this response, Foley remained engaged in the debate until April 2005, when the Perth scientists, in their last posting, had brought him to the brink of defeat. They were demanding evidence that genetic material claimed by Gallo to represent the HIV genome could be shown to have come from purified 'HIV', and to be capable of giving rise to infectious viral particles. After 842 postings, lasting 26 months, the correspondence was abruptly halted by a new editor at the BMJ. If Foley had such evidence, it remains unseen.

Even mainstream Aids scientists admit that what they take to be the genome of HIV is a 'consensus' construct, rather than established fact, though they maintain this has to be the case because the virus is so variable.

Squelching dissent

The HIV/Aids industry will go to extraordinary lengths to protect its belief system. There was and is 'an insatiable need to squelch dissent', as Lawrence Solomon, of Canada's Consumer Policy Institute, has put it in the context of other scientific controversies.

In October 2019 this even took the form of the retraction by the journal *Frontiers in Public Health* of a peer-reviewed article published five years previously. The retraction came about not because of any errors, but because the information was reaching too many people!

The article, 'Questioning the HIV-Aids hypothesis: 30 years of dissent', first appeared in September 2014 under a 'Hypothesis and Theory' tagline. The author was Dr Patricia Goodson, a highly respected professor of health education at Texas A&M University. Within days, the journal received several formal complaints. At that point the editors decided to allow the article to stand, but to classify it as an 'Opinion', and to have it linked to several invited critical commentaries. The aim was 'to ensure that all readers understand that the causal link between HIV and Aids cannot be called into question'.

Over the months and years that followed, however, while the critical commentaries went largely unheeded, the original paper continued to attract attention. By the time of the 2019 retraction, it had received more than 91,800 views and was still being shared on social media. The commentaries, in contrast, had fewer than 19,000 views between them.

In announcing the 2019 retraction, the *Frontiers* editorial office said that with a new chief editor in post – Dr Paolo Vineis, of Imperial College, London – new complaints had been received, and it had now been decided that the article 'presents a public health risk by lending credibility to refuted claims that place doubt on the HIV causation of Aids'.

Imperial College, of course, was the source of Covid modelling exercises that not only proved wildly inaccurate but were critical to selling the disastrous concept of lockdowns to the world.

Growing pressure for reform

In such ways, the work of the Perth group and other 'dissident' scientists has been ruthlessly suppressed for decades. Thus it is that with more than 130,000 papers predicated on the HIV theory having been published in the scientific press, contrary claims sound outrageous, even today. And yet more than 35 years after Gallo's announcements, there is still no HIV vaccine, and no 'cure' for the supposed infection.

Damaging misunderstandings about 'HIV' persist. Health care priorities in many parts of Africa are still subject to gross distortions because of the activities of the HIV/Aids industry, who have a continuing, post-colonial presence on the continent. In December 2020, for example, the BBC World Service reported that a new, strawberry flavoured anti-retroviral tablet 'suitable for children living with HIV', including babies, was about to be rolled out in several African countries.

In July 2022 *The Lancet* carried an article urging greater use, particularly in sub-Saharan Africa, of 'pre-exposure prophylaxis (PrEP)' drugs that are claimed to reduce HIV transmission among people who are well, but who might be at risk. These drugs have encouraged gay men to have unprotected sex and may well be contributing to the spread of genuine infections such as Monkeypox, declared 'a public health emergency of international concern' by WHO in July 2022. Almost all cases – 98 per cent – are among men who have sex with men, typically young and with multiple partners.

At the time of writing, fears are even being expressed that 'HIV' may be making a more general comeback. Prince Harry has entered the fray, urging everyone to get an 'HIV' test. Dutch researchers say they have identified a new 'HIV' strain. President Biden has announced a White House plan to 'end the HIV/Aids epidemic by 2030'.

The truth is, there is no 'HIV/Aids' epidemic, and there never will be a vaccine or cure, because there is no 'HIV'.

The case that the corruption surrounding Aids science set the stage for the exploitation and mishandling of Covid is gaining ground, thanks especially to Robert Kennedy Jr.'s best-selling *The Real Anthony Fauci: Bill Gates, Big Pharma, and the Global War on Democracy and Public Health.** The abuse of power now evident has awakened many to the idea that something is deeply rotten in the state of medical science.

Even so, as with Covid, suppression of dissident views on Aids causation has been so far-reaching that many people do not even know such critiques exist. I hope the account that follows, the largely unknown story of the 'HIV/Aids' precursor of the Covid crisis, will add to the growing pressure for reform, and to efforts to stop such disasters from happening again.

The book takes the reader through my gradual conversion from HIV zealot to unbeliever, marshalling much detailed evidence along the way. My summary of the Perth group's work, the culmination of years of trying to help them to be heard, is included as an appendix. It can also be seen at their website through the link below.**

In a way, I am more troubled by the monstrous wrong the group suffered as individuals at the hands of scientists and others who should have known better, than by the global repercussions of the mistakes surrounding Covid and Aids. Biophysicist Eleni Papadopulos-Eleopulos, who tirelessly led the

* Skyhorse Publishing, 2022

** *http://www.theperthgroup.com/HIV/NHSummaryVLNOFinal.pdf*

group's efforts to dismantle the belief in 'HIV' for nearly four decades, died on 19 March 2022, aged 85. She was an unsung hero.

With Covid, at least the internet made it possible for contrary views to reach millions, despite Facebook, YouTube and Paypal as well as most mainstream media blocking scientific and medical challenges to the ruinous lockdown measures and mass experimental vaccine rollout.

One voice that could not be ignored was that of the UK's Lord Sumption, historian and former Supreme Court judge. In an interview, he was asked: 'There will be people listening who admire your legal wisdom but will also say, "He's not an epidemiologist, he doesn't know how disease spreads. He doesn't understand the risks to the health service if this thing gets out of control." What do you say to them?'

He replied: 'What I say to them is that I am not a scientist but it is the right and duty of every citizen to look and see what the scientists have said, and to analyse it for themselves, and to draw common-sense conclusions. We are all perfectly capable of doing that, and there's no particular reason why the scientific nature of the problem should mean that we have to resign our liberty into the hands of scientists. We all have critical faculties and it's rather important, in a moment of national panic, that we should maintain them.'

Critical faculties are impeded when in order to 'save lives', mass media unquestioningly align themselves with official propaganda. In the decades over which the Perth group were mounting their critique of the 'HIV'/Aids theory, the censorship was just about total.

Even with Covid, most people were bludgeoned into fearful obedience through public health messaging on billboards, apps, newspapers, radio and television. Alternative media channels such as Odysee, Bitchute and Telegram gave a voice to some of the doctors, scientists and others who challenged the official accounts, but the information they shared reached only a limited audience.

Emergency physician Dr Val Turner, a central figure in the Perth group, says it is younger people who are rekindling interest in 'HIV'/Aids. 'They are the ones who do not yet know what sort of questions they are not supposed to ask,' he says, citing a quote from Bertolt Brecht's *Galileo:* 'The aim of science is not to open the door to everlasting wisdom, but to set a limit to everlasting error.'

Aids and Covid are both signal examples of the almost infinite error into which scientists can lead us when they forget this aim, and become carried away by unreasoning emotion and self-serving intentions.

In both these public health disasters, the self-correcting process for which science is justly famed, failed to operate. Now, after years of obfuscation and denial, there is at last a stirring of conscience within the scientific community, and perhaps even the beginnings of a return of the critical faculties Lord Sumption has urged us to use.

As Leonard Cohen sang:

Ring the bells that still can ring
Forget your perfect offering
There is a crack in everything
That's how the light gets in

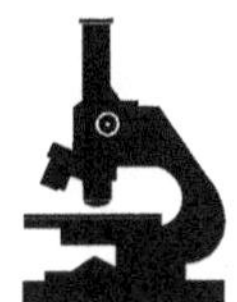

AIDS: THE FAILURE OF CONTEMPORARY SCIENCE

How a Virus That Never Was Deceived the World

Comments on first publication in 1996

'The emotional response to the HIV story, especially by the scientific/medical community, never ceases to amaze...It is a pleasure to read Neville Hodgkinson's thoroughly researched, well-argued book on the emotive topic of HIV and Aids.'
– Beverly E. Griffin, director and professor of virology, Royal Postgraduate medical School, Hammersmith Hospital, London

'Superb...full of new information. Research by Hodgkinson converted an initially orthodox HIV-Aids follower to an HIV sceptic who would give up his prestigious job as science correspondent at the Sunday Times to write the book of his life. Hodgkinson proved to be the scientist among the science correspondents, noticing the growing list of exceptions to the rules of a virus-Aids hypothesis. It is the hallmark of a real scientist to follow the exceptions, because in science the exception does not confirm the rule – it breaks it. In his book Hodgkinson breaks with the HIV-Aids hypothesis and opens the stage for new and productive solutions of the Aids epidemic.'
– Peter Duesberg, professor of molecular biology, University of California, Berkeley, USA

'A masterful and sagacious account of the history and science of the HIV/Aids dissident movement since 1981...will probably be one of the most remarkable books in history'
– Dr Valendar Turner, Aids analyst and senior consultant in emergency medicine, Royal Perth Hospital, Western Australia

'Well-written and immensely important'
– Dr Gordon Stewart, professor emeritus in public health, Glasgow University, and former World Health Organization adviser on Aids

'If WHO estimates are to be believed, millions of Africans should be in the grave by now, killed by Aids; and a heterosexual spread of the disease should be killing millions more around the world. But the apocalypse hasn't materialised. Now a new book...has nailed all the nightmare scenarios about Aids firmly in the coffin. It is a riveting read, but the Aids establishment will not be pleased.'
– Baffour Ankomah, New African magazine

'This excellent book requires you to review your fundamental assumptions about the nature of Aids and its relationship with HIV, and also the appropriate way to prevent and treat the disease.'
– Dr Rupert Holms, Institute of Immunology, Moscow

'A challenging book that will radically alter the way you think about Aids and about the Aids establishment...shows how science has come adrift from its intellectual moorings and is drifting dangerously in the murky waters of big business, big government and popular delusion.'
– Ian Young, Torso magazine

'Hodgkinson's brilliantly clear book contains the best of lucid journalism, readable science and step-by-step explanations on the subject...Books like this don't come along often.'
– Huw Christie, Editor, Continuum

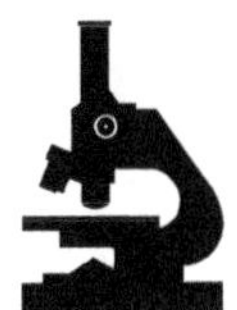

PREFACE, OXFORD, DECEMBER 1995

Last April, I was invited to give a talk at a Wednesday morning seminar held at the Kobler Clinic in London, a leading centre of Aids treatment and research. The title was 'HIV/Aids: Some Unanswered Questions'. The seminar room at the clinic, which forms part of the showpiece Chelsea & Westminster Hospital, was packed with an audience that included leading Aids physicians as well as research nurses, health counsellors and social workers. I was received coolly but courteously, and by the end of the one-hour meeting I felt the mood was generally appreciative.

That may have been not so much because of the information I shared, as because I seemed less of a monster than some workers in the field had come to expect. Even one year previously, I could never have expected such an invitation. A series of articles I had written over a two-year period, reporting on a scientific challenge to the HIV theory of Aids, had brought prolonged, high-level and often passionate criticism, nationally and internationally.

The articles highlighted inadequacies in the theory that Aids, the most emotionally-laden diagnosis of the times, was caused by a deadly new virus, HIV. While not offering any clear-cut alternative theory, the articles featured claims by a small group of scientists that the disease was not behaving as would be expected if the cause really was a new microbe. The way the syndrome developed within individuals, and the pattern of spread within society, suggested its origins might be better explained by a variety of exceptionally risky circumstances in the lives of those affected, rather than by a single germ.

These reports were greeted with accusations of extreme irresponsibility. In the minds of many, HIV and Aids had become inextricably linked. To challenge HIV's role in the disease meant weakening public and personal resolve to fight the spread of Aids, thus imperilling thousands or millions of lives. In addition, to question HIV as an 'equal-opportunity' virus meant risking a damaging backlash on its victims. The criticism came from highly respected individuals and organisations within the worlds of politics and the media, charities and religion, as well as science, medicine, and the gay community. It was a controversy unprecedented during my 30 years in newspaper journalism.

At times I felt very isolated. This had a positive side for me. It fuelled inquiries that carried me across several continents, and deep into the wonders of molecular biology, in order to meet and learn from a small group of generous-hearted individuals who had also found themselves at odds with mainstream science over HIV's role in Aids. The longer I have studied the issue, the more convinced I have become that these different viewpoints have much to offer in terms of hope for a more successful approach to Aids. I am grateful for having had the chance to study and write about these people. I have distilled their ideas and experiences as clearly as I could and shall be pleased if others can now give them a hearing.

There was a downside to the intense controversy. I sometimes fell into the trap of becoming over-reactive and self-righteous. Such reactions blunt one's sensitivity to the feelings of others. I was struck by the sincerity with which Dr Brian Gazzard, a senior London Aids physician and researcher, spoke at the seminar of the hurt felt when treatment uncertainties and difficulties were attributed to drug company agendas. Although money has played a big part in sustaining the HIV story, I do not believe it was ever a primary motivation with any of the players.

A gay man at the seminar asked how I would feel if I realised I had caused hundreds of thousands to die. Pretty bad, I said. When I added, defensively, that I didn't think a newspaper could have that kind of influence, most swiftly disagreed.

But was the influence for better or for worse? It ought to be born in mind, I said, that the HIV hypothesis itself might have cost thousands of lives. This caused puzzlement, and I was asked what I meant. If the theory was wrong, I said, the neglect of other ways of thinking or lines of research meant thousands had been denied information or treatment that might have saved them. For example, if anal sex, or drug use, played important roles in their own right, regardless of any new virus, then failure to address those behavioural aspects would have boosted the epidemic, and would still be doing so.

Although the 'safer sex' drives have had a valuable impact in the gay community, many HIV-positive gay men believe that since HIV is the cause of Aids and they are already infected, they have nothing to lose by continuing to use drugs and to have unprotected sex with HIV-positive partners. To interpret an 'HIV' diagnosis in that way may be lethal. Similar serious mistakes have been made with harmful chemotherapeutic drugs targeted against HIV. Their use would never have been contemplated if the HIV paradigm had not convinced doctors and patients there was no other rational choice.

Coming to terms with these mistakes is going to be difficult, but will eventually strengthen science and society. This book is not an exercise in trying to apportion blame. On the contrary, writing it has been a healing experience, in which the siege mentality that had started to trouble me gradually faded until I arrived back at a point of respect for all involved.

Hans Eysenck, the eminent psychologist, once defined neurosis as an inability to follow the carrot or the stick. He was referring to the difficulties wounded individuals encounter when they lose their ability to respond to life's signals (often because of having received too much stick and not enough carrot). Perhaps the same can apply to institutions as well. This book suggests that an institutional neurosis – a prolonged failure to respond appropriately to the emergency represented by Aids – has gripped the great body of human endeavour we call science for more than a decade. It is causing much suffering, and ought to be brought to an end.

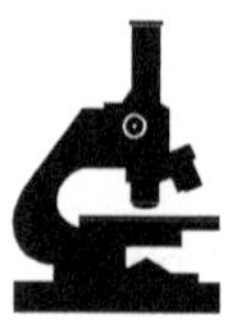

ACKNOWLEDGEMENTS

I am immensely grateful to numerous *Sunday Times* colleagues for their unflinching support during storms of criticism over the HIV critique, and in particular to Andrew Neil for putting such enormous trust in me. Special thanks also to Tony Rennell for his encouragement to keep going when my stamina was failing, and to Lois Rogers for loyally weathering front-line medical hostility over the newspaper's reports. I am indebted to Joan Shenton, Michael Verney-Elliott, Hector Gildemeister and others associated with the Meditel team for first making me see the need for a rethink on Aids; to Peter Duesberg, Harvey Bialy, Charlie Thomas, Phil Johnson and the rest of the *Reappraising Aids* editorial board for providing so much rich fuel for that rethink; to Gordon Stewart for allowing me to document his marathon struggles with the scientific establishment over Aids; and to Eleni Papadopulos-Eleopulos, Val Turner and Stefan Lanka for tutoring me so patiently in the techniques of molecular biology in order that I could accompany them on their journey to the roots of the HIV phenomenon. Consistently brilliant journalism by John Lauritsen and Celia Farber, meticulous work at *Continuum* by Huw Christie and Molly Ratcliffe in the wake of Jody Wells's pioneering contribution, and Serge Lang's inclusion of me on his "cc list", all provided sustenance and inspiration at times when self-doubt might otherwise have made me falter. Finally, very special thanks to David Godwin for suggesting the writing of this book, and for keeping a watchful and encouraging eye on its development.

One impulse from a vernal wood
May teach you more of man,
Of moral evil and of good,
Than all the sages can.

Sweet is the lore which Nature brings;
Our meddling intellect
Misshapes the beauteous forms of things
We murder to dissect.

Enough of science and of art;
Close up these barren leaves
Come forth, and bring with you a heart
That watches and receives.

– **William Wordsworth,** *The Tables Turned*

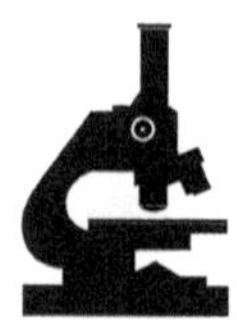

1: THE PROCRUSTEAN BED

Procrustes was a cruel giant in Greek mythology who trapped and tortured weary travellers on the road to Athens. He enticed them into his house by telling them he had a wonderful bed that suited everyone, no matter what their size. But once inside, they found there was a terrible price to pay: those travellers who were too short for the bed were put on a rack that lengthened them, and those who were too large had the bits of themselves that didn't fit sawn off.

On 26 September 1991, an extraordinary challenge to conventional thinking about Aids was published by the science journal *Nature*. More than seven years after it had been accepted by most doctors and scientists around the world that a new, lethal microbe, which came to be known as the human immunodeficiency virus (HIV), was the cause of the syndrome afflicting many homosexual men and putting millions of other people at risk, research evidence indicated that the true causes were at the very least much more complicated than the virus theory had hitherto allowed.

The article, headed 'Aids Research Turned Upside Down',[1] described several fresh, mutually consistent findings. In one, experimenters injected mice with immune system cells - those cells responsible for protecting the body against infectious organisms and other unwanted invaders – taken from another mouse strain. The treated animals were not exposed to HIV in any form, yet they became HIV-positive: that is, they developed antibodies against proteins thought to belong to the virus and to indicate its presence (antibodies are substances that help rid the body of foreign proteins, called antigens).

The other finding came from experiments with a monkey virus, SIV, thought to be the simian equivalent of HIV. Although SIV is harmless in animals living in the wild, laboratory animals can become sick when injected with cells containing it. As a step towards finding a possible vaccine against HIV, researchers at the National Institute for Biological Standards and Control in Hertfordshire, England, took some monkey immune system cells (T-lymphocytes, or T-cells) and infected them with SIV. They then injected the inactivated preparation into four macaques. The scientists were encouraged to find that three of the animals became protected against later challenge with SIV.

The puzzling aspect was that two out of four monkeys injected with identical cells that had not been infected with SIV were similarly protected. The 'sensation', as *Nature* described it, was that the essential difference between the monkeys who became protected and those who did not had nothing to do with antibodies to a virus. Rather, just as with the mice, the immune response appeared to have been triggered by the foreign T-cells. The monkeys who stayed well had ten times more antibodies against components of these cells than the unprotected monkeys.

Hunting through past records, the researchers found similar results from experiments with forty other animals. Those who became protected against SIV were those who developed a high level of antibody against foreign immune cells. A related discovery was that mice bred to be susceptible to auto-immune disease, in which the body reacts to its own tissues, spontaneously make antibodies to one of the key 'HIV' proteins — again, without any exposure to HIV.

The *Nature* article, written by John Maddox, the journal's editor, concluded that 'until confirmed (or otherwise), these developments must cause heart-searching throughout the world's programmes of Aids research'. People would be wondering whether the search for a vaccine against HIV should be replaced by programmes to induce tolerance of its protein components (so as to damp down immune system over-reactivity). The hunt for mechanisms of the adventitious infections characteristic of Aids and of Kaposi's sarcoma (one of the original Aids-defining diseases) would be given pause. 'Even the epidemiologists would be set back on their tracks.'

John Maddox's many years at the helm of *Nature* have been distinguished by periodic flashes of prophetic brilliance, and this was one of them. Four years on, the vaccine programme has thrown up more questions than it has answered and after ten years' work is considered by many scientists to be heading nowhere. Despite several highly speculative theories on offer, there is still no firm evidence on how HIV could be doing the damage attributed to it, and efforts to defeat it with anti-viral drugs have often done more harm than good. The epidemiology of Aids – in particular, the statistical evidence linking HIV-positivity with the disease – is also nothing like the clear-cut picture it once seemed to be.

Furthermore, although Maddox did not face this issue, the animal findings implied a need to call into question the reliability of the HIV test, and even to challenge the conventional view of what a positive HIV test means. If animals test HIV-positive (or SIV-positive) in response to manipulations involving a certain category of immune system cells, without any virus being present, then perhaps HIV-positivity in humans does not mean that a person is infected with a virus. Maybe, instead, as in the animals, HIV-positivity can signify that a person's immune system has been challenged by exposure to foreign cells. Alternatively, also as in the animals, perhaps the challenge sometimes comes through an autoimmune process, in which cells within one's own system have become confused and can no longer discriminate between friend and foe, 'self' and 'non-self'. Either way, the mechanism could still be harmful, perhaps life-threatening, but the implications for prevention and treatment, and for the public health, would be very different from those that have accompanied the 'deadly new virus' idea.

If it became established that there was indeed a serious flaw in the HIV test, capable of causing people to test positive for a virus when they were not infected with that virus, the next question should be: how many false positives of that kind existed? Was it just a marginal effect, or was it widespread? Even more fundamentally, were we sure that *any* HIV-positive people were infected with this new virus? Did HIV actually exist, the way the scientific community had presented it to the world?

In his article, Maddox confined himself to discussing one very specific theory which says HIV may not kill cells directly, but instead triggers a self-destructive auto-immune process. Nevertheless, he revealed the unease that the findings provoked in him by beginning and ending his commentary with favourable references to a critique of the HIV theory mounted by Professor Peter Duesberg, a molecular biologist at the University of California at Berkeley.

Duesberg, once a golden boy of virology, California's scientist of the year and recipient of a $350,000 'outstanding investigator' award from the National Institutes of Health, had been arguing for several years that HIV was harmless and could not possibly be doing the damage attributed to it. He had first been ignored, then pilloried for his views, then deprived of his research funds. But he was 'probably sleeping more easily at night now than for five years, since he first took up cudgels against the doctrine that Aids is caused by the retrovirus HIV,' Maddox wrote. 'Now there is some evidence to support his long fight against the establishment (among which, sadly, he counts this journal).' After describing the new developments, the article concluded: 'None of this would imply that HIV is irrelevant to Aids, but that an immune response to foreign cells, most probably lymphocytes, is also necessary. Duesberg will be saying, "I told you so."'

Credit is due to *Nature* for having shown an awareness, over a period of years, that some of the questions being asked about HIV deserved examination. As recently as December 1993, Maddox acknowledged in an editorial that the effort to understand the causation of Aids 'has been a profound disappointment to the research community'.[2] He went on: 'Almost ten years have passed since HIV was first recognised, but the evidence that it causes Aids is still epidemiological. The mechanism of the pathogenesis of the disease has not yet been uncovered (although parts of Duesberg's "challenge" have been met) so that the evidence necessarily seems circumstantial.'

However, as if some of the possibilities raised by the 1991 research findings were too awesome to consider, Maddox shrank back from the deeper implications of the research – that HIV-positivity might mean something quite different from what the world had been led to suppose. In fact, by bringing Duesberg into the argument, he set loose something of a red herring, which was quickly pounced upon by other commentators.

In a follow-up article, *Science* magazine, *Nature's* main rival, took Maddox strongly to task. *Science* agreed that the monkey vaccine trial findings had forced researchers to reconsider some of their approaches to developing an Aids vaccine for humans, and Ronald C. Desrosiers, of the New England Regional Primate Centre in Southborough, Massachusetts, acknowledged that the experiments suggested the immune response was caused by some component of the T-cell line the animals were vaccinated with, rather than by SIV. 'It's going to be scientifically interesting and important to sort out what's going on here,' Desrosiers said.

But if researchers were uncertain what to make of the findings, said *Science*, they had a very different reaction to Maddox's interpretation that the results vindicated Duesberg. 'In general, I'm pretty mild-mannered, and I was furious' about Maddox's article, said David D. Ho, director of the Aaron Diamond Aids Research Centre at the New York University School of Medicine. Numerous other researchers contacted by *Science* failed to see any connection between the new studies and the stand taken by Duesberg. And that went for Duesberg, too: 'Those studies have nothing to do with [my position],' he was quoted as saying. Geoffrey Hoffman, of the University of British Columbia, the main author of the mouse study and proponent of the auto-immunity theory, told the magazine that just because it might be possible for an Aids-like disease to occur without HIV, that did not mean it typically does. 'We have nothing in common with [Duesberg]'s idea that HIV has nothing to do with Aids,' Hoffman said.

So how did Maddox explain why he leapt to that conclusion? *Science* asked. 'I'm not for a minute saying Duesberg is right in all points,' the beleaguered editor told his rival. 'But I feel sorry that *Nature* has not done more to give his view prominence. It would have hastened the process by which the scientific community is coming around to the view that the pathogenesis of Aids is more complicated than the baby-talk stories we were all given a few years ago.'

Those were brave words, but it must have been an uncomfortable time for Maddox, who three years later was to declare in an interview that he 'got into a lot of trouble' for saying Duesberg had some cogent questions that might now have been answered by the auto-immunity argument. 'A lot of people wrote in and asked why I had given house room to the man's ideas,' he said. It was a sadly missed opportunity, and later, like a reformed heretic, Maddox was to become prominent in denouncing those, including Duesberg, who continued to question the HIV hypothesis.

Nevertheless, the *Nature* article is important. It stands as the first and as far as I know the only one in a mainstream scientific journal to approach what I now believe to be the roots of an enormous mistake in the handling of Aids.

A Mass Illusion

Ten years of reporting on HIV and Aids, and three years of deep involvement in a controversy over Aids causation, have led me to the conclusion that a decade ago we became ensnared in a mass illusion surrounding the issue. It came about originally because of a misinterpretation of biochemical events by scientists racing to find a microbial cause for the syndrome. The illusion was powerfully promoted by a gay community who also desperately wanted to be able to blame a new virus for Aids, rather than face the likely contribution of the wild lifestyle characteristic of the gay liberation years. Furthermore, religious and political leaders, public health officials, charities and the media found in HIV a ready-made, relatively uncontroversial target for expressions of feeling and morality: on the one hand, compassion towards the victims (although as John Lauritsen, a leading gay journalist, was later to write, 'To pretend that the behaviour of PWAs [People With Aids] has nothing to do with their being sick is to kill with a false kindness'); and on the other, a missionary-like condemnation of 'unsafe' sex, although the consumerisation of sex through condom campaigns risks deeply damaging effects on health and happiness. In addition, the illusion suited the recipients of the billions in research moneys that the HIV hypothesis drew forth.

Stretching or disregarding facts to fit a comfortable theory – or to avoid the discomfort of admitting error – has been a human weakness since ancient times, but there has rarely been a more dramatic example, or one with such far-reaching consequences, as that surrounding the theory that the collection of immune deficiency diseases known as Aids is caused by a deadly new virus called HIV. How this particular Procrustean bed came into existence, enticing almost all the world to lie on it, despite a paucity of scientific evidence, and how it was sustained vigorously for more than a decade, despite numerous findings that contradicted it, is the subject of this book.

The story has no specific villain. Many have profited from the HIV paradigm, but there has been a collective quality about its rapid acceptance and promulgation that makes it more of a social phenomenon than a crime demanding retribution. Many have also suffered, including not just the numerous victims of an unwarranted HIV 'death sentence', and the gay men and others who have died because of false beliefs about the nature of their illness, but also doctors and scientists whose consciences have been troubled by the gap between their own observations and instincts, and what they were told to believe by the church of science.

A few have persistently raised their voices against the conventional view, withstanding considerable pressures to be quiet, and becoming outcasts because of their refusal to lie on the bed of conformity. They have sacrificed time, energy, professional standing, wealth and even health for the sake of their doubts, beliefs and convictions, but they have kept their integrity, and they are the stronger ones today. Their stories provide a framework for examining the various challenges made to the 'deadly virus' theory since Aids was first described in 1981, and the response to those challenges from the worlds of science and medicine.

A reader new to the HIV-Aids controversy may be outraged to find me referring with such apparent certainty to 'illusions' surrounding the subject. After all, has not the World Health Organization declared that 30-40 million people world-wide will be HIV-infected by the end of the century, that Aids cases in Africa soared from 2.5 million to 4 million during 1993, and that cases in Asia increased eight-fold, from 30,000 to 250,000, over the same period? Haven't numerous scientific and medical bodies declared HIV to be 'beyond reasonable doubt' as the cause of Aids?

It is true not merely that most of the world's doctors and scientists accepted the HIV theory, but that the theory itself has more merit than some of its critics have acknowledged. It led to greater caution over the quality of blood supplies. It boosted 'safer sex' precautions, which, despite the 'condom culture' disadvantages, must have reduced the burden of disease in some, even if not in the way HIV protagonists believed.

Furthermore, a novel phenomenon *was* identified at an early point in the epidemic, related to immune system over-activation and, potentially, to Aids, by French researchers headed by the Institut Pasteur's Professor Luc Montagnier, and by an American team led by Dr Robert Gallo, of the government-funded National Cancer Institute. Their observations were a worthwhile achievement.

The interpretation of those observations as signifying the presence of a new virus, which caused the collapse of the immune system seen in Aids by gradually destroying all the body's T-cells, went beyond what was proven at the time, but very quickly became established as dogma. This book looks at some different interpretations of the same facts, with the help of the hindsight provided by much that has happened since.

One reason for the success of the virus concept was Gallo's skill in marketing it. He was helped in this by Reagan administration officials who, having belatedly awoken to the severity of Aids, were desperate to be seen to be doing something tangible and who acclaimed the virus 'discovery' as a victory for American science – thereby also setting in train a long-running and distracting dispute with French scientists over who had found it first. But Gallo's real coup was the simultaneous publication in *Science* on 4 May 1984 of four papers from his laboratory. 'Getting one paper in *Science* is a lot,' Gallo was reported as saying. 'Getting two is fantastic. Getting three is a record. We had four at one time.'

The first described the development of a cell system for continuously producing a cytopathic (cell-killing) retrovirus, which Gallo called HTLV-3, from patients with Aids and at risk of Aids. The second claimed detection and isolation of the new virus from forty-eight such patients. The third presented a case to the effect that the microbe was a member of a species of retrovirus Gallo had previously claimed to have isolated, the HTLV family. The fourth described the development of a blood test for the virus, which was to come to be known as the 'HIV test', and which subsequently swept the world.

Problems over the accuracy of claims made in these papers emerged almost immediately, but were eventually documented in meticulous detail on 19 November 1989 in a book-length special report, 'The Great Aids Quest – Science Under the Microscope', by John Crewdson in the *Chicago Tribune*. Crewdson summarised the story as one of 'misstated data and secret experiments, phantom viruses and disappearing genes, unreproducible results and muddled lab notes, mislabeled cultures and misleading photographs'. For him, the special interest lay in demonstrating how Gallo misrepresented his lab's early experience with a sample sent from France. The result was that it seemed he had come first in the race to find an Aids virus, when in fact the French sample played a fundamental part in his own lab's work. But as we shall see, Gallo may well have been right to challenge the French claims to have discovered a new virus. Where he went wrong was in making and successfully promoting similar claims on his own behalf.

New Approach Needed

I have been on a long journey of inquiry myself. As medical correspondent of the *Sunday Times* during the second half of the 1980s, I was responsible for many articles that accepted and promoted the prevailing view of HIV as the universally accepted cause of Aids, and reported warnings that because it was a virus either new or newly spreading within humanity, almost everyone could be at risk. It was not until 1992, now playing the somewhat different role of science correspondent, that a special set of circumstances made me aware that a serious scientific challenge had been mounted to the orthodoxy. Somewhat reluctantly, because of all I had previously thought and written about HIV, I checked out the arguments and many of the references and the responses given by the mainstream to the dissident voices. After some weeks, in April 1992, colleagues decided that the case for questioning HIV's role was compelling enough to be put before a national newspaper audience for the first time.

We were not convinced at that time that HIV had no role in Aids, let alone that the microbe which thousands of scientists had spent years studying could be a figment of their collective imagination. But since then the evidence has mounted to the point where I have reached the view that the HIV theory does not fit the facts as they have now been established. A false paradigm of Aids causation is harming patients, the public, the public purse, and the image of two great professions. A new approach is urgently needed to establish the true causes of the conditions known as Aids, and how to prevent and treat them.

There has been official acceptance that ten years of intensive research into HIV – research currently costing $1.3 billion a year in the US alone – has raised more questions than it has answered. The focus on anti-HIV drug therapies has proved fruitless. It has 'masked an ignorance of many basic facts about how HIV works', as *Nature* put it in a 1994 editorial. In the same issue, the journal published an article in which the late Dr Bernard Fields, chairman of the department of microbiology and molecular genetics at Harvard Medical School, argued that the very definition of Aids research should be broadened, to include research on diseases that might at first glance seem to have little relationship to Aids.

Science, in a February 1995 report recalling Fields's article, said it had touched a nerve 'because it crystallised what many Aids researchers were themselves beginning to admit: they still lacked a basic understanding of how HIV works, and as a result, have yet to discover a drug or vaccine that can outwit the virus'. In the same article, reporter Jon Cohen described renewed optimism among Aids researchers after the publication of studies purporting to answer one of Duesberg's original objections to the HIV hypothesis, that there was nothing like enough virus present in Aids patients to account for the decline in their immune system. But the studies, despite being trumpeted by *Nature* as 'an embarrassment for Duesberg' because they 'resolve the paradox', amounted to little more than a mathematical game, in which it was speculated that billions of virus particles were indeed produced every day, and billions of cells infected, but that they could not be detected because they were destroyed at the same rate by the immune system. I shall be describing arguments which challenge the fundamental assumptions behind these calculations. The papers may come to be seen as one of the final, desperate flings by orthodoxy to breathe a little more life into a dying theory.

One sign of a failing paradigm is an increasing complexity in the arguments used to support it and, in the case of a medical hypothesis, increasing complexity in proposed treatment regimens. Single-drug therapy cannot succeed, according to a *Nature* commentary[3] discussing the mathematically deduced 'virological mayhem', because a patient without symptoms can harbour at least 1 million genetically distinct variants of HIV, and for an Aids patient the figure is said to exceed 100 million variants. 'Against this background, monotherapy cannot succeed. Only combinations of drugs have the potential to outgun the virus.'

Thus, HIV is kept in the mainstream's frame, but is acknowledged to be 'A Most Clever Virus', as *US News & World Report* headlined an account of the 1993 international Aids conference in Berlin. The article, subtitled 'Aids researchers are humbled by HIV's microscopic artifices and wiles', attributed the 'false promises and disappointments of all efforts to treat Aids' to HIV's supposed ingenuity. It concluded: 'More than any time since the discovery of HIV, researchers are openly expressing a sense of frustration. They are not even clear on what more they must know about the virus to win the battle against Aids.' A similar refrain was heard at the 1994 international conference in Yokohama, Japan. There was open acknowledgement that a vaccine against HIV, originally thought likely to be available within a couple of years of the announcement that the virus had been identified, has not just proved difficult to develop but is still not even on the horizon.

Predictions of HIV's spread, based on the 'new virus' theory, have turned out to be not just inaccurate but completely ill-conceived. In countries such as the UK where relatively careful testing and screening programmes have been established, estimates of the numbers of people testing HIV-positive are lower than they were seven to eight years ago. An anonymous screening survey published in 1993 came up with an estimated total of 23,000, hardly an epidemic in a nation of 55 million people, and a half to a third of estimated totals quoted by experts during the second half of the 1980s. Aids cases outside the original 'risk groups' – that is, where no special risk has been identified – are almost non-existent in such countries: a cumulative total of sixty-three in the UK in the ten years to the end of 1992, out of an overall total of nearly 7,000 cases; and sixty-six out of 37,600 in New York City, where from the start the health department has put considerable effort into investigating the background to cases. In the US as a whole, latest estimates (as of November 1995) put the total number of people testing HIV-positive at between 630,000 and 897,000, lower than a previous, long-standing Public Health Service estimate of around 1 million people.

Unvalidated Test

The situation as I have come to understand it is far more hopeful for patients than the HIV paradigm allows. HIV-positivity does not signify infection with an inevitably fatal virus, as so many have been led to believe. Since *Nature* first touched on the seemingly paradoxical animal test results, powerful evidence has accumulated that the HIV test does not signify infection with a virus at all, harmless or otherwise. It should definitely no longer be used.

I shall be describing the work of scientists who have shown that the antibody proteins which it detects are not specific to a particular virus, but rather an indication that the immune system has been challenged by one or more of a variety of stimuli. I shall also be describing evidence that when that challenge is removed, the risk of Aids recedes dramatically. The ever-increasing time span said to lie between 'infection' and Aids – it has grown from an initial estimate of between one and five years to a recent projection that 15-20 per cent of HIV-positive people will still be healthy after twenty-five years – does not reflect improved understanding of HIV, but a fundamental flaw in thinking. For the most part, for narrative purposes, I shall abide by the convention that HIV exists as a genuine viral entity, although even that assumption will ultimately be challenged.

The information and arguments set out in this book should not be taken as criticism of those who, in good faith, have promoted the HIV theory, believing it to be both true and desperately important. In particular, the arguments should not detract from our admiration for those many people who, touched by the plight of Aids victims, have given of their time, money and energies to try to help. That includes many scientists, doctors and other health professionals. Around the world, thousands have benefited from their generosity and care.

As well as attempting to describe what has happened, however, the book will look at how and why the illusions surrounding HIV and Aids arose, and how they could have been sustained for so long. Academics are beginning to address this question. David Mertz, a philosopher of science at the University of Massachusetts, Amherst, says HIV is an 'entity of convenience' that met the needs of powerful groups: researchers competing for personal and national prestige after the failure of the US 'war on cancer'; gay civil rights campaigners 'who wanted to remake Aids as an "equal opportunity killer"'; and the right wing, 'who wanted an agent to concretise the "wrath of God" that they fantasised as visited upon gays'. Professor Hiram Caton, head of the school of applied ethics at Griffith University, Brisbane, Australia, says that after the orthodox view has collapsed – which must happen 'because it flunks the practical tests...the hype will exhaust its credibility' – we will then have to come to terms with an awful fact: 'The Aids epidemic was a mirage manufactured by scientists who believed that integrity could be maintained amidst the diverting influences of big money, prestige and politics.'

In recent years, I believe we have been witnessing a kind of group mental pathology concerning Aids, affecting opinion leaders in the scientific and medical professions. It is such that the closer critics have come to unmasking the illusion, the more agitated the 'patient' becomes. After investing so much money and energy and professional credibility in HIV, many doctors, scientists, politicians, gay activists, charities and religious organisations involved with the fight against Aids have been finding it hard to adjust to the reality as it has gradually emerged. Challenges to the HIV theory, and to the predictions and treatments associated with it, have often been greeted with emotion bordering on hysteria. Contrary views have been marginalised, authoritative critics silenced, persistent 'dissidents' ignored or abused. At one point, after a series of *Sunday Times* articles exploring the case against HIV, *Nature* even contemplated organising pickets of the newspaper's offices in the hope of persuading it to end its 'perverse' reporting on the issue.

Because of its devastating nature as well as its association with sex and drugs, Aids touches strong feelings in almost all of us. This has made it easy for people and groups with opposing viewpoints to accuse one another of ignoring facts in order to favour some fixed viewpoint. Despite a right-left concordance on the peril of Aids in the mid-1980s, many people believed that the *Sunday Times,* for example, was pursuing a right-wing agenda when at the end of the decade it first challenged the claims that a heterosexual epidemic was imminent and that everyone was at risk. (It is unfortunately true that in the UK, a definite political divide developed in newspaper coverage of this issue, with those on the right proving much more ready to discount claims of heterosexual spread, and those on the left much more ready to promote them.) When, as science correspondent, I began to set out the case for questioning the HIV theory, it was readily assumed that my reports reflected some editorial slant, although the reality was that at first I had to fight hard within the office to have the idea that HIV might not be the cause of Aids taken seriously. I was surprised and eventually wearied by the vehemence of the attacks, and at the lack of considered response to information which I felt to be of life-and-death importance.

I shall examine suggestions that lack of integrity is a key issue in the generation and maintenance of the HIV myth, but not in the sense of obvious corruption. On the contrary, many of those who have been most active in the fight against Aids live with the sense that for once in their lives they have been doing something really worthwhile. The fight seemed to make it possible for them to demonstrate aspects of their own potential as human beings which were otherwise denied expression.

Identity Crisis

Michael Baumgartner, a Swiss man working in the field of Aids, says that despite gay liberation and the 'gay pride' movement, homosexual men are particularly liable to grow up feeling deeply unsure of themselves and their place in the world. He sees this as being partly due to the extreme polarisation of gender identity that has been prevalent in most western societies, and partly because of taboos surrounding homosexual sex. In addition, he says, homosexuality has become falsely identified with promiscuity because of the politics of gay lib. He believes these factors help to explain why the gay community in general, and not just those who have led a promiscuous lifestyle, have tended to embrace and cling determinedly to the virus theory, rather than accept that behaviour might be of primary importance in causing Aids.

Baumgartner, who came out as a gay man nearly ten years ago and has served as an Aids chaplain at San Francisco General Hospital, says: 'The fact of the matter is, a lot of gay men are ruining their lives. It's not a big proportion – maybe 1 per cent in the US – of male homosexuals overall, but if you look into who gets Aids, it's in certain risk groups. Being in the closet is the first major health risk – constantly hiding. But then, maybe as a reaction, there is the fast life, partying every night, having very little rest, not eating properly, working to be better than other people, using recreational drugs, sexual stimulants.

'A lot of people say homosexuality is a lifestyle. It's not, it's a way of being, and within that there are many different lifestyles. But Aids suddenly made what people called a homosexual lifestyle associated with death. That was not tolerable. It was much preferable to blame a virus, that can hit anybody.

'Then, over the years, HIV took on another value. Because one could present it as a threat to the general population, homosexuals became important as "cross-carriers", Jesus-like figures. We were going to die, but our lives would be the sacrifice that led to a cure that would benefit the rest of the human race. We would establish Aids organisations who would teach safer sex messages to everyone, and although it might be too late for us, the organisations would be there to care for the others as well when they needed it.

'So gay men need HIV and Aids, as an ongoing, life-threatening disease, because it fits their unacknowledged image of themselves as a tragedy, and so they can have an established role, health-wise and help-wise, in society. They will only be able to understand HIV and Aids when they reorganise their understanding about themselves. When they redefine gayness, and redefine their self-identity, the facts will fit. Until then, they may know the facts, but they cannot believe them, because they don't fit their picture of themselves.'

I find this a powerful thought, and wonder how many others – politicians, doctors, scientists, businessmen, charities, civil servants, and journalists, including myself – fell into a similar trap, of having their judgement distorted by the feeling that for once they were doing something really worthwhile, something redeeming and fulfilling, by becoming parties to the fight against HIV. I suspect it was this, rather than greed or ambition, that led so many to lie on the HIV bed, and to be so reluctant to climb off it even after it should have become clear that it was demanding more and more compromises of the intellect.

Human beings have a strong need to feel they have a place in the world. It is a need that speaks to our essentially benign nature, whose natural expression automatically earns us that place. But sometimes we become cut off from the goodwill that is our essence, and the need shows itself in weak instead of positive ways. Without realising what we are doing, we become dependent on 'giving' such that our actions are not genuinely altruistic, but instead express our neediness. In such circumstances the recipient of our 'giving' has to play the same game, and becomes dependent on its continuation. This 'co-dependency' has been well described in terms of dysfunctional family relationships, but it can happen on a mass basis as well. It binds together large groups of people who need to be caring with other groups who feel themselves to be in need of that care. I believe the HIV story provoked just such a phenomenon, at an institutional level.

At an individual level, in terms of both courage and compassion, the Aids crisis did also often bring out the best in people, both patients and their helpers. This book presents a new challenge: in the light of all the information now available, and through the eyes of a variety of observers, to experiment with different ways of looking at the syndrome, and see if there may not be benefit in adopting a different explanation from the one we have lived with for so many years.

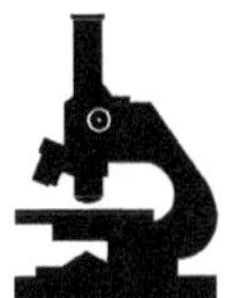

2: WHEN TWO ROADS DIVERGED

The idea that a lethal microbe, the Human Immunodeficiency Virus, is the cause of the collapse of the immune system seen in Aids has been with us for so long that it is hard to recall that anyone ever thought differently. Yet when the syndrome was first reported in the American urban gay community during the early 1980s, two schools of thought about its origins competed for dominance.

One, that rapidly gained the strongest currency, was the forerunner of the HIV story. It held that the outbreak bore the hallmarks of being caused by some as yet undiscovered transmissible agent, probably a virus; a germ that had struck out of the blue, and was unrelated to the lives of its victims except in so far as it was probably spread sexually or by the use of a needle contaminated with someone else's blood or secretions. According to this single-virus theory, even one sexual encounter with an infected person could lead to Aids. That meant that although having many sexual partners would increase one's chances of being infected, luck was also playing a big part. In time, all sexually active people could become at risk.

Many doctors and scientists, especially if they were already working with viruses, naturally warmed to this theory. It gave them a clear-cut aim that brought the fight against Aids right into their territory. They could track down the virus, then prepare drugs and vaccines against it, just as they had done so successfully with polio and smallpox, for example. So when Robert Gallo declared in 1984 that HIV was the probable culprit, the world scientific community breathed a collective sigh of relief and almost immediately rallied to the cause of defeating this new enemy of mankind. World-wide, the single-virus theory became the basis for research and public health efforts to curb the spread of the infection and thus, it was thought, to fight the disease.

But from the start, another way of looking at Aids was available. One of its most articulate and tireless exponents was Michael Callen, who was diagnosed as suffering from the full-blown syndrome in 1982 in New York City and spent the following twelve years struggling to persuade the scientific community, as well as fellow homosexuals, not to stop asking questions about the cause, or causes, of Aids. 'I don't have the answers; I only have the questions,' he told me when I met him in London in 1992, soon after I had begun to examine the HIV critique. But when I asked him what had caused the breakdown in his own system if it had not been HIV, his reply was shocking in its directness.

'You try having 3,000 men up your butt by the age of twenty-six and NOT get sick,' he said. 'And I was a baby! I knew the first wave of people with Aids: they were founders of what we called the 10,000 club; they had had 10,000 or more different sexual partners.' Callen said that among homosexual men in general, only a small minority had 'pigged out' on sex in this way. But he insisted it was within this 'brotherhood of lust' that most of the homosexual Aids cases were to be found. The single greatest risk factor for contracting Aids was a history of multiple sexual contacts with partners who were themselves having multiple sexual contacts. The Gay Liberation years of the seventies had brought unprecedented opportunities for gay men to have sex with each other, as well as unprecedented peer pressure to take advantage of these newly won freedoms, and he and others had subscribed to the idea that the more sex a gay man had, the more liberated he became. Although the lesbian and gay political agenda was much broader than sex, he was only interested in the part that dealt with pleasure. 'Never before had so many men had so much sex with so many different partners.'

In Callen's view, it wasn't just a matter of having too much sex. It was true that the immune systems of passive partners in rectal intercourse were indeed compromised by the sex act itself, especially when it involved repeated exposure to secretions from many different partners. There was also a hazard from the cumulative effects of drugs used habitually to drive this sexual merry-go-round. But the main problem, he believed, was that the men who had become a part of this fast-lane gay life, which operated on an international basis, had concentrated among themselves just about every sexually transmitted microbe available. They were a diseased group, repeatedly infecting one another; one didn't have to look beyond the way of life they had been leading to find an explanation for Aids.

Callen owed this way of thinking, and with it, he believed, the many precious years of life that were to follow his Aids diagnosis, to a New York City doctor, Joe Sonnabend, who became one of the first to identify the new syndrome when he saw and reported several cases of Kaposi's sarcoma among young gay men attending his practice in Greenwich Village. From the start, Sonnabend began to formulate a multifactorial theory about what might be causing Aids, based on what he knew about the lifestyles and disease histories of the gay men who were getting the new disease. In an early study among his patients, he found that those who were monogamous had normal immune system function; those who occasionally ran in the fast lane had minor degrees of immune dysfunction; and those such as Michael Callen with a long history of sexually transmitted disease were profoundly immune-deficient. He believed Aids probably developed in other groups through a similar multifactorial process, although the specific infections and other immune-suppressing factors might be different from those seen in gay men.

Callen had been plunged into depression by the first reports of what was then known as GRID – Gay-Related Immune Deficiency – in the *New York Native* in the spring of 1981, and by his own diagnosis the following year. In his 1990 book, *Surviving Aids,*[1] he describes how he could still remember himself on a subway platform at rush-hour, frozen in place, 'reading for the first time about a new, lethal, sexually transmitted disease that was affecting gay men'. With his history, both sexual and medical, there was no question in his mind that he would get it.

By late 1981, at the age of twenty-six, he was already experiencing mysterious fevers, night sweats, fatigue, rashes, and relentless, debilitating diarrhoea. When a doctor walked into his hospital room in June 1982, after he had collapsed from dehydration, and announced that 'it's GRID all right', a part of him felt strangely relieved. 'You have cryptosporidiosis,' the doctor said. 'Before GRID, we didn't think cryptosporidiosis infected humans. It's a disease previously found only in livestock.' While he was still trying to take in the fact that 'I had a disease of *cattle!*' as he put it, the doctor went on: 'I'm afraid there is no known treatment... all we can do is try to keep you hydrated and see what happens. Your body will either handle it or...it won't.'

This was a depressing outlook, because already at that time the predominant medical and social view of GRID was that the appearance of unusual diseases such as cryptosporidiosis, even though these were potentially lethal in their own right, was due to the ravages of some as yet unidentified killer virus that was slowly and inexorably destroying the immune system. 'Because they hadn't even identified any such virus in 1982, I felt helpless,' Callen wrote. 'And I knew that even if an Aids virus was eventually found, there probably wouldn't be a treatment for it within my lifetime, because there weren't many effective treatments for other viral infections. Believing that a killer virus was responsible for my illness made my survival prospects seem grim and sapped my will to put up a fight.' Since a reduction in cell-mediated immunity – an important branch of the body's immune defences – is a classic sign of severe depression, Callen's outlook was poor indeed.

Fighting Back

He fought back. A first step was to face squarely just how much sex, and how much disease, he'd had. From 1973, when he came out as a homosexual, to 1975, he only got mononucleosis and non-specific urethritis (NSU). In 1975 he had his first bout of gonorrhoea. 'Not bad, I thought. I'd had maybe 200 different partners and I'd only gotten the clap twice.'[2] But from there, it all began to snowball. 'First came hepatitis A in 1976. Then more gonorrhoea and NSU. In 1977, amoebas [intestinal parasites] – and hepatitis B. More NSU and gonorrhoea. 1978: more amoebas. And my first case of shigella [which causes dysentery]. And of course more VD. Then in 1979, hepatitis yet a third time: this time, non-A, non-B. More amoebas, adding giardias this time. And a fissure. And my first case of syphilis. And of course more gonorrhoea [penile, anal and oral]. In 1980: the usual gonorrhoea, shigella twice, and more amoebas. By 1981, I got some combination of venereal diseases EACH AND EVERY TIME I had sex.' Added to that list were herpes simplex types I and II; venereal warts; salmonella; chlamydia; cytomegalovirus (CMV); Epstein-Barr virus (EBV); mononucleosis; and finally cryptosporidiosis, and the diagnosis of Aids. There were also colds, sore throats, flu, rashes and other infections too numerous to count, which at the time he did not connect to his promiscuous sex life.

Promiscuous is a dangerous, emotive word that touches sensitive buttons in most of us. It is especially dangerous used in relation to a group of people who have suffered greatly from 'inhuman stereotypes', to use Callen's phrase, dumped on them by a society in which guilt over sex is near-universal, although far from universally acknowledged. 'Prior to the gay liberation movement, gay people looked in the mirror of American culture and never – not once – saw our image accurately reflected,' Callen wrote.[3] 'It's easy now, when lesbian couples attend high school proms and openly gay people are elected to Congress, to forget what it was like to be homosexual before gay liberation – particularly if you didn't live in a major city on either coast.' For the first seventeen years of his life, he had never travelled outside a sixty-mile radius of the small Indiana town where he had been born, and he was fourteen before he even heard the word that instinctively he knew must be the most horrible thing anyone could be. He was playing cards with three girls when the oldest narrowed her eyes, pointed at him, and declared: 'If you don't stop acting like a girl, you're going to turn into a homosexual.' Looking it up in a psychology textbook, he found it in the chapter on deviance alongside murderers, paedophiles and kleptomaniacs. Doctors, priests – everywhere he turned, he heard similar messages, 'that men who felt like I did were pathetic psychopaths who hung out in public rest rooms writing lurid notes to each other on toilet paper'.

Not until his first year at Boston University, when he chanced upon a meeting of a gay student group, did he find gay liberation and learn that there were millions of others like him. 'It was life-changing to discover that the horrible things mainstream society was saying about us – things I had internalised – were not true.'

He came out with a vengeance, and promiscuity formed a part of that revenge. At first he had been promiscuous because that was the textbook picture, the only information he had about gay men. But then he proudly and defiantly celebrated the promiscuity of which mainstream society so disapproved. In a lecture he attended on the eve of the age of Aids, one of his favourite authors, Edmund White, co-author of *The Joy of Gay Sex*, proposed that 'gay men should wear their sexually transmitted diseases like red badges of courage in a war against a sex-negative society'. He remembered nodding his head vigorously in agreement and saying to himself: 'Gee! Every time I get the clap I'm striking a blow for the sexual revolution!'

It was a matter of microbiological, not moral, certainty that lifestyles such as this should have led to concurrent epidemics of numerous pathogens. 'Unwittingly, and with the best of revolutionary intentions, a small subset of gay men managed to create disease settings equivalent to those of poor third-world nations in one of the richest countries on earth.'

The reason he felt it so important to dwell on promiscuity, Callen wrote in *Surviving Aids,* was that he believed he was still alive because at a crucial point in his illness he was willing to confront some of the harsh realities about the life he had led. He became convinced he had overloaded his immune system once too often; that as Sonnabend proposed, it was the repeated assaults on the immune system by a *variety of common* sexually transmitted infectious (and other non-infectious) factors that, over time, were resulting in a profound, sustained immune deficiency.

In a speech given early in 1983 at a meeting to discuss GRID, Callen, then aged twenty-seven, said his 'conservative' estimate of having had sex with more than 3,000 different partners was arrived at by taking a long, hard look at his patterns of sexual activity — 'something I advise every concerned gay man to do'. He had been having gay sex, he said, in 'tearooms, bathhouses, bookstores, backrooms and movie houses since I came out at seventeen'. These were the institutions, described vividly by Randy Shilts in *And the Band Played On,*[4] that formed a $100m sex industry across America and Canada, spawned by the gay liberation movement of the 1970s. Like Callen, gay activists had told themselves that the businesses serviced men who had long been repressed, and were perhaps now going to the extreme, but that it was all part and parcel of political liberation. Bathhouse owners were often gay political leaders as well, and some of their profits went to help support activist groups. But the institutions were a horrible breeding ground for disease. They were hot and steamy. They hosted multiple sexual liaisons, driven by drugs. And as if anal intercourse was not microbiologically hazardous enough in itself, infections were made a virtual certainty through the practice, popular at the time, of rimming, described by medical journals as 'oral-anal intercourse' and by a best-selling gay sex book as 'the prime taste treat in sex'. Cases of persistent intestinal infection, known to doctors as the Gay Bowel Syndrome, had increased by 8,000 per cent during the 1970s in San Francisco. A Denver study found that an average bathhouse patron risked a 33 per cent chance of walking out with syphilis or gonorrhoea. Another study found that 94 per cent of sexually active gay men showed evidence of CMV infection, and 7-14 per cent of gay men tested at a venereal disease clinic were actively infected, with the virus present in their semen.

Callen estimated that he went to the baths at least once a week, sometimes twice, and that each time he had a minimum of four partners 'and a maximum of... well, let's just use four. And let's not count this last year because I have stopped promiscuity entirely.' So that was nine years of active promiscuity, fifty-two weeks in a year, times four people a week – a total of 1,872. 'And that's just the baths. I also racked up about three men a week for five years at the Christopher Street Bookstore, so that's another 780 men. Then of course there was the MineShaft [a New York gay night spot]; the orgies; the 55th Street Playhouse; the International Stud backroom; the Amsterdam Bookstore; trips to similar establishments in San Francisco, Los Angeles, Atlanta, Boston, Europe. You see my point.'

Not just anyone developed Aids, Callen said. In a Centres for Disease Control (CDC) study of the first 100 gay men with Aids, their median number of lifetime sexual partners was 1,160. 'That number indicates a very specific type of gay person with a very specific lifestyle,' Callen said. 'In plain English, only excessively promiscuous gay men like me are developing Aids.' As the National Cancer Institute had reported the previous year, 'Taking all of the apparent epidemiological observations together, a growing accumulation of risk factors is suggested rather than spread in the classic sense of contagion... The syndrome is occurring mainly in a specific subset of homosexual men, possibly, but not exclusively defined by the number of sexual partners.'

Callen said he always got into a lot of trouble when he used the words 'excessively promiscuous' among clinically healthy gay men – 'that is, gay men who are not yet showing symptoms of Aids'. But when he met in groups with other Aids victims, no one ever had any trouble understanding what he meant. 'The sexual history of every Aids victim that I have spoken to has been consistent with mine. Every Aids victim I have read about or met has had many lifetime sexual partners (most in excess of 1,000) and each man has had the correspondingly long list of sexually transmitted infections which attend the promiscuous lifestyle.

'Of course, not all of us tell the CDC the truth. Some Aids victims see no reason to tell others – particularly some heterosexual CDC interviewer – the true extent of their sexual excess. Yet you will continually hear rumours of monogamous or sexually celibate gay men (whatever that means) who have developed Aids. Let me assure you, this simply is not true. There are none. I reiterate: each Aids victim has a long history of many sexually transmitted infections and this fact can be verified by an examination of their blood for evidence of antibodies to diseases prevalent among the sexually promiscuous and by a review of their medical files.'

Callen said his views were based on his own reading in the medical and lay press, discussions with various researchers, discussions in support groups with other gay men with Aids, and his own experiences as an Aids sufferer. 'My sense from talking with other Aids victims is that the 1,160 median number of lifetime sexual partners that the CDC study has found is probably an underestimate. But let's use that figure for a moment. There would, of course, be no particular health consequences from having sex with 1,160 *healthy* people. But as a simple function of mathematics, disease rises exponentially when so many people are having so much sex with each other. The real issue is that so many common diseases have become epidemic on the gay circuit. Clearly, having sex with 1,160 people, when a large percentage of them at the time of sex are sick with CMV and other infections, has led to more serious health consequences. Promiscuity has finally led to the development of a profound and apparently self-sustaining state of immune suppression in those of us who have so abused our body's defences.

'Sometimes I believe that even the gay researchers and those affectionately known as "clap doctors" do not grasp the magnitude of the promiscuity I am talking about. If on a typical evening at the baths one has sex with four people, each of whom has had sex with four people, each of whom has had sex with four people, the cumulative health effect will be an explosion of disease. This is exactly what has happened. My Aids is simply the logical result of having been sick so often and having continually exposed myself, through promiscuity, to the whole array of common diseases epidemic on the gay circuit.

'So many people have a knee-jerk defensiveness to use of the word "promiscuity". Some say the word has no meaning – that it is not exact enough to be useful scientifically. They believe that when I decry promiscuity, I do so from some vague morality or some discomfort with sex or my own gayness. Though it seems strange that someone who has had sex with over 3,000 men could be accused of having problems with sex or with his gayness, this is nevertheless often the charge. Let me assure you: I don't have problems with sex or my gayness; 1 have problems with DISEASE. I am sick of being sick. And not just sick with Aids, but sick of the myriad of common infections to which so many promiscuous gay men have grown so accustomed.'

That speech, in early 1983, reflected the position as Callen saw it at the time. After the introduction of the HIV test, the definition of Aids was to be constantly widened and, as we shall see, more and more people were pulled into an HIV/Aids diagnosis, including many for whom promiscuity formed no part of their background. But Callen was concerned with how Aids was occurring in gay men, and in subsequent years he remained convinced that Aids would never be understood until it was put in the context of the gay sex explosion of the 1970s. Understanding the correct theory was critical, he said, because each theory had different consequences for treatment and prevention, because the political and social consequences of the two theories were so different, 'and because in the end, only one theory will prove to correctly explain why Aids is occurring in some gay men'.

'We Know Who We Are'

A few months before this impassioned speech, Callen had written a remarkable article with another Aids sufferer, Richard Berkowitz, on the background to the epidemic, at that point only about two years old. Published in the *New York Native* in November 1982, it was called 'We Know Who We Are: Two Gay Men Declare War on Promiscuity'. The article declared there was 'overwhelming evidence' that the health crisis was a direct result of unprecedented promiscuity on the urban gay sex circuit. Denial of this fact 'is killing us,' it said, and would continue to do so 'until we begin the difficult task of changing the ways in which we have sex'. It went on:

> Those of us who have been promiscuous have sat on the sidelines throughout this epidemic and by our silence have tacitly encouraged wild speculation about a new, mutant, Andromeda-strain virus. We have remained silent because we have been unable or unwilling to accept responsibility for the role that our own excessiveness has played in our present health crisis. But, deep down, we know who we are and we know why we're sick.

There was no evidence for the 'new or mutant virus' theory. Aids was not 'spreading' the way one would expect a single-viral epidemic to spread. In their review of medical literature, and in conversations with Aids victims and their doctors, the authors had encountered no evidence that non-promiscuous gay men were contracting Aids, although it was certainly possible that an individual with few sexual partners could be at risk if those partners were themselves highly diseased. 'If one partner in a couple is monogamous and the other is not, the effect of disease transmission will be similar for both partners.'

As for Aids cases reported in drug abusers, haemophiliacs and Haitians, there were different logical explanations for risk of immunosuppression in each of these groups, and therefore no need to postulate a single virus as the common cause. Diseases associated with profoundly depressed immune responses had been noted in intravenous drug abusers for years. By sharing needles, they often exposed themselves to common viruses from others' blood. By injecting these viruses directly into the bloodstream, they bypassed the body's front-line defences. And it did not help that these abusers often ingested narcotics which were further immunosuppressive.

Haemophiliacs periodically received blood transfusions, obtained from many different donors, and so continual re-exposure and reinfection with common viruses might also have led to the Aids that had been occurring in that community. Haitians, due to generally poor sanitary conditions, were also frequently exposed and reinfected with a variety of tropical viruses endemic to the region.

Further, review of autopsy reports in the United States and Europe going back thirty years indicated cases which bore a striking resemblance to Aids, even though verification was impossible as the tests which detected immune deficiency had only recently come into use. 'It now seems quite likely that Aids has occurred in the United States and other countries before, but has only recently been recognised.'

The article also noted that 'the heroic hunt for mutant viruses' had been a response in previous epidemics when doctors had found that their usual weapons against disease were ineffective. In the winter of 1978-9, there was an outbreak of fatal respiratory infections among children in Naples, Italy. Initially, a new virus was blamed. But eventually 'Naples disease' proved to be the result of immune system depression caused by 'socio-economic factors such as malnutrition and family size, and a transitory immunosuppression due to vaccination'.[5]

On the basis of their analysis, which was backed by considerable scientific evidence, Callen and Berkowitz warned fellow gay men not to expect the arrival of a vaccine or drug treatment for Aids. The need of the hour was for someone to connect the new syndrome to behaviour and lifestyle, especially as these were factors that could be susceptible to change. 'While a fatally disorganised gay leadership scrambles for a way to present promiscuity in a manner palatable to a generally unsophisticated heterosexist world (and an understandably defensive gay community) gay men are dying unnecessarily.'

They expected controversy. No one was naive enough, they said, to believe that providing a clear warning about the dangers of promiscuity would bring about its end. Promiscuity had spawned an industry 'which has a stake in keeping us promiscuous, even if it kills us. Where is the money that we've spent on pleasure over the last thirteen years, now that we need it for our survival?'

The authors were also aware of the potential political ramifications of making the link between promiscuity and Aids, but felt that should not be allowed to get in the way of the facts. 'Unfortunately, those who would say that promiscuity is related to the incidence of Aids would appear to be correct. This is a statement of scientific fact, not moralistic bluster. Those who fear linking promiscuity with the present epidemic should consider the far more dangerous implication already circulating in the national media: that gay men are carrying and spreading a fatal, cancer-causing virus.'

Disease had changed the definition of promiscuity. What ten years previously was viewed as a healthy reaction to a sex-negative culture now threatened to destroy the very fabric of urban gay male life. 'What we have in the 1980s is a positive political force tied to a dangerous lifestyle. We must recognise the self-hating short-sightedness involved in knowingly or half-knowingly infecting our sexual partners with disease, only to have that disease return to us in exponential form.'

Today, in 1995, after thirteen more years of the death and suffering caused by Aids, I find it striking that most of the observations and predictions made in the *Native* article have been confirmed by harsh experience. Yet our society has still not come to terms with the truths it contained. There is no vaccine in sight. There is no effective drug treatment available. The syndrome is killing thousands, but it remains almost exclusively confined to the original groups whose lifestyle puts them at risk of immune suppression, regardless of HIV.

The gay community was rightly concerned about what it describes as 'sexual fascism' among those who were uncomfortable with their own sexuality. It had seen plenty of examples of hostility being dressed up as a concern for morality, most notably in Nazi Germany but with echoes down through subsequent decades in the behaviour of some right-wing, 'moral majority' or religious fundamentalist groups. But gay activists who had spearheaded the linking of gay sexual identity with promiscuity were also compromised, along with their sympathisers on the left. In their minds, a new killer virus *had* to be the cause of Aids, and all those who suggested otherwise were obviously working from some hidden anti-sex or anti-gay agenda. What they did not realise was that the killer virus theory also met the needs of the moralists for a sacrificial witch hunt. The needs of both these subgroups came together to create an enduring 'group fantasy', as the psychiatrist Dr Casper Schmidt has described it,[6] 'a trance state which is noticeable in a certain suspension of logic in the lay press and the medical literature'.

Fierce Reaction

Callen and Berkowitz were not prepared for the ferocity of the reaction their article provoked. It caused such a stir that Chuck Ortleb, the *Native's* publisher, 'refused to ever publish another word by us', according to Callen. That was despite the *Native* carrying four critical articles and several letters which, the pair said, misrepresented their views, refused to deal with the science as presented by their hypothesis, and centred around 'such tedious and distracting digressions as "tone", "guilt", "panic and paranoia", "morality" and "blaming-the-victim".'

One of these articles, 'In Defence of Promiscuity', slated the pair for having a 'superior tone'. Another, 'Guilt and Aids', objected to the 'vehemence of tone', and claimed that 'the real message' Callen and Berkowitz imparted was their feeling of guilt. In another issue, a medical doctor linked them with 'the right which in our time has been strongly associated with religious fundamentalism', described them as 'not unlike religious converts', implied that they were 'sex-negative propagandists' out to exploit the Aids epidemic, and referred to their 'vigilante impulsivity'. An attack in another journal referred to them as the 'Callen/Berkowitz/Sonnabend axis' and claimed that they had urged promiscuous gay men to 'follow along in self-flagellation'.

In an article submitted and rejected for publication in the *Native* –their third unsuccessful attempt to respond to the criticisms – Callen and Berkowitz declared themselves suspicious of the motives of those who continually raised the issue of guilt, pointing out that it had not once been used in their own previous writings. 'The fact is that neither of us has experienced a moment of guilt about our own promiscuous behaviour. We are, however, capable of accepting some responsibility for the role that promiscuity and the illnesses which have resulted from that lifestyle appears to have played in the development of our present life-threatening illnesses. We believe that the prudish responses of some readers to *any* frank discussion about certain sexual lifestyles show more about their *own* guilt than about any guilt we supposedly feel. Most shocking to us is the implicit notion that anyone who talks about having many sexual partners must somehow feel guilty. Neither of us has problems with our gayness or with sexuality; we have problems with disease.'

They felt that the 'incredible' resistance to the immune overload theory stemmed from those who felt it 'blamed the victim' for Aids. But issues of blame and guilt were irrelevant to the development of any disease. It would be pointless to 'blame' a smoker for developing lung cancer, or for the smoker to waste time feeling guilty. 'But it would not be inappropriate to state that the smoker must bear some responsibility for his condition.' Few gay men could have predicted 'that the result of overloading our immune systems with so many common diseases would result in a disease syndrome as devastating as Aids. But being victims of a disease does not preclude the possibility that particular habits of an individual may have encouraged the development of a particular disease.'

Callen and Berkowitz complained that the attacks on their 'tone' were attempts to obscure the fact 'that no one had bothered to discuss the *science* underlying our hypothesis. We now believe that most of the controversy resulted from the simple fact that we reached different conclusions than those sanctioned by a visible and vocal majority of gay "leaders". We anger some gays because we are unwilling to join the "new germ" bandwagon.'

The president of the New York Physicians for Human Rights, for example, had betrayed the underlying cause of his anger when he stated:

> They also reject the idea that there is a previously unrecognised germ causing the epidemic... It's all our fault, they seem to say; there is no new germ at all, it's just us gays being promiscuous, doing all this damage to ourselves. But they go further. They seek to discredit the other theory, the new germ theory.

'We sought to "discredit" the "new germ theory",' Callen and Berkowitz wrote, 'precisely because we do not believe sufficient evidence has been produced to support it; furthermore, we believed at the time – and continue to believe – that the new germ theory has dangerous political ramifications for the gay and other disenfranchised communities presently affected by Aids.' The theory offered a simplistic solution to a complex phenomenon. It painted gays in the familiar role of victims. It deflected attention from public scrutiny of the commercialised sex circuit of bathhouses, backrooms, bookstores, and so on. It raised the hope that there would be a vaccine. It created hope 'that any changes we must make in the way we socialise will only be temporary'.

The immune overload theory, by contrast, 'shifts public attention away from a sense of random and raging contagion and identifies specific risk factors. If the immune overload theory is correct, the common link between all affected Aids groups is that each is being repeatedly re-exposed and reinfected with common viruses. The task then becomes to figure out precisely how each different group is exposed, and it is unlikely that the methods will be the same for the different groups. Though poor sanitation, malnutrition, drug abuse and contact with blood products "contaminated" with many common viruses may constitute the risk factors in other groups, multiple sexual contacts in settings where common viruses have reached epidemic levels would constitute the risk factor in gay men'. This way of looking at Aids might seem less preferable than a 'new germ' theory at first, but it would diffuse panic over some random epidemic 'by relieving those who are neither poor, abuse drugs, require blood products or are promiscuous' from worrying that they were going to catch Aids. That included the majority of gay men who did not lead the 'fast lane' urban lifestyle. Because gay leaders had been unwilling to admit that there were different gay lifestyles, that majority had been forced to share the stigma and fear of Aids.

They went on: 'For those of us who are ill, for those who wish to avoid developing Aids and for those physicians faced with the burden of treating patients with techniques and medications of unproven efficacy, the issue is not what *may* be causing Aids; rather, the issue is what is *most probably* causing Aids. We do not wish to limit speculation or research; we simply wish to prevent premature "authoritative" endorsement of the single virus theory.'

Undaunted by the fire-storm of protest over 'We Know Who We Are', in May 1983 Callen and Berkowitz published 5,000 copies of a forty-eight-page booklet called *How to Have Sex in an Epidemic: One Approach.* It was one of the first, if not the first, publications to introduce the concept of safe sex (the 'r' was added to 'safe' later, Callen wrote in *Surviving Aids,* to appease conservatives who maintained there was no such thing as risk-free sex). Widely disseminated, the booklet was based on Joe Sonnabend's multifactorial theory and emphasised interrupting the transfer of bodily fluids, later to become an accepted standard of Aids risk reduction. But even this advice drew harsh criticism from gay leaders when it was first proposed. They argued that to focus attention on the diseases common among promiscuous gay men was to 'shout guilt from the rooftops'.

'When I say that I had a hand in inventing safe sex, it startles most people because it's now so much a part of our ethos, especially for gay men, that they have to stop and imagine that it needed to be invented,' Callen told me in London a decade later. 'But this was two years before the HIV theory. Aids involves infectious and non-infectious immunological assaults, but controlling the infectious assaults is most crucial. Things like the rectal introduction of semen will not in and of themselves cause Aids, but they modify the body's ability to respond properly to an immunological assault.'

Ill-effects of 'Killer Virus' Theory

Within a year of Callen and Berkowitz failing to persuade the *Native* to publish their response to the attacks on 'We Know Who We Are', a single virus, HIV, became accepted as the cause of Aids. To many, that rapid acceptance by the scientific and medical communities meant the argument was over. However well-meaning the interventions by those who had argued otherwise, they had been wrong. The world had to get on with the job of countering the enormous threat posed by HIV.

As the years passed, however, Callen continued to maintain that the widespread acceptance of the HIV hypothesis did not make it true, and that the evidence in its favour had never amounted to scientific proof. So many groups of people, he felt, had wanted a 'killer virus' to be on the loose that the HIV theory had been allowed to enter scientific lore without adequate examination. In December 1987, he wrote in the PWA (People With Aids) Coalition newsletter: 'The cause of Aids remains unknown. There. I've said it! It's heresy, I know, but as far as I can tell, the sky hasn't fallen in.' The following year, he wrote in similar vein:

> Belief that HIV has been proven to be 'the cause' of Aids has many of the characteristics of religion: as 'revealed truth', it's not wholly rational, but emotionally reassuring and certainly influential. I often compare my attempts to generate debate on the cause (s) of Aids to walking into a fundamentalist revival meeting and asking those present at least to *consider* the possibility that God doesn't exist. There are blank looks of incomprehension. (But of *course* HIV is the cause of Aids!) Some shake their heads and grimace as if to say they must not have heard me right. When I persist in stating my belief that the cause or causes of Aids remain

> unknown, this initial incomprehension turns to either pity or contempt. ('Poor boy; he must have Aids dementia.') Or I'm lumped in with the *New York Native* theory-of-the-week group or with the CIA/conspiracy theory loonies. ('Oh, you're one of *them.'*)
>
> HIV breeds a form of scientific nationalism: you're either for it or against it. And like America, one must apparently love it or leave the Aids debate.

Few gay leaders, he said, seemed to have thought through the harmful social consequences resulting from the unproven notion that gay men – once thought to be merely morally contagious – were now, by the HIV hypothesis, literally contagious with a new killer virus. When one had told Congress in 1983 that Aids was 'a steaming locomotive aimed at the general population', the strategy was apparently that the only way to get an adequate research response from homophobic Americans was to scare them with the notion that they were going to get Aids too. But all sorts of discrimination could be traced to the notion that gay men and other groups were carrying a killer virus. 'Although most Aids discrimination is odious, it's also easy to understand. Humans seem to have an almost instinctual fear of those who are sick and, given the press HIV has been receiving, I'm not sure *I'd* want to be around someone carrying such a killer virus. The best analogy is probably rabies. PWAs – indeed all members of risk groups – are now treated with the horror reserved for mad, frothing dogs. (Prison guards' and policepersons' obsessive fear of being bitten by people carrying HIV fits this analogy nicely.)'

Another ill-effect of the killer virus theory was that if Aids was something being done to you, there wasn't much you could do for yourself to prevent its inexorable march. 'Countless first-wave PWAs said, "Well, I have Aids, so what does it matter if I stop smoking, stop drinking, stop getting sexually transmitted diseases etc." Many became quite passive in the belief that "the virus" would have its way with them no matter what they did. By contrast, the notion that Aids was the result of repeated assaults on the immune system suggested to some of us that if we figured out what those results were and stopped them, we might theoretically recover before the immune deficiency became self-sustaining.' Belief in HIV could be disempowering. Those who saw HIV behind every rash, ache, pain and neurological oddity were often sapped of the fighting spirit which seemed necessary to have a chance of beating Aids.

Women and children who were getting Aids in America were also marginalised and disempowered by the simplistic notion of a single killer virus. They were from a very specific socio-economic class: poor blacks and Hispanics. A multifactorial explanation of their illness would have been threatening to some political interests, as it would have forced an examination of their poverty, the reasons for it, and the health consequences of it. A 'killer virus' made it unnecessary to examine the social conditions from which the disease was springing. 'So we find ourselves in a situation where the New Right – which would have wished to avoid the suggestion that cuts in programmes for maternal care and the failure of drug treatment programmes might have been contributing to rising infant mortality – preferred for its own reasons the same explanation for Aids that gay men favoured for very different reasons.'

Aids meant day-to-day management of uncertainty, Callen added. Because of that, 'when I and others suggest that the one central "fact" of Aids may not be true, we unleash a storm of emotions. So much seems to depend on our believing that HIV has been *proven* to be the cause of Aids that we label as the anti-Christ those who suggest otherwise... If you'll pardon the paraphrase, the religion of HIV has become the opiate of the masses. And it's keeping us from asking some important questions.

'I often wake in the middle of the night and wonder: what if *I'm* wrong! What if HIV is every terrible thing they say it is? Well, all I can say is, they haven't convinced me yet. If it's so obvious that HIV is pathological, it ought to be pretty simple to produce proof that even a layperson can understand. And in any event, I have tried to present my multifactorial views in such a way as not to exclude the possibility that HIV may play a role in Aids. Although right now it remains my suspicion that HIV is probably only rarely, if ever, pathogenic, I am not so arrogant that I would assert that as fact.'

Even though HIV's dominance of scientific thinking on Aids seemed to have shown that the Callen and Berkowitz stand was wrong, the specific predictions they made on the basis of the multifactorial model have been largely vindicated. We now know that in the western countries at least, predictions based on the 'deadly new virus' model, that everyone was at risk and millions would soon be testing HIV-positive, were wildly inaccurate. Even in the United States, Aids has left many geographical areas and population groups virtually untouched, and they will probably remain so, according to a 1993 National Research Council panel report. Instead, says the report, the syndrome has remained largely confined to 'socially disadvantaged' groups of people. Callen and Berkowitz were making the same point back in 1982-3, but nobody was able to listen.

The same is true of their predictions about the possibilities of long-term survival. The 'deadly new virus' theory meant nothing could be done to save patients other than strive for a vaccine and anti-viral therapy. When very sick men died of Aids within months of their HIV diagnosis, it was assumed that the outlook would be similarly grim for all those who tested HIV-positive. But that too was quite wrong. The scientific and medical mainstream has had to keep extending its estimates of the likely time lag between 'infection' and death, as many HIV-positive people remain stubbornly well. It was no surprise to those holding the multifactorial view, however, that people who were able and willing to remove some or all of the damaging risk factors from their lives stood a chance of halting or reversing the damage to their immune system.

The worst aspect of the mainstream approach, Callen said at a 1992 conference in Amsterdam, was that it had failed to provide answers to the fundamental question of what people could do to stay alive. This was 'the most damning evidence that the HIV hypothesis has produced nothing of value for people like me,' he said. 'If the hypothesis had produced any therapies that actually extend life or improve the quality of life, I would be less crazy about attacking it. But in fact, not only has it in my opinion not produced any therapies of value, it has produced therapies that – I believe – are making people sick and shortening people's lives, and ruining the quality of whatever time they have left on Earth.' He was referring in particular to the anti-viral drug AZT, once embraced by orthodoxy as the 'gold standard' of Aids treatment, but which from his own observations among gay men, and from his reading of the scientific literature, left most people worse off than if they hadn't started it at all.

Secrets of Long-term Survivors

I shall be looking in more detail at the tragic story of AZT later in this book. For the moment, suffice it to say that in researching his 1990 book *Surviving Aids,* Callen interviewed nearly fifty people who had lived for many years not just after being pronounced HIV-positive, but after an Aids diagnosis. He found that only four had ever used AZT; three of those had since died, and one was dying of AZT-induced lymphoma. But the overwhelming majority of long-term survivors had somehow managed to resist the enormous pressure to take AZT.

The pressure did not just come from doctors, Callen told the Amsterdam meeting, but from a certain segment of Aids activism that seemed driven by a 'drugs-into-bodies' mentality. 'I feel my Aids activist friends who are in the forefront of this frenzy are very misleading to people with Aids, who are frightened and desperate. They only seem to talk about two possible outcomes of taking experimental drugs: one is that it works and one that it does not work. There is a third, apparently much more common possibility, which is that you will be worse off than if you did nothing at all. And nobody likes to talk about that because it is so unpleasant.' He had seen the devastation wreaked by AZT, watching with horror as friends with Aids 'turn the colour of boiled ham from AZT poisoning, endure the melting away of their muscles, become transfusion-dependent, and experience drug-induced psychosis'. Yet his perception of a person diagnosed with Aids in 1992 was that 'they would sell their grandmother into slavery to get a slot in the latest drug-of-the-month clinical trial'.

Another feature of the long-term survivors was that they rejected the predominant scientific view that HIV-positivity meant inevitable decline of the immune system towards an early death. They were passionately committed to life, believed in the possibility of survival, and tended to surround themselves with people who would love and support them. They all mentioned making major lifestyle changes, including in their sex lives, and in most cases they had given up drugs and alcohol. They had also 'dabbled' with dietary changes.

They all talked about what they called 'emotional house-cleaning'. Usually after they had survived their first major opportunistic infection, it represented a crisis to them and they did some soul-searching. They either repaired relationships, or ended them. And all but two – Callen himself, who professed himself 'a pretty high profile, rabid atheist', and one other – talked about a rebirth of spirituality in their lives. Half had returned to the religions of their childhood – 'although none in a fundamentalist, judgmental way' – and half spoke more generally of the sense that there was a meaning to suffering, and a life after death. This gave them a sense of purpose in the here and now. 'They were not done with life yet. They had a reason to stick around.'

Perversely, because their survival challenged the predominant view of HIV and Aids, some had to face abuse simply by virtue of being alive. 'One that I interviewed had received death threats from the lover of someone who had died from the disease that he had survived. What often happens, and certainly has been the case with me, is that people are so threatened by your survival that they find some way to say that you must not really have had Aids to begin with, since everyone knows that everyone dies of Aids.'*

When I met him in London in 1992, shortly after the *Sunday Times* had devoted two pages to setting out the scientific critique of the HIV hypothesis, Callen knew that death was approaching. Yet there were still people for whom his survival, in the light of all he had argued for and stood for, was so challenging that they were either claiming he had never had Aids, or pretending he was already dead. Just before leaving for Europe, he had been for a radiation treatment for his Kaposi's sarcoma and on returning to his home, two reporters called.

* In the January 1989 *PWA Newsline,* Callen wrote: 'As long as I am the dancing PWA bear, producing tears on cue so the hat can be passed, no one questions my right to represent myself as a PWA. But when I take controversial positions – when I assert that AZT doesn't work; when I argue that HIV may not be the cause of Aids; when I argue that the gay community should take some action against bathhouses – then enemies re-circulate the rumour that I don't really have Aids. Rather than deal with the merits of my arguments, they attempt to knock me out of the debate by undermining my credibility. It's called fighting dirty. But my real crime is that I'm not dead. I've actually been asked not to talk about the fact that 15 per cent of us seem to have survived full-blown Aids for five or more years. It's bad for fund-raising, we're told; or it might undermine attempts to convince the federal government that more money is needed to fight Aids.'

'They both said, independent of each other, "Boy, I had a hard time tracking you down!" One had called the big Aids service group in Boston and been told that I'm a fake, don't bother calling him. And the other had been told the same thing from Project Inform in San Francisco. That is the level at which people fight against AZT heresy and HIV heresy. The same people who have consistently spread the rumour that I am a fraud and shouldn't be listened to, then turn around and spread the rumour that I have died. Twice a year, like clockwork, I get a spate of calls from reporters asking me to confirm or deny whether I have died.'

Callen felt the origins of this behaviour lay ten years back, in the premature closure of debate on Aids aetiology. That was also the turning point that he believed would be responsible for his death. 'And believe me, I screamed loudly at the time, as did Joe Sonnabend and others. It was perfectly fine to announce HIV, perfectly fine to research, it and characterise it and sequence it, but assertions were made that the evidence was a lot stronger than it was, and it became impossible to get funds to research alternative aetiological hypotheses.

'When I read your article, I had two back-to-back reactions. One was, I chuckled. I had made a bet with myself, that I lost: I didn't think I would live long enough to see an article that serious in a mainstream publication. I have been labouring in these trenches for more than ten years now, and the abuse that has been heaped upon anybody who calls into question HIV orthodoxy, the religion of HIV …I just didn't think I would live to see it seriously raised.'

He didn't quite articulate the other reaction, but it was not humorous. 'It made me…my health is precipitously declining. I don't want to sound overly dramatic, but I have seen a lot of Aids. I have lost more than 137 friends. I know what Aids looks like, and I know what the decline looks like and feels like, and I am in that stage right now. It suddenly made me…if we could somehow have held our ground in 1984, and simply kept the door open, it's entirely possible that treatment research based on a multifactorial conceptualisation of Aids might have by now produced treatments that would save my life, or at least extend my life. Maybe you are hearing a decade of bitterness. It's been impossible for anyone to get funding for any treatment unless you can explain some rationale, some mechanism, linking it to HIV.

'I am profoundly anaemic. I have spots on my lungs and we are at our wits' end about what they might be. They have cultured an obscure strain of mycobacterium. I've just had a catheter pulled out of my arm. I am 14lb underweight. I used to get my Aids complications discretely, one problem at a time, and I could turn the full force of my energy and concentration towards them. Now I am getting them three at a time, and I am at that horrible Aids stage where the treatments are causing me more problems than the symptoms, and they are giving me drugs to counteract the side-effects from the treatments. That is a vicious cycle that ultimately kills people, but in every instance so far I have not had any choice.

'A lot of people are concerned when I talk this way. I haven't given up – I very desperately want to live. I am simply trying to send signals to my friends and those around me that I have moved into a new level of medicalisation, a new level of energy drain. I am staying engaged, keeping up with the literature. My brain is still popping and crackling like a fire; my body is not. My body arrives about five seconds after my will – I'm on digital delay. That's very hard for me. There is this super-PWA mentality that I have been promoting. I have other long-term surviving friends who did the same thing, and then they had trouble when they started to die – people wouldn't let them. People would say, "You can't; too many people use you as a model, an image." And I will not go through that. I feel I've been at this disease a very long time.'

'I Will Die from All the Dallying'

Michael Callen finally died in January 1994, a decade after most of his Aids contemporaries. He was thirty-eight. The previous July, while battling fulminant KS of both lungs, he wrote to me at the *Sunday Times* of his pleasure at seeing AZT conclusively discredited, after a careful, four-year Anglo-French trial had shown it to do more harm than good in HIV-positive people. But he was still bitter at the scientific community's continuing failure to appraise the question of whether what had come to be called 'the Aids virus' actually caused Aids. Back in about 1986, he recalled, 'I was being driven literally insane by my persistent refusal to speak the language of HIV. I would continually correct people who said "the Aids virus" when they meant HIV, etc. Finally, I reluctantly learned to speak the foreign language of HIV – hopefully without too much of an accent. Now, I simply quietly translate what people say to me into a multifactorial conceptualisation. My point is that they have so tautologically controlled the language that it's virtually impossible to raise the question of whether the "Aids virus" actually "causes" Aids.'

His letter continued:

> Naive poor midwestern boy that I was, I thought this battle would be fought according to the rules of science. It came as quite a shock to discover that the true discourse of Aids is theological. There are received truths; papal bulls (papal bullshit, more like it), and various sects and denominations who launch jihads against one another. It's an unholy holy war. All the standard rules of science, at least as I understand them, have never been followed. Eg, reproducibility. Joe Sonnabend introduced me to the ideas of Karl Popper and his fascinating theory of falsifiability. But falsification is contrary to human nature. It's asking a lot for someone who has proposed a hypothesis to then immediately set about trying to knock it down. But science is supposed to be sceptical; adversarial; contentious. But Aids science certainly isn't. Maybe I just had a naive understanding of how science is 'supposed' to work.
>
> When I was being driven MAD by the debate (or non-debate), I took refuge in reading up on prior scientific controversies. I have discovered many that have fascinating parallels. There is, of course, the famous incident where Max Pettenkoffer drank a vial of cholera bacilli with no ill-effects in a failed effort to disprove the germ theory of disease. And I just finished reading 'The Malaria Capers' by Robert S. Desowitz. He tells the fascinating tale of the search for the cause of malaria. It's absolutely parallel to Aids. Everything was proposed at one time or another, and each 'camp' ferociously defended its theory. In the end, they were all wrong.
>
> But historically, what I would say I have found is that it often turns out that BOTH camps were right. Applied to Aids, that would mean that some role for HIV in some cases of Aids may indeed one day be proven. It seems settled, to me at least, that the presence of cases of what clearly is Aids in people who definitely do not have HIV proves two things: (1) HIV is not

> and cannot be the sole cause of Aids; and (2) there are probably multiple causes, of which HIV might be an important element in some cases.
>
> I hope this clarifies the muddy waters of my thought. Chemotherapy is frying what's left of my brain, so I don't know if this is terribly lucid or helpful. I have enormous amounts of material stretching back to 1982 about the public debate about aetiology, and the vicious attempts to silence any such speculation...[it] reads like a heart-breaking chronology of stupidity.
>
> Thanks again for your courageous stand. Good luck. Please persist, long after I'm dinner for worms.

Far from being unhelpful, I felt that the letter contained a unique distillation of sense, intelligence and compassion. This time, he stated clearly what the 'non-debate' had meant to him personally. 'I will die from all the dallying. Two roads diverged in 1984 and I still believe in my gut that we took the wrong road, and that the only way to get it right is to admit first that we got it spectacularly wrong and start anew.'

Looking back, I realise my own reporting on Aids – while true to what mainstream science was saying – was spectacularly uncritical in the 1980s. I feel I owe a debt towards Michael, and many others, and I hope that this book will help bring about the fresh look at Aids that he wanted.

What of Richard Berkowitz, co-author of the 1982 'We Know Who We Are' article, co-founder of the People With Aids Coalition, and with Callen a self-confessed victim of 'excessive promiscuity' and Aids? It is heartening to be able to report that he is alive and well, as of 1994 when I called him in the US. He summarised his own story in an article entitled 'Still Kicking After All These Years', published in *QW* magazine in August 1992 – exactly ten years after he joined the very first support group in New York City for gay men with Aids.

He had walked to that first meeting, on a hot August night in 1982, 'like a man on his way to the gallows'. But ten years later, he had never felt better in his life.

> Recently, I bumped into an old friend on the street. As soon as our eyes met, he blurted out, 'I thought you were dead!' His words startled me... To

> my old friend it was clearly a miracle that I was alive. But I don't believe in miracles – I believe that knowledge is power.
>
> I made radical and unpopular choices ten years ago which I now firmly believe saved my life. These choices were based on the multifactorial theory of Aids. Now I see change in the air because a growing number of scientists have begun to say something I have always believed: *You cannot get Aids just from HIV.*

Recalling the 'We Know Who We Are' article, he said the response of the gay community had been absolute contempt. 'It seemed to me then (and it still does now) that if you want to be regarded as a Good Gay Man in the Age of Aids, then repeat after me – and mean it: *1. "The Aids virus causes Aids." 2. "It only takes one time." 3. "Gay men with Aids were just unlucky."*' But now, all that might be about to change. The HIV theory's painful failure to produce anything of value in terms of treatment or therapies was suggesting to more and more scientists that HIV could not be the single cause of Aids.

> When I walked home from that first support group meeting...I felt more hopeless than before I went. Everyone in the group led me to believe that I was a ticking time bomb and that there was nothing I could do about it. They told me that, until I accepted the fact that I had caught the new killer Aids virus and it was only a matter of time until I would die, I was in a state of unhealthy denial. Without a shred of hope, I understood why some of the men in that support group continued going out to the baths and backrooms (safe sex had not yet been invented).
>
> The next day, I went to see my doctor, Joseph Sonnabend, who had urged me to go to that support group. He told me that it was possible to explain my condition without there being any new killer virus. He told me that *common* viruses, which unfortunately had reached epidemic proportions among sexually active urban gay men, could explain my night sweats, swollen glands and fatigue. He told me that my history of repeated infection with common viruses, most notably cytomegalovirus, could explain why I was immune deficient. Most important of all, he told me that if I stopped exposing myself to further viral infections, my immune system might actually heal...

> Finally stopping having sex made me a very angry and unpleasant man, but I knew in 1982 that a tidal wave of death was about to engulf the community I loved and I was grateful for my early warning.

After publication in 1983 of the safe-sex manual which he co-authored with Michael Callen, Berkowitz 'fled the Aids debate', wearied by the vehement resistance to the multifactorial theory – a resistance that was to continue for the next decade. Now, encouraged by the fact that a debate about 'co-factors' and other views of Aids causation had begun to appear in the mainstream media, he felt compelled to share his experience. 'I have known for a long time how much gay men hate the multifactorial theory because it requires scrutiny of the urban gay male promiscuity of the 70s – and the powerful right wing in this country would love a few more excuses to try to justify and spread its hate. But at the same time, I firmly believe that the reason I am here today (and able to continue fighting those right-wing forces) is that I faced what I believed was a painful, ugly truth and figured out what to do about it by discovering safe sex.'

He felt 'queasy' about telling his story, he said, particularly in the current climate of sexual McCarthyism ('Does *he* have "it"? Do *you* have "it"?' 'He looks like he *must* have "it".') fostered by the killer Aids virus theory. However, 'no matter how much we gay men worship our own Doctor Daddies, the unavoidable truth is that there are still no experts when it comes to this disease...Not everyone who believes in the multifactorial theory is anti-gay or self-hating. In my case, the multifactorial theory stopped my time-bomb ticking.'

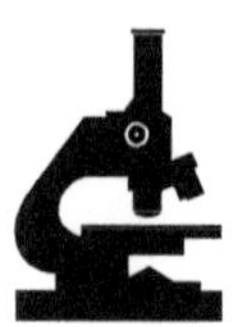

3: AN EDITOR IS SILENCED

Joe Sonnabend's face is an open book, and for once it was glowing with triumphant pleasure. He had just sat through a dramatic 'emergency' session at the July 1992 International Aids Conference in Amsterdam, Holland, concerning a cluster of Aids cases in which scientists had failed to find any trace of HIV. The session was called after an article about the eleven cases in *Newsweek* had raised the possibility that some other as yet undetected virus might be the cause. A report from the United States of a sixty-six-year-old woman with severely weakened immunity — her only evident risk having been a blood transfusion forty years earlier – added to the state of alarm.

In fact, Luc Montagnier, who headed the French team that first claimed isolation of a new virus linked to Aids, had been reported by me three months previously as saying his laboratory was occasionally seeing clear-cut cases of Aids in which no trace of HIV could be found. At the emergency session, a series of doctors stood up from the floor of the packed conference room – once 'licensed' to speak out openly by the official announcement that such a phenomenon was real – to testify that they too had patients who fell into this mysterious category.

It was no mystery to Sonnabend. He had long argued that Aids was more likely to be caused by repeated exposures to a variety of infectious and toxic challenges – as most of his New York City patients had experienced – than by a new virus. He accepted that HIV existed and that it might contribute to this burden; in his view, however, while the presence of antibodies to HIV signified that a person was at risk, it was probably not because of HIV in itself. Rather, the antibodies were a marker of a variety of immunosuppressive risks that could be present in patients' lives, allowing HIV to be expressed as an opportunist, when the immune system defences were depleted. He saw no evidence for Aids being caused by a single agent.

He had other reasons to be pleased about the emergency session. One was that it confirmed a prediction he had made many years previously that difficulties would arise with the way the Centers for Disease Control (CDC) were defining Aids. Essentially, back in 1984, an Aids case required the diagnosis of one of a number of diseases thought to indicate a deficiency in the patient's immune system cells, *in the absence* of any known cause for the deficiency. The diseases included opportunistic infections – those which a healthy immune system readily controls, but which may run riot in an immunocompromised body – and Kaposi's sarcoma.

Sonnabend, who qualified medically in South Africa and had a scientific background in virology with Britain's National Institute for Medical Research, was the founding editor of *Aids Research,* the first scientific journal devoted to the syndrome. In the second issue, published in early 1984 – before the press conference that launched the virus that was to come to be known as HIV – he co-authored a prophetic article emphasising that the Aids definition was one of exclusion, in which all cases of cellular immune deficiency not accounted for by known mechanisms became Aids cases. 'This is tantamount to declaring that only one unknown cause of cellular immunodeficiency remains to be discovered – the cause of Aids,' the article reasoned. The CDC's definition 'almost demands the existence of a single Aids agent, as this appears to be the only unifying hypothesis to explain the appearance of an identical disease (by definition)' in the disparate groups in which it had been seen. In reality, what the various groups had in common was an immune deficiency that was unexplained. It did not follow that identical disease mechanisms were operating in them all.

For example, it had been shown that some haemophiliacs suffered unexplained immune system disorders, but these might have an environmental cause, such as the repeated administration of blood concentrates made necessary by their condition, rather than exposure to a new infectious agent.

Some apparently healthy homosexual men had also been found to have immune system changes, whose magnitude was related to the number of sexual contacts with different partners. That might be because of their exposure to sperm and seminal fluid from many different men, as well as from repeated sexually transmitted viral and other infections so common in that population. The article pointed out that semen and sperm were well documented as a cause of immune system abnormalities in anal intercourse, when the proteins involved permeate the colon's thin lining and enter the bloodstream. (In vaginal intercourse, the vagina has a thick wall that restricts such invasion to its intended target, the womb.) There are antigens – foreign proteins capable of stimulating an immune response – expressed on cells in the ejaculate that are shared by cells of the immune system, raising the possibility that repeated exposure could set up an immune reaction in the body against one's own immune cells.

Drug addicts, another group seen to be at risk of Aids, might be suffering immune cell deficiencies because of a directly damaging effect of opiates on T-cells, for which they have an enormous affinity, as well as because of malnutrition and the transfer of blood-borne infections through shared needles. Similarly, an understanding of Aids in less developed countries should take into account changes in economic and social conditions such as intense overcrowding, an increase in common infections, failure of malaria eradication programmes and malnutrition; all were possible contributing factors.

Having described a variety of difficulties in the study of Aids, Sonnabend set out three possible explanations for what was going on. The essence of Aids was that the clinical conditions seen were a consequence of an underlying disorder of the immune system. But what was the cause of that underlying disorder?

The single 'Aids agent' theory blamed a unique microbe, presumably a virus, transmitted sexually and by blood, that was so deadly that it caused Aids without the need for other factors. Proponents of this 'Mack truck' model often stated that time was the only co-factor. This was a hypothesis built on a set of hypotheses: that the same disease is occurring in disparate groups, that it is spread by contagion between the groups and that the disease is new in all groups.

A second theory held that a unique 'Aids agent' was responsible, but that it only caused Aids in conjunction with other factors, which could be infectious or non-infectious. According to this view, the groups were linked by a single infectious agent, but they could be made susceptible to that agent by different co-factors operating in different risk groups.

A third hypothesis proposed that there was no specific 'Aids agent', but that instead, multiple factors, both infectious and non-infectious, interacted to produce the disease. According to that view, the disease might develop in different ways in different groups, although the outcome might be similar. If this idea were to hold, some explanation of the recent appearance of the syndrome would be needed, as well as some mechanism to explain how the disease developed and how the syndrome could be transmissible from person to person. Whenever an apparently new disease appeared, it was reasonable to look for a new influence, such as a novel biological or physical agent; but another way to generate newness was to recombine old influences in a new way.

Lifestyle Changes

In this and other scientific articles published at about the same time, Sonnabend described a model of Aids causation which clearly favoured the third, 'no specific agent' option. He documented the adverse effects on the immune system of homosexual men, the most intensively studied group, arising from lifestyle changes which became apparent in the late 1960s. These changes had brought a subgroup of men into sexual contact with large numbers of different partners in settings that meant repeated exposures to a combination of infectious and non-infectious factors: semen, with potential ill-effects as described above, drugs, and infection with various sexually transmitted diseases. 'Such conditions were met in New York City, San Francisco, and Los Angeles in the mid-1970s.' The model was testable, and lent itself to a formal epidemiological analysis, to see both how those affected had interacted with such an environment, and how the various biological effects generated by these exposures interacted with one another.

Sonnabend paid particular attention to cytomegalovirus (CMV), a member of the herpes family, which had become present as an active infection in the semen of up to 35 per cent of sexually active homosexual men in big US cities during the previous decade. Each bout of infection had several adverse effects on the immune system, some of which could last for weeks or months and possibly longer. Anal exposure to the large 'dose' of the virus from semen was probably the biggest risk.[1] To dismiss the possibility that CMV played a significant role in Aids – as some had done – on the grounds that everyone was infected with the virus was not appropriate, in conditions where individuals were repeatedly exposed rectally to the massive amounts of CMV that could be found in semen.

Syphilis and hepatitis B were also highly prevalent in this same pool of men, and Epstein-Barr virus (EBV) played an important role in immunosuppression. Most people had also been exposed to EBV, but reactivated infections, as well as producing specific symptoms, also contributed to disorder in the immune system.

Sonnabend argued that none of these factors was likely to prove fatal on its own, and that even after an Aids diagnosis the disease might prove reversible if the assaults on the immune system were reduced. However, after prolonged exposure to their combined effects, the system became so overburdened, and so confused by cross-reactions between antibodies formed in response to the promiscuous gay lifestyle, that a self-sustaining and possibly progressive condition became established. The process had features characteristic of positive feedback systems. For example, if the ability of lymphocytes to clear CMV-infected cells passed a certain point, an expansion of total CMV activity in the body would result in yet further immune suppression. An additional viral infection might precipitate the initiation of a vicious circle of this kind.

In short, Aids was not a disease of gay men as such – indeed, since Aids was first recognised it had rapidly become apparent that the risk for developing the syndrome was not uniformly shared by all homosexual men. It was occurring in a subgroup whose lifestyle changes of the past ten to fifteen years might provide sufficient explanation for their immune system disorder.

Some recent changes had also occurred in the environmental exposures of other risk groups. An important change in the lives of haemophiliacs over the previous decade had been the availability of pooled commercial Factor 8 preparations that could be self-administered.

Among drug addicts, an important change might be the setting in which drugs were used, with increased likelihood of blood being transferred (as with needle sharing). Similarly, an understanding of Aids in less developed countries would have to take into account changes in economic and social conditions.

By 1985, HIV had been adopted by the scientific mainstream as the sole and sufficient cause of Aids, and Sonnabend published letters and articles in *Aids Research* predicated on this belief. However, he continued to keep other options open. For example, the summer 1986 issue of the journal carried an article by three French researchers who, while accepting that Aids and related disorders resulted from infection with the virus, and from progressive destruction of the T4 lymphocyte pool, nevertheless questioned the relationship between these events. The conventional view at that time was that the virus was killing T-cells directly. But with apparently fewer than one in 10,000 T-cells infected at any time, that seemed an inadequate explanation to the French. They proposed instead that Aids was a viral-induced auto-immune disorder, directed against the immune system itself. In mounting a defence against the virus, the immune system was also setting in train a sequence of events that led to the gradual destruction of the T4 cells. For prolonged periods, the losses could be made good, but when destruction finally outweighed regeneration, the T4 cell pool was progressively reduced, leading eventually to opportunistic infections. By this reckoning, rather than try to spur the immune system into fresh activity, it might be better to try to damp the system down.

A similar hypothesis from researchers in Houston, Texas, was published in the following issue. It suggested that once HIV infection was acquired, progression of disease would depend on continuous T-cell activation either by antigens such as sperm, or by other viruses. The more the T-cells were activated, the more they were attacked both by the virus and by the immune response against it, leading to progressive immune deficiency.

Sonnabend considered it important to give space to these modified HIV theories, as well as to articles that addressed Aids causation from non-HIV viewpoints, because they kept open a variety of treatment and research strategies. In particular, they kept alive the possibility that HIV-infected people could exert some control over their situation. If HIV required co-factors in order to cause Aids, removing those co-factors might prevent the syndrome, even in HIV-infected people. That would not just be a more hopeful message to give patients, it also fitted Sonnabend's medical philosophy, based on his clinical experience, which told him that the terrain was as important as the germ and that disease was usually the outcome of a multiplicity of factors acting simultaneously.

'It Was Completely Crazy'

When Mary Ann Liebert, *Aids Research's* publisher, had invited Sonnabend to launch the magazine late in 1982, she could hardly have found a better-qualified person. After training as a doctor in Johannesburg, he had studied at the Infectious Diseases Unit at the Central Middlesex Hospital in London before becoming a member of the Royal College of Physicians of Edinburgh in 1961. From then on he had worked continuously as a research virologist, including seven years at NIMR in London, where he did pioneering work on interferon, an anti-viral substance secreted by lymphocytes, and four years at Mt Sinai Medical School in New York City as associate professor. His curriculum vitae totalled eight pages of distinctions and honours, and he 'had a list of articles and scientific publications worthy of a Nobel Prize', despite 'his poorly shaven stubble, his old basketball shoes and his shabby jeans', as the French author Dominique Lapierre neatly summed up Sonnabend's appearance in his story of the fight against Aids.[2]

In the late 1970s Sonnabend served as director of New York City's Bureau of VD Control, a job that brought him into contact with the Centers for Disease Control in Atlanta. He also did voluntary work at a gay clinic for sexually transmitted diseases before setting up in 1978 as a community physician in Greenwich Village, at the heart of New York City's gay quarter. He was still specialising in STDs, and retaining access to a hospital research laboratory.

An epidemic of disease was already spreading through the gay community at the time, terrifying to Sonnabend, who felt many of the young men coming to him for treatment of their latest bout of the 'clap' were asking for serious trouble. The problem was not just the gonorrhoea, the syphilis, the parasitic infections; there were drugs that could deal with those. But people were coming in time and again for a shot of penicillin, then going straight back to the bathhouses. Some even requested continuous antibiotic treatment as prophylaxis. They thought Sonnabend was being old-fashioned and moralistic when he told them such behaviour could lead to major problems. But in 1978-9 some were suffering from persistent fevers, swollen lymph glands, chronic skin eruptions, and multiple viral infections that would not clear up.

'It was completely crazy,' Sonnabend told Dominique Lapierre.[3]

> A number of doctors had set themselves up in this particularly sensitive area and were treating a succession of cases of gonorrhoea, syphilis and parasitic infections. At that time antibiotics were a universal panacea. Syphilis was cured with one or two injections of penicillin. It cost only 25 or 30 dollars. No one was doing any detailed research, and the very idea of research was totally alien to the majority of practitioners. The most tragic part about it was their refusal to adopt an educational role with their patients. The slightest suggestion, the least warning about the dangers their lifestyle was exposing them to, could be taken as a moral judgement. It was the best way of losing your clients. In any case, irrespective of whether they were doctors in the field or representatives from the Centers for Disease Control in Atlanta and the federal Department of Health, they all thought that it was useless, indeed futile, to try and change people's behaviour, that the only realistic approach was to cure them as quickly as possible. They would rather say to people: 'You keep on wrecking yourselves and we'll pick up the pieces.'

Some of his patients boasted ten to fifteen doses of gonorrhoea, others suffered from repeated outbreaks of herpes. 'It was staring us in the face: the human body could not be subjected to so many onslaughts without something fundamental beginning to give way.' The picture Sonnabend paints of that time refutes the generally held view that Aids struck 'out of the blue' in an otherwise healthy gay population.

However, by early 1981 it was clear to Sonnabend that something dramatically new *was* happening, and he was alerting colleagues to it for some months before the first announcement in the medical press. He was seeing his first cases of pneumocystic pneumonia, a parasitic disease known mainly to modern medicine as a complication in the treatment of children with leukaemia whose immune systems have been suppressed by chemotherapy. He also had cases of Kaposi's sarcoma, a rare cancer whose purplish lesions affect the skin and internal organs, including the lungs, and which for the most part had previously been seen only in old men. Yet these diseases were affecting mainly young men in their twenties. A new syndrome of immune deficiency was present; medical history was unfolding before him. Yet he knew it must be associated with aspects of the lives some of his patients had been leading and which had long been worrying him. He felt a mixture of alarm and excitement. His many years in research, alongside his current clinical experience, put him in an ideal position to contribute to an understanding of what was going on.

Sonnabend drew blood from thirty of his gay male patients, and sent it for analysis by a former colleague, Dr David Purtilo, at the University of Nebraska, a pioneer in the technique of counting T-cells and relating the count to immune system function. Ten of the samples came from men who were known to Sonnabend as highly promiscuous (Michael Callen, who was one of them, referred to them proudly as the 'sluts'). Ten were in monogamous relationships with their male lovers, and the third group were the ones Callen called 'weekend dabblers'.

Purtilo did not know which were which, but the T-cell counts correlated precisely with their sex lives: while the monogamous group had healthy immune systems, and those who dated around were somewhat depressed, the 'sluts' had extremely low counts. This research, the first of its kind, was published in the *Lancet* in early 1982. The last sentence spelled out a clear message: promiscuity was depressing the immune system. Sonnabend wrote an article for the *New York Native* giving the same warning. He said the fast-lane gay lifestyle was killing people. They had to stop being so promiscuous. Having hundreds or thousands of partners was making them very sick. 'If you don't stop fucking around, you'll die,' he told one of his immuno-deficient men. He began to tell all his gay male patients of the dangers they faced, advising them to wear condoms, and to stop crazy practices like fisting – inserting the hand and even the arm into another man's anus – and rimming, oral-anal contact.

Gay leaders gave him the same reception they were soon to give Callen and Berkowitz for their 'We Know Who We Are' article in the *Native*. There was a barrage of protest. He was seen as blaming the new 'gay disease' on the gays themselves, despite his insistence that he just wanted to save lives. There was even uproar among his patients. It seemed that hardly anyone wanted to know the facts.

Rejection by the CDC

If the patient did not like the medicine, that was something doctors were used to handling. But worse was to come. Dr James Curran, who headed the VD prevention division at the Centers for Disease Control in Atlanta, came to see Sonnabend as part of his efforts to track the cause of the new syndrome. He too did not seem to like what he heard.

Sonnabend told him of the patterns emerging from his research: that the gay men at risk had a long history of syphilis and gonorrhoea and various other infections, that they had been part of the fast-track promiscuous gay lifestyle, with all that entailed. But according to Sonnabend it was as if he were talking to someone whose mind was already made up on different lines. Curran seemed somewhat annoyed with Sonnabend, and left him with the impression that he should carry on treating the patients, and leave the theorising to the professionals.

The previous year, Curran had spotted the importance of a cluster of five cases of pneumocystic pneumonia that Drs Michael Gottlieb and Joel Weisman had seen in Los Angeles, cases that were to become the first report on the epidemic when published in the CDC's *Morbidity and Mortality Weekly Report (MMWR).* With colleagues, he had briefly wondered if there might be an environmental cause – maybe a bad batch of nitrite inhalant drugs, the 'poppers' that had come into widespread use as an aid to gay sex. Those getting the new diseases all seemed to have a history of snorting poppers. On the other hand, some 5 million doses of the inhalants were sold in the United States in 1980; everybody in the gay community was using them. The idea soon fell out of favour. A study to test it was proposed by Dr James Goedert, of the National Cancer Institute, but was never properly funded or followed through.

The other major hypothesis discussed from the outset, far more frightening, was that it could be an infectious disease: that there was a new contagion spreading immune deficiencies and death in the gay community. Like Sonnabend, however, Curran had noticed how the victims seemed to be a particular type of gay man, which conflicted with his experience of epidemic illness. Randy Shilts described Curran's early puzzlement on this point:[4]

> Curran was...struck by how identifiably gay all the patients seemed to be. After years of working with the gay community, he knew that you couldn't tell homosexuals by looking at them. These clearly must be patients who put a high personal stake in their identification as gay people, living in the thick of the urban gay subculture. They hadn't just peeked out of the closet yesterday. It was strange because diseases tended not to strike people on the basis of social groups. Epidemics could be restricted geographically, like the Legionnaire's epidemic of 1976, hitting a group of conventioneers at a particular hotel in Philadelphia. Diseases might appear in a group bound together by physiological similarities, such as women who had physical reactions to Rely tampons and suffered from Toxic Shock Syndrome. To Curran's recollection, however, no epidemic had chosen victims on the basis of how they identified themselves in social terms, much less on the basis of sexual lifestyle. Yet, this identification and a propensity for venereal diseases were the only things the patients from three cities - New York, Los Angeles, and San Francisco - appeared to share. There had to be something within this milieu that was hazardous to these people's health.

Shilts also described how in the week before publication of the *MMWR* report, CDC staffers debated how to handle the gay aspects. Some of the workers in the venereal disease division had long experience working with the gay community and worried about offending the sensitivities of a group with whom they would clearly be working closely in the coming months. 'Just as significantly, they also knew that gays were not the most beloved minority in or out of the medical world, and they feared that tagging the outbreak too prominently as a gay epidemic might fuel prejudice.' So the report appeared not on page one of the *MMWR* but in a more inconspicuous slot on page two. Any reference to homosexuality was dropped from the title, and the headline simply read: *Pneumocystis* pneumonia — Los Angeles. 'Don't offend the gays and don't inflame the homophobes. These were the twin horns on which the handling of this epidemic would be torn from the first day of the epidemic,' Shilts wrote.

In retrospect, one can see that the idea that a new virus was to blame, although frightening, had the attraction of meeting both those requirements. If promiscuous gays had just been unlucky in being afflicted first, it relieved them of having the syndrome identified with their way of life. And since a new virus would not discriminate, but eventually put all sexually active people at risk – with time the only co-factor, as leading scientists around the world would soon be saying – there would be no basis for a homophobic reaction. Homophobes would have plenty else to think about.

The 'new virus' theory also had a powerful proponent at the CDC in the person of Dr Don Francis, a young but already eminent epidemiologist who had helped rid the world of smallpox. In June 1981, after hearing that victims of the new syndrome showed depletion of their T4 cells, Francis had called Dr Max Essex, with whom he studied virology at the Harvard School of Public Health in Boston, to declare his belief that a new virus capable of being sexually transmitted was at the root of the problem. It could even be a retrovirus, he said – one of an obscure subgroup of viruses thought likely by Essex to have a considerable role in human disease. A big research effort to link retroviruses with cancer during President Nixon's 1970s 'war on cancer' had proved a resounding failure, but with one apparent exception: Robert Gallo, the National Cancer Institute researcher, who claimed he had shown that a retrovirus caused a leukaemia common in Japan. Essex was to become a close collaborator with Gallo in the search, apparent discovery and promotion of a retroviral cause of Aids.

Francis had studied the mechanisms of what was believed to be a leukaemia virus in cats, and right from the start of the new epidemic had concluded that it bore the hallmarks of a similar disease in people. Both feline leukaemia and the new gay disease involved opportunistic infections that were apparently taking advantage of an immune system weakened by some primary infection. In cats, the leukaemia virus knocked out the cats' immune systems and left them open to various cancers. Clearly, some similar virus was doing the same to the gay men, and they were getting cancer too. Secondly, feline leukaemia had a long latency period, before the ill-effects were seen. The new disease must work the same way, which would account for how it was now killing people in three cities before anybody even knew it existed. The more familiar viruses under discussion, such as CMV, were unlikely to be the cause. They had been around for years without killing people.

For these various reasons, by the time Curran came to see Sonnabend the CDC was predisposed to finding a more specific aetiology than he was proposing. He seemed unimpressed with the 'clap doctor's' research. For Sonnabend, fired with enthusiasm to draw on his clinical and research experience in the fight against the syndrome, Curran's attitude was an infuriating put-down. 'I've never forgotten that. Absolutely never forgotten that,' Sonnabend says. He was to suffer a similar frustration with the biomedical establishment after he had discovered from a search of the medical literature that pneumocystic pneumonia, the most frequent cause of death in people with Aids, could be prevented with prophylactic drug treatment. Sonnabend and other community doctors began protecting their Aids patients this way from 1982 onwards, but it would take a few years more before the treatment became widely accepted (mainly as a result of campaigning by people with Aids).

Aids Research Coup

Despite the unfortunate encounter with Curran, by late 1982 and early 1983 Sonnabend's star of fortune appeared to be rising. Liebert, the publisher, called to ask him to launch *Aids Research,* an invitation he was thrilled to accept. Dr Mathilde Krim, an old friend and research colleague, began working with Sonnabend at her laboratory at the Memorial Sloan-Kettering Institute for Cancer Research. Krim also saw Sonnabend through a difficult financial patch, backing his research first from her personal funds, and in 1983 through the Aids Medical Foundation (later to be called the American Foundation for Aids Research, or AmFAR) of which she was the founder and chairman.

Aids Research published some ground-breaking material. As well as pioneering the concept that the disease probably involved an autoimmune process, as far back as 1983 it had an article proposing that cyclosporin, the immune-suppressing drug used as an anti-rejection agent in transplant patients, could be an appropriate treatment in Aids. Eleven years later, at the international Aids conference in Japan, there was to be excited discussion over the same theme. Another paper drew attention to a theory that Aids was a new form of disease caused by the agent responsible for syphilis. Years later, the idea is still the subject of academic discussion (Sonnabend says he does not find the arguments compelling, but he thinks syphilitic infection may contribute to the immune suppression seen in Aids). Another article reported prolonged survival in Aids patients treated for CMV infection.

In a further article that may have contributed to Sonnabend's undoing, *Aids Research* challenged attempts by the NCI's Robert Gallo and Harvard's Max Essex to attribute Aids to the Human T-cell Leukaemia Virus, HTLV-1, which Gallo had discovered. A paper by Essex, published in *Science,* purported to show that with coded sera (a 'blind' study), about 35 per cent of Aids sera tested positive for reactivity with HTLV-1-infected cells. Sonnabend was suspicious and staged a similar trial with samples from his own Aids patients, sending the sera to laboratories in three different countries. None came up with a single positive result. Sonnabend published an account of this refutation himself after *Science, Nature* and several medical journals refused to take it.

Another blot on Sonnabend's copybook occurred in February 1985, when he became the first scientist to come close to accusing Gallo of promoting the French discovery, originally called LAV and later HIV, as his own, HTLV-3.

He was not to be a thorn in Gallo's side for much longer. A few months later, Mary Ann Liebert took him out to lunch and apologetically produced a bombshell. She said she had arranged some meetings involving biotechnology companies, and Max Essex had been a part of that. He had told her that the journal would have no chance of success unless it changed direction – it should concentrate on retroviruses. She had decided that he was right; Sonnabend had to go.

The journal was renamed *Aids Research and Human Retroviruses.* The new editor was Dr Dani Bolognesi, of Duke University, who was collaborating with Gallo in an effort to develop both a vaccine and a drug against 'the Aids virus'. Gallo had originally encouraged Bolognesi to get involved in human retroviruses shortly after the discovery of HTLV-1, and he and co-workers had been the first in the United States to extend and confirm Gallo's results.

Duke University is located near Research Triangle Park in Durham, North Carolina, an area housing some large pharmaceutical company research enterprises. One of these is Burroughs-Wellcome. Bolognesi knew one of its scientists, David Barry, later to be vice-president in charge of research, and the two men had become interested in investigating some of the drugs the company had sitting on the shelf as possible antiretroviral agents. One, in particular, which had failed as an anti-cancer agent after being investigated under a National Cancer Institute grant many years previously, was identified by Barry as worth a try. In the early 1970s, work at the Max Planck Institute in Gottingen had shown that the agent inhibited an animal retrovirus believed to be linked to the development of leukaemia.

In September 1984, Bolognesi asked Gallo to a meeting with him, Barry and Dr Samuel Broder, then director of the NCI's clinical oncology programme. The eventual outcome of the meeting was the development of the drug AZT. Despite grave concerns by many scientists, including Sonnabend, that its action was such as to risk long-term toxicity in return for short-term benefits, the drug was to be given singular support by US and British government institutions and was to earn hundreds of millions of pounds for Burroughs-Wellcome and the American company's British parent, the Wellcome Foundation (which has since been taken over by Glaxo, another pharmaceutical giant).

Bolognesi removed all but two of the old editorial board of *Aids Research*, and installed in their place a team favourable – to put it mildly – to the Gallo approach. Apart from Gallo himself, David Barry was there, along with Sam Broder and Max Essex. The board also included NCI epidemiologist Dr Bill Blattner, a key collaborator in Gallo's work. There were also NCI staffers from within the heart of Gallo's team: Mikulas Popovic, a Czech scientist, molecular biologist Flossie Wong-Staal, and George Shaw, a postdoctorate graduate who worked with Wong-Staal.

The board had international representation. From London, there was virologist Robin Weiss, who had worked with Gallo back in the 1970s, and had been involved in an embarrassing mistake concerning claims over the discovery of the first human retrovirus – it turned out to be a mixture of monkey retrovirus contaminations. Weiss, of the Institute of Cancer Research, did some early work on LAV/HTLV and was co-developer of Britain's first blood test, manufactured under an exclusive licence by Wellcome Diagnostics.

There was Arsene Burny, of Belgium, a close friend of Gallo's and expert on bovine leukaemia virus; Guy de Thé, from Lyons, France, who had been involved in HTLV-1 studies in the Caribbean and Africa; and Gerhart Hunsmann, of Gottingen, who had done studies of HTLV proteins in monkeys. Luc Montagnier of the Institut Pasteur was also listed, along with David Klatzmann, who worked with Montagnier in Paris, and immunologist Daniel Zagury of the University of Paris, a friend of Gallo's and part of a group, which included Gallo, seeking to develop a vaccine against HIV.

Dr Anthony Fauci, who had also done work on HTLV-1, was there; he now coordinated Aids work for the National Institute for Allergy and Infectious Diseases, a neighbour of the NCI's at the enormous National Institutes of Health complex in Bethesda, just outside Washington. Fauci was later to take charge of federal Aids funding for several years.

Margaret Fischl, principal investigator in AZT trials that rapidly earned the drug a 'shotgun wedding' licence, was also appointed, as were Dr Martin Hirsch, of the Massachusetts General Hospital clinical centre, a co-investigator in the trials; Paul Volberding, a retrovirologist heading the Aids clinic at San Francisco General Hospital, and later to become a leading advocate of early AZT treatment for HIV-positive people; and Thomas Merigan, another Aids drug trial principal investigator.

James Goedert, of the NCI's environmental epidemiology branch, was another board member. Goedert had leaned towards the poppers theory of Aids in the early days, but by 1983 his 'conversations with Jim Curran thoroughly committed him to the idea that a new infectious agent was causing the syndrome'.[5] The last of a collection of blood samples he had been building up since 1981 from gay men in Washington and New York were used to support Gallo's HTLV-3 hypothesis.

Also on the board were a group who had collaborated with Gallo in the clinical and scientific work that gave HTLV-3 its scientific launch, in May 1984, through the *Science* collection of papers: Jerome Groopman of the New England Deaconess Hospital in Boston, Dr Robert Redfield of the Walter Reed Army Institute in Washington, DC, Barton Haynes of Duke University (who had also worked on HTLV-1 with Bolognesi), Bijan Safai of the Sloan-Kettering Memorial Hospital, Mark Kaplan of Cornell University and James Hoxie of the University of Pennsylvania.

Others included Hilary Koprowski, another Gallo friend and collaborator, who had helped develop polio vaccine; William Haseltine, a Harvard researcher closely aligned to Gallo, who worked on HTLV genes, as did Stephen Petteway, of Du Pont, manufacturers of a leading HIV blood test;

and Paul Luciw, of the University of California at Davis, who had contributed to the early molecular biology of the HTLV viruses.

It was an unashamed HTLV coup. The journal was to be a vehicle for retroviral research and treatment approaches. Robert Gallo's associates were not just in the driving seat, but taking almost every place on the coach. Topics listed in a flyer for the renamed journal comprised natural history of infection and disease progression, improved diagnostic procedures, viral pathogenesis, molecular and cellular aspects of virus infection, vaccine approaches, antiviral agents, and development of immune-restorative approaches.

There is nothing intrinsically wrong with having a narrow focus, especially when you believe, as Gallo did, that you have found the cause of Aids, and indeed a group of viruses that he believed would eventually be seen to be associated with many other diseases. He was a man with a mission: he wanted to shed scientific light on these microbes and alert the world to their dangers.

To Sonnabend, however, it was agonising to see science, and medicine, lose the one journal which, while not short of articles on retroviruses, was looking at wider themes as well in the context of Aids, for most of the mainstream journals had already closed the door on non-HIV approaches. Why couldn't Gallo and company have started a journal of their own? 'At that time I felt it was a very bad thing,' he said later. 'Not just for me, but because I knew that when I went, that was it: these articles wouldn't be published anywhere else. I received a letter from Dani Bolognesi, which spelled my name wrongly, asking me to be on the editorial board; I politely declined. I knew something bad was happening. It was turned into something that represented a particular viewpoint. It was not a conspiracy, just the way HIV was marketed, and not just by Gallo but by the institutions who sent out press releases and press kits from a particular viewpoint.'

Sonnabend still had a prominent role through the Aids Medical Foundation, which had been formed around him at the suggestion of one of his patients to raise funds for his research, since he had no other institutional backing. It had grown in strength, and by 1986 was raising funds for a variety of research projects and researchers. Sonnabend was the scientific committee chairman, and as far as he knew, nothing went out from the foundation's offices in Park Avenue that he did not see. 'In a sense, I had made it my own institution,' he said. 'I didn't think anything was happening other than what I knew about.'

But one day he picked up the phone and took a call from a journalist responding to a press release from the foundation that Sonnabend had not only not seen, but would never have approved. It had said that society faced an emergency: scientists now believed nobody was safe from the deadly virus that was causing Aids. 'I was appalled. There was certainly no evidence for such claims, and I felt the consequences would be absolutely dreadful,' Sonnabend said. 'There would be general hysteria, and if people felt a fatal disease was spreading from homosexual men, there could be violence against them as a visible group. I called Mathilde [Krim] and told her she should think about the consequences of doing such a thing. I then discovered that my foundation had hired a publicist as a fundraiser, someone who came from radio. He was a pushy, aggressive person, who orchestrated the whole campaign. There were cover stories in the international magazines saying this explosion into the general population was about to happen.

'Instead of being independent, as it started out, the foundation had become a funding agency raising money for the same things as the government. If you are at all threatening to the way things are perceived, you are not going to be able to raise money. If you have a person like me criticising Dr Gallo, you are a liability. In effect, I was fired, on the issue of heterosexual spread. I didn't think I could fight this, so I resigned.'

HIV Antibodies a Consequence, Not the Cause

Sonnabend continued to try to keep his alternative model of Aids causation alive. In his scientific writings, he explained why he believed the widespread association established between HIV antibodies and Aids might be an effect of the disease, not a cause. It was accepted that HIV was a virus that could be maintained in cells in a latent state, and the activation of latent micro-organisms, whether harmful or not, was characteristic of Aids. So the expression of HIV, leading to the production of antibodies, might simply be a consequence of the immune disorder resulting from the true cause or causes of Aids, whatever those might be. HIV's widespread presence in groups at risk of Aids was a consequence of those groups having been exposed to the spread of *all* infectious agents that can be transmitted by blood or semen. In 1987, Sonnabend made a specific prediction based on this alternative model: that HIV, in its latent state, would be more widespread in the population than either Aids, or HIV positivity.

In some of his writings, Sonnabend expanded on factors that he felt were probably important in causing Aids within the gay community, all of them arising from the cumulative effects of the unprecedented sexual promiscuity that had developed among a subgroup of homosexual men since the late 1960s. In particular, he showed that CMV and Epstein-Barr Virus (EBV) infection and activation can both have dramatic effects on lymphocytes.

One type, known as the B-lymphocyte or B-cell (so-called because of its origins in the bone marrow), is responsible for producing antibodies – molecules that attack and eliminate infectious organisms or other unwanted invaders ('antigens'). Every B-cell has a unique gene which gives it a very specific protein receptor, known as an immunoglobulin, on the surface of the cell, like a space docking unit with a precise configuration that will recognise only an equally specific spacecraft (the antigen). If the B-cell's receptor meets an antigen that succeeds in 'docking', a torrent of activity may follow. Given the right signals from certain regulatory cells, the B-cell divides rapidly and gives rise to armies of antibodies, all tailor-made to destroy the invader alone and not other parts of the body.

A second type of lymphocyte, known as the T-cell or T-lymphocyte (this one gets its name because of being processed by the thymus during its development), comes in four main groups. Abnormalities in two of these, known as T-helper cells and T-suppressor cells, have been known since the beginning of the Aids epidemic to play a part in the disorder.

T-helper cells direct much of the immune response. They do not attack microbes themselves. Instead, they produce chemical signals (cytokines) which activate the immune system. One set of signals stimulates production of cytotoxic T-cells, which kill infected cells, a process known as cell-mediated or cellular immunity. Another generates signals that induce mainly antibody production: once it has recognised a specific invader, it stimulates the appropriate B-cell into manufacturing the antibodies needed to see the invader off. It is a part of the checks and balances within the system that the

B-cells, and cytotoxic T-cells, will normally only activate when given the go-ahead by a T-helper cell.

A further, remarkable, twist to the story is that alongside the foreign antigen, the T-helper cell normally needs to have a 'friendly' protein presented to it, one that it recognises as unique to the self, before it can trigger these defensive actions. It is as though the invader has to be handcuffed by a police escort who says, 'I am on your side, but this one isn't,' before the defending forces can be put into action. These escorts play a big role in the body's ability to distinguish friend from foe. The genes that carry the code for producing them are located in a region on one of the chromosomes called the major histocompatibility complex (MHC), and the agents themselves are known as MHC proteins. They form an important part of the control machinery that limits the immune system's destructive potential. MHC molecules have been found to be prominent in purified 'HIV' preparations and probably play a significant part in the immunological disorder seen in Aids.

The T-suppressor cells, again as their name indicates, are another mechanism of putting the brakes on the immune system. They also work in a specific way, probably by inhibiting the action of helper cells specific for the same antigen as themselves.

It was a strange coincidence that at about the time the Aids epidemic began in gay men, the technology became available for routinely differentiating and counting helper cells (also known as T4 or CD4 cells) and suppressor cells (also known as T8 or CD8 cells) on a large scale, and from very early on abnormalities were seen in Aids patients. Generally, healthy people have two helper cells to one suppressor cell, but this ratio was reversed in Aids. It was also found to be reversed in many homosexual men who did not have Aids, however, and Sonnabend has pointed to studies showing that CMV and EBV both cause a diminishing ratio of helper to suppressor cells, as well as other immunosuppressive changes, that are maintained for as long as the infections persist. In the case of CMV, the aberrations can persist for up to a year following a single primary infection.

Gallo had originally believed that HIV was causing Aids by directly killing T4 cells, removing the ability of these key players in the immune system to do their job properly, and hence leading to the appearance of cancer and rampant opportunistic infections. After it became clear that so few of the cells were actively expressing HIV that this was impossible, another mechanism suggested was that the immune response against HIV becomes an auto-immune response against the T4 cells, because of a similarity in their surface proteins.

Sonnabend argued that there was no need to invoke HIV in such a mechanism. Instead, multiple assaults on the immune system arising from anal intercourse could provide an adequate explanation. There was evidence that the MHC proteins which, as described above, play an important part in controlling immune system reactivity can act as receptors for sperm. Immune responses have also been demonstrated to the cellular components of semen. So Sonnabend postulated that repeated exposure to semen from many different men was causing the immune system to lose sight of which proteins belonged to the self and which to others, eventually leading to the appearance of antibodies and killer cells which destroyed the body's own T-cells. Anti T-cell antibodies had been repeatedly described in Aids. (It is also now known that some HIV-positive people have cytotoxic T-cells which kill activated but uninfected T4 cells.)

He reasoned that since homosexuality was not new, whereas Aids was, it was unlikely that semen in itself could do all the damage (although there may never have been a time previously when the male body was exposed to semen from thousands of different partners). Rather, the proposal was that immune responses to semen could provide a background of immune suppression, promoting repeated viral infections; and when this process had gone on for too long, the accumulated effects were such as to cause a switch to an irreversible and self-sustaining condition, independent of promiscuous behaviour. So the disease developed from the combined and cumulative effects of sustained or repeated exposure to multiple factors, rather than following an incubation period after infection with a single agent.

The details of this model were confined to an attempt to explain the development of Aids in homosexual men. Analogous models could be developed for other groups. However, although Aids was a new phenomenon, at least in its epidemic form, among homosexual men, that could not be said with confidence for the other groups. Before 1982, diagnosis of pneumocystic pneumonia required an open lung biopsy, and so it would not have been routinely detected in any group.

Sonnabend concluded one account of his multifactorial model with a comment that, as he acknowledged, went beyond what was traditionally regarded as appropriate in a scientific communication. He felt it to be justified because, as he put it, 'the potential for adverse social effects of a particular scientific proposal appeared so great'.

The problem was that if groups already bearing a heavy burden of stigmatisation were perceived to carry a lethal virus capable of spreading to and decimating the population at large, 'the danger of consequent brutalisation of such groups is only too real'. The situation was even more perilous when there was a test purporting to identify apparently healthy individuals in those groups who were carrying the virus. 'Because of the potential for the abuse of individuals identified as a source of contagion, it is especially important to make the distinction between hypothesis and scientific fact. Few would question the inappropriateness of creating public policy on the basis of mere conjecture. Unfortunately, in the case of Aids such a distinction has not been made.'[6]

There were other adverse consequences arising from the acceptance as fact of the theory that HIV caused Aids. Research on other causative factors had not been pursued; aspects of the disease process apparently unrelated to HIV had not been explored; treatment models other than anti-retroviral approaches had not been developed; and strategies for managing Aids patients had not been worked out because of the belief that an effective anti-retroviral approach would make such considerations redundant.

As HIV's dominance of Aids treatment and research approaches continued unabated, Sonnabend's tone grew angrier. In a 1989 article, 'Fact and Speculation About the Cause of Aids'[7] he complained of how in 1984 Margaret Heckler, the US Department of Health and Human Services Secretary, had 'ceremoniously propelled' the contention that HIV was the cause of Aids out of the realm of speculation into that of proven fact with her public pronouncement that US government scientists had discovered 'the probable cause of Aids'. 'Today we add another miracle to the long honour roll of American medicine and science,' she had told a press conference in Washington, DC. 'Today's discovery represents the triumph of science over a dreaded disease.' A blood test would be available within six months, and a vaccine ready for testing within two years.

'Thus, overnight, a new orthodoxy came into being,' Sonnabend commented. It had been unruffled by the subsequent discovery of a second purported cause of Aids in a second, distinct retrovirus, which came to be known as HIV2. He went on:

> The premature acceptance as fact of a contention that more properly belongs in the realm of speculation has had a number of far-reaching consequences – let alone the painful fact that it has provided virtually no help to people with Aids, despite a massive investment and six years of intensive work on the biology of the HIVs and the chemotherapy of infection with these viruses...it has justified the almost total commitment of resources to the study of the HIVs and of treatments to counter them.

In this paper, Sonnabend spelled out in detail how the close association of HIV positivity with Aids could be explained without attributing any significance to the virus as the cause of Aids. In order to make this clear, he first outlined some relevant points about the biology of retroviruses such as HIV, and of the immune response.

A retrovirus consists of a core made of ribonucleic acid (RNA) surrounded by a protein coat; and around that, an outer protein coat derived from the membrane of the cell in which the virus was produced. Antibodies are made against the protein components of the virus, not the RNA, although the latter contains the genetic instructions that can direct the cell to make viral proteins.

When the body is exposed to the virus, it does not necessarily make antibodies to it. If very little virus enters the body, cells may become infected but there will not be enough virus protein present to stimulate the immune system into mounting an antibody attack. When retroviruses enter a cell, they are disassembled and their genetic information is first transcribed from RNA into DNA, then integrated with the DNA of the host cell. This viral DNA may remain completely dormant. When that is the case, no viral proteins are made and the only indication that the cell contains viral material may be the detection of viral DNA by a variety of techniques, including the recently developed polymerase chain reaction (PCR).

For many years it had been an article of faith among Aids experts that following infection with HIV, the virus multiplied until enough viral protein was present for the body to start producing antibodies. There was said to be a 'window' period of about three months during which an individual became increasingly infective, despite being HIV-negative. Then the immune system mounted an antibody reaction, and the infected individual became reactive on the HIV test. A graphic representation of this course of events was shown at Aids conferences around the world in the mid-1980s.

But this picture was hypothetical. There had never been an animal model to prove it, or any other scientific validation. There was therefore '*absolutely* no basis to justify this authoritative depiction of the course of infection. It is yet another example of speculation being presented as fact that has typified presentations on Aids,' Sonnabend wrote.

It was just as likely that infection was followed by very limited viral replication, insufficient to trigger an antibody response, but where the viral DNA was maintained in the cell in a dormant or latent state. In such a case, the individual would remain negative on the antibody test, but might show the presence of HIV by a genetic detection technique such as PCR.

If, however, the mechanisms maintaining latency were disturbed, or the infected cells were otherwise activated, at some later date – it might be decades later – then the viral DNA would start producing viral proteins, to be assembled into viral particles and released into the bloodstream. If that process went on for long enough, the immune system would respond by making antibodies to the proteins, and the individual would seroconvert – that is, become HIV-positive.

Sonnabend cited several mechanisms that had been shown to trigger into action the cell DNA associated with HIV production. Chemical mediators such as interleukin-1 and tumour necrosis factor, both generated during the course of many different infections, could do it, as could antigens displayed on the surfaces of foreign cells such as from semen and other people's blood. Herpes viruses had also been shown capable of directly activating latent HIV.

Furthermore, there were also likely to be mechanisms whereby cells in a healthy immune system kill cells that start to produce HIV, limiting virus production. A damaged immune system might not be able to exercise that restraint. Sonnabend urged Aids scientists to seek the presence of such anti-

HIV cell-mediated responses in people who were negative for the HIV blood test.

So here was a very plausible explanation as to why so many promiscuous gay men, as well as those with Aids, could test HIV-positive without HIV necessarily playing any causative role in Aids. Because of their lifestyle, most of these men had encountered HIV Some of them had also at some point been subject to the repeated infections, viral reactivations and multiple rectal inseminations which had been shown capable of bringing HIV out of latency.

Add to that the fact that Aids patients and most promiscuous gay men were immune-deficient, and so unable to block HIV activation directly with a cellular response, and one could see clearly why the second line of defence, the production of antibodies against HIV proteins, had so often come into action. By this way of thinking, HIV-positivity was a consequence and not a cause of Aids. It was just one example of the activation of latent micro-organisms – a hallmark of Aids and the decline of the immune system that led up to Aids.

Sonnabend noted that these mechanisms would operate in all the Aids risk groups. Needle-sharing intravenous drug users and blood transfusion recipients were all exposed to the foreign cells, and to some extent also to the infections, that could activate HIV. Tumour necrosis factor was also present in tropical infections, particularly malaria, and was detectable in the blood of needle-sharing intravenous drug users.

One important conclusion from this analysis was that risk factors for infection with HIV should be separated from risk factors for the appearance of HIV antibodies in the blood (seroconversion). The latter should be thought of as an event separate from infection, and with its own determining factors. In some circumstances, there might be a risk of both happening at once, such as if someone was transfused with blood massively infected with HIV. Anal intercourse could constitute a risk for infection if the semen contained HIV; but even if the semen was not infected with HIV, it could also constitute an independent risk for seroconversion. This could happen in a number of ways: by activating latently infected cells in the lining of the colon, or further afield if cells in semen entered the blood or lymphatic systems; and by serving as the vehicle for infection with other viruses, notably CMV, which had been shown capable of triggering activation of latent HIV.

The risks for infection with HIV, although overlapping with the risks for seroconversion, would extend more broadly. In other words, one might become infected with HIV in ways that are more casual than the contacts required to become HIV-positive and develop Aids. There was already epidemiological evidence suggesting that this was the case. For example, Aids appeared to be spread by an insertive sexual partner and by injection of blood; women seemed to transmit Aids to men with difficulty, if at all. But it would be difficult to comprehend how HIV (as distinct from Aids) could have been preserved in nature if it were only transmitted by an insertive sexual partner or by blood transfusions. The likelihood was that HIV could be transmitted more easily than Aids, from women to men as well as from men to women, and that when the virus was transmitted *without* risk behaviours for Aids, the individuals concerned would neither risk becoming HIV-positive nor developing Aids.

If HIV was not the cause of Aids, one might also expect that groups other than those at risk for Aids would be found to carry HIV by the new genetic techniques such as PCR, while remaining HIV-negative. 'Should this be found, for example, in health care workers, laboratory personnel working with HIV, or household contacts of Aids patients, there will undoubtedly be an initial panic that Aids is indeed spreading out of the groups at risk; but in fact, such findings must bring further into question the causative roles of the HIVs in this disease.' Finally, Sonnabend predicted that if this analysis was correct, 'there should be small numbers of people with Aids who have not been infected with the HIVs'.

He concluded:

> I have attempted to show why the contention that HIV causes Aids should be returned to the realm of speculation. The costs of inappropriately accepting that the cause of Aids has been firmly established to be HIV have been enormous, in time wasted and lives lost. Some of the areas of neglected research have been outlined. The cause or causes of Aids remains unknown, and thus all hypotheses, including HIV, must be pursued.

Predictions Confirmed

How have Sonnabend's arguments stood up in the six years following this May 1989 article? Several of the predictions based on the multifactorial model he described have been confirmed.

We now know that a decline in T4 cells seen in HIV-positive haemophiliacs can be greatly slowed and commonly halted or reversed when patients are put on to a high-purity form of their Factor 8 treatment. The old treatment, a concentrate made from pooled extracts of thousands of people's blood, contained large quantities of immunosuppressive materials. The new, introduced in 1988, contains only the protein haemophiliacs need to correct their clotting disorder. It is clear from studies comparing the outcome of treatment with the old and new Factor 8 that the impurities, not HIV, were responsible for the decline previously attributed to the virus. Sonnabend had speculated on this possibility as far back as 1984. The failure to attend to it has been responsible for much needless worry, and inappropriate and damaging treatment.

The stabilisation and recovery now seen in the immune systems of many HIV-positive haemophiliacs provide powerful support for Sonnabend's suggestion that HIV is an opportunistic infection rather than a killer in its own right. It also means that a positive result in the HIV test should not be regarded as a sentence of death. If the pressure on the immune system that led to the expression of the 'HIV' genes can be lessened or removed, the clinical course in such HIV-positive patients may be no different from that in seronegative patients (in fact, some of them revert to seronegative).*

Second, there has been striking confirmation of Sonnabend's prediction that some groups of people, such as drug addicts or health care workers, might be found to have been exposed to the virus without developing antibodies or necessarily being at risk of Aids. At the Eighth International Aids Conference in Amsterdam in 1992, a study showing widespread and

---

* More details of the evidence against the HIV theory provided by the experience of haemophiliac patients – and of the extraordinary resistance of many doctors and scientists to this evidence – are contained in Chapters 7, 8 and 13.

undetected exposure to HIV was presented by Dr Gene Shearer, chief of the cell-mediated immunity section of the National Cancer Institute in the US.

Shearer's colleague, Dr Mario Clerici, had investigated four risk groups of HIV-negative people with a test designed to see if their immune system had ever encountered HIV. The test involved seeing how T-helper cells responsible for triggering a cell-mediated killing effect against viruses – as opposed to those that trigger antibody production – responded to synthetic HIV proteins. A strong response, held to indicate previous exposure to HIV, was seen in 65 per cent of the gay men tested; 45 per cent of injecting drug users; and 75 per cent of a group of health care workers involved in a needle-stick accident that might have exposed them to infected blood, but who did not become HIV-positive on the antibody test. Eleven out of twenty-one babies born to HIV-positive mothers showed a similar response, although it was less pronounced, as did ten out of 155 people who were not thought to have had any special risk of encountering HIV.

The revolutionary nature of these findings, in relation to the conventional view of HIV and Aids, was made clear by an article in *New Scientist* the following week. Phyllida Brown, who has done much careful reporting on Aids research over a long period, referred to Shearer and Clerici having 'dared to think something that, to many scientists, has been unthinkable: that there might be a successful immune response to HIV'. The article went on:

> Could the T cells have mounted an attack on the virus that was enough to protect against infection? Are these people (and, presumably, many others like them who have not been studied) the immune 'success stories'? Suppose that, by studying only the immune responses of infected people, we have been looking only at the immune 'failures' until now?

Shearer was not clear at the time whether the immune mechanism involved was preventing HIV from infecting cells in the first place, by killing the virus before it could enter cells, or keeping the infection latent within cells. Evidence presented at the same conference by an Israeli scientist, Dr Tamar Jehuda-Cohen, supported the idea that in many cases the HIV genes *are* present in the cells, but remain inactive. Jehuda-Cohen, a clinical immunologist working with Ethiopian immigrants, sought to identify exposure to HIV in the wives of HIV-positive men. Three out of fourteen wives were HIV-positive on the antibody test; and a further seven gave a positive result for the presence of HIV genetic sequences using the PCR test. Findings among children born to HIV-positive mothers were similar, Jehuda-Cohen said. Most were HIV-negative, but the PCR test showed some clearly had the virus. 'It is a latent, dormant, silent infection in these people. There are definitely people who carry the virus in this way.' She said she had met resistance from some leading figures in the international Aids field to her calls for studies to establish how widespread this 'silent infection' was. 'But it is not a reason for panic. I think it's wonderful news. It means that getting infected or being exposed is not equivalent to being doomed.'

Apart from altering our attitude towards HIV, the findings could have important implications for vaccine development (assuming that a vaccine approach continues to be pursued). If there is a successful natural cellular immune response to HIV, candidate vaccines could be sought that stimulate the cellular part of the immune system, rather than the antibody-producing part. Shearer and Clerici have even speculated that stimulating antibodies could be harmful, since studies have indicated that these two arms of the immune system may inhibit each other.

The late Dr Jonas Salk, the originator of polio vaccine, who was also present at the Amsterdam conference, was working on just such a cellular approach, designed to improve the immune system's ability to keep the virus in check. He believed it might have been with us for centuries and normally coexisted peacefully with us. 'It could be in a quiescent state in an individual for decades, and then become activated under the influence of stress, or advancing years,' he told me. 'The important thing is to keep it in a non-pathologic form. I wouldn't care if it was neatly tucked away in the genetic material, as long as the immune system was prepared to deal with it if it became activated.' He said he had been attempting to achieve a 'live-and-let-live' situation, 'as distinct from chemical treatment intended to poison the virus. I don't want to destroy the HIV, just let it be there but without causing harm.'

At the time of writing, more than three years have passed since the Amsterdam conference but these important findings of cellular elimination or control of HIV have hardly begun to penetrate public awareness. Gene

Shearer says there are now about twelve papers that have reported evidence of cellular immunity. Furthermore, at least two studies, one in France and one by Shearer's group, have looked for and demonstrated the activity of cytotoxic (cell-killing) T-lymphocytes, which are found only when infection has actually taken place – that is, the virus has not just paid a passing visit, but has definitely infected some of the host cells.

The main targets of these killer cells, which have been described as 'professional assassins that kill cells outright',[8] are body cells infected with viruses, which they destroy before the virus can proliferate (they also play a part in killing cancer cells). They have surface receptors that make them specific for a particular antigen – in this case, they are targeted against HIV antigens. The antigens are expressed inside infected cells, and then presented alongside a characteristic protein marker of the major histocompatibility complex (MHC) - the 'escort' proteins referred to above that help the immune system distinguish friend from foe. Cytotoxic T-cells need to see their antigen alongside a class 1 protein, which is found on all body cells. This restriction ensures that the T-cells confine their activity to killing any infected cells in which viral protein begins to appear on the surface, rather than being 'distracted by futile skirmishes with free viruses, which they cannot kill'.[9] However, cytotoxic T-cells also go into action against cells from another individual, whether from blood, semen, or cells in a transplanted organ.

Like B-cells, cytotoxic T-cells become primed by an encounter with a particular target and carry this memory with them, so that they can respond rapidly if they meet the same invader again. Also as with B-cells, however, they are regulated by the T-helper and T-suppressor cells which, as we have seen, are present in abnormal proportions as Aids develops, with helper cells no longer being predominant.

Shearer and Clerici now suspect that when healthy people become exposed to HIV, particularly at a low level of virus, their immune system is capable of mounting a successful cell-mediated reaction. This includes the priming of a cytotoxic T-lymphocyte defence mechanism to ensure that to the extent that some cells have become infected, the virus is not allowed to break out of those cells and spread through the body. Such a priming mechanism may help to explain why some people, such as certain groups of African prostitutes with multiple exposure to HIV-positive men, and the wives of some HIV-positive men who have continued to have unprotected sex, have been seen to remain HIV-negative over many years.

For those who believe HIV is the prime cause of Aids, this mechanism might also help to explain why the syndrome has remained almost exclusively confined to the so-called risk groups who have immunocompromising factors in their lives other than HIV, and the lack of spread outside those groups. If the immune system was busy coping with a variety of onslaughts at the time it first encountered HIV, it would be more vulnerable to widespread initial infection as the virus would be more free to replicate. Similarly, subsequent events in the immune system could increase the virus's freedom to express itself. Malnutrition, and parasitic infections such as malaria, for example, have both been demonstrated to depress cellular immunity profoundly. One theory holds that the multiple parasitic infections to which promiscuous gay men were exposed through anal intercourse and related practices may have provided exactly the right conditions for HIV to break loose of the natural restraints on it and become pathogenic within such hosts.

This description of events, if true, would be very different from the idea the world lived with so long, that HIV was a 'new killer virus' set to attack just about everyone with an active sex life in time.

But there is another way of looking at the same data. The work by Shearer and Clerici and others is demonstrating that the 'HIV' phenomenon is far wider than indicated simply by the number of people who test HIV-positive. It is also demonstrating that HIV-positivity may by its very nature be associated with an impaired immune system, in which the immunodepression is a cause of the person becoming HIV-positive, rather than an effect. That does not on its own rule out the possibility that HIV, when allowed to multiply, subsequently sets in train the devastation of the immune system seen in Aids (though ten years of work in numerous laboratories around the world have failed as yet to show how it could do that). But the demonstration that healthy people can 'carry' HIV as a harmless passenger provides powerful confirmation of Sonnabend's longstanding, unheeded warning to the medical and scientific professions not to jump to the conclusion that because HIV antibodies were almost always detectable in Aids patients, but not in healthy people, that made it the cause of Aids. As far back as July 1984 he was writing to *Nature* that with at least two other similar viruses (Gallo's

HTLV-1 and HTLV-2) having apparently also been recovered from Aids patients, 'it suggests that they are more likely to represent opportunistic infections or reactivations from latency'. The letter added presciently: 'Aids is indeed a tragic disease...This tragedy can only be compounded by premature interpretations of the role of the new viral isolates with the promise of a vaccine, and a diminished focus on other possible aetiologic factors.'

There are other important implications of this different way of thinking about HIV, foreshadowed in Sonnabend's writings. For example, when someone becomes HIV-positive, it does not mean they have necessarily been given the virus by their current sex partner. They might have been infected previously, and the virus brought out of latency by some subsequent immune challenge.

Secondly, it implies that the important event in becoming HIV-positive may not be exposure to the virus in itself, but the cumulative burdens on the immune system that permit activation of the HIV genes. This means that people in risk groups, including those who already test HIV-positive, should not consider avoidance of HIV transmission as the only step they can take to protect themselves or others. The general reduction of toxic, infectious and immunogenic challenge to the immune system could be expected to play a big part in the prevention of Aids. Thus, it would be quite wrong for two HIV-positive people to have unprotected sex in the belief that they had nothing to lose.

Anger – and Vindication

I met Joe Sonnabend in May 1992 at an 'alternative' Aids conference in Amsterdam which preceded by a couple of months the main international event. Called 'Aids: A Different View', the symposium – the first to challenge HIV – brought together about 200 scientists, doctors and patients who were for the most part united by the belief that the role of HIV in Aids had been over-simplified or exaggerated.

At that point, he was very angry. He had seethed for years over the way HIV was marketed to the exclusion of other hypotheses; over his dismissive treatment at the hands of the CDC in the very earliest days of the epidemic, when he felt he had so much to tell that would be so important to the future handling of Aids; over his dismissal from the editorship of *Aids Research*; over the promotion by government as well as commercial agencies of AZT, a drug whose toxicity was such that he regarded its long-term use as unethical; over the manufacture and spread of the myth of heterosexual Aids; over the billions that had gone into the search for a vaccine to protect the world against this non-existent threat; and over the deaths of nearly 300 of his patients in the twelve years since the beginning of the US epidemic.

Eight years after HIV was identified, he said, he still had nothing substantial to offer as treatment. 'It's strange for me now to be at a meeting where issues we were discussing eight years ago are being resurrected. But this is not just a discussion among detached scientists. I have no words to express my anger at what has happened. I know that if many, many promising leads apparent at that time had been explored, we might well have developed effective treatments.' The tragedy was a result of the total concentration of research funds on HIV and the 'criminal' suppression of other research possibilities. 'The Aids research establishment are responsible for this tragedy. The marketing of HIV, through press releases and statements, as a killer virus causing Aids without the need for any other factors, has so distorted research and treatment that it may have caused thousands of people to suffer and die.'

It wasn't just the loss and suffering among patients that enraged him. He was still acutely troubled by the scene nine years previously when he had resigned as scientific committee chairman of the Aids Medical Foundation because they insisted on putting out press releases 'telling the world there was going to be a heterosexual explosion, and everyone is going to die'. He went on: 'It was unbearable. I couldn't stand what they were doing. They were going to destroy marriages, relationships, lives – they were freaking out entire populations. There was no evidence for it then, and there isn't now. But the idea suited the agenda of many groups.

'People who wanted to promote family values liked it, because it was nice to say extramarital sex could be lethal. Others liked it because they could promote celibacy before marriage. Gay men liked the idea, because they could avoid thinking about the behavioural part. For them, a killer virus that would not discriminate became a way of saying that promiscuity was less important. Even in Africa, with a killer virus theory, it was easy for politicians to say our economic policies, and the fact that many people live in squalor, have nothing to do with this disease. And for scientists and health workers, there were going to be a lot more funds for fighting a virus that was a threat to everyone, than for a condition affecting special groups. Yet promising leads that pointed in different directions were shut down. Those decisions were criminal; not only on the part of the scientists involved but the governments that supported them.'

Two months later, back in Amsterdam at the International Aids Conference, Sonnabend's anger had at least temporarily given way to the joy of vindication after the emergency session at which his May 1989 prediction that 'there should be small numbers of people with Aids who have not been infected with the HIVs' was dramatically confirmed. It wasn't just the pleasure of being proved right. It was also seeing Jim Curran, now head of HIV/Aids at the CDC, who ten years previously had been so dismissive of Sonnabend's multifactorial thinking, getting visibly tied up in knots as he tried to find words to describe the eleven Aids cases in which scientists had failed to find any trace of HIV.

Attacked for not having alerted doctors previously to six such 'anomalous' cases being studied by CDC experts, Curran said the reason was that since HIV was not present, they could not be called Aids. The patients' symptoms and backgrounds were Aids-like, with persistent decline of the immune system, resulting emergence of opportunistic infectious diseases, and risk factors in most of the patients' histories such as blood transfusions, homosexual intercourse and drug abuse. 'This is not Aids caused by something else,' Curran said. 'Aids is severe immune depression caused by HIV1 or HIV2. Do the patients have HIV1 or HIV2? Our six cases, we are quite convinced, don't.'

The CDC would now call for HIV-negative cases to be reported, he said. But he was still struggling. 'It's particularly hard in the era of Aids to call for anything that looks like Aids. These things are automatically labelled Aids without HIV…it's immunodeficiency.'

Dr Martien Brands, a Dutch GP who organised the 'alternative' conference the previous May, told Curran that the confusion arose because of a mistaken view of what the disease entailed. 'Originally Aids was defined as what it is, a syndrome with many possible causes,' he said. 'You have made from the

Aids paradigm a definition of HIV disease. You should now change your definition of Aids.' Curran, however, insisted that in 'people who are proven not to have HIV infection, these cases are not Aids'.

After listening to a series of doctors testify at the meeting that they, too, had cases supporting the 'heresy' of Aids without HIV, Sonnabend declared: 'This is the moment I have waited eight years to see.' The CDC had created an absurd situation, he said. In the past, many cases of immune suppression had been listed as Aids without an HIV test, on the basis that they were in risk groups for HIV-positivity. 'So if these HIV-negative patients had not been tested, they would have been legitimately diagnosed as Aids. But because they tested negative, they cease to be Aids. It is an unbelievable muddle. The truth is, we don't know what is causing this disease.'

In a recent attempt to rehabilitate the HIV theory, and with it, the scientific profession's reputation,[10] Dr Steven Harris took Aids sceptics to task for creating too wide a definition of Aids, and then claiming that thousands of HIV-negative cases had been identified. But Harris was also misleading. He stated in a review article published in the rationalist journal *Skeptic* that after a 'massive' search the CDC had only been able to find fewer than 100 people without HIV infection across the country with severely depleted T4 (CD4) cell counts. He justified the CDC's decision to call these cases 'idiopathic CD4 lymphocytopenia (ICL)' (meaning 'people with low CD4 counts for which we have no explanation') on the grounds that they 'were found not to come from the Aids risk groups. They did not use illicit drugs, had not been exposed to blood products, and had no evidence of sexual behaviour which would have exposed them to a special infection risk...What the sceptics had forgotten (or hoped their readers would not notice) was that the immune deficiency of people with ICL did not seem to be *acquired*. What justification was there, then, for calling it Aids?'

This was puzzling, because Curran had clearly stated in Amsterdam that risk behaviours *were* present among the six exhaustively investigated CDC cases he described at that time. They were also identified in four out of the other five cases he had referred to, which had been described in the *Lancet* by a group of New York City researchers. So I checked the references given by Harris. It turned out that they were from the book of abstracts of workshop and poster presentations at the 1993 Berlin Aids conference. But the data did not support his claim that the ICL cases did not come from risk groups. On the contrary, the CDC's ICL task force, who conducted their survey of such cases between August and November 1992, reported risk factors present in nearly half of seventy-eight adult cases identified. Seven were homosexuals, thirteen were haemophilia patients, eight were transfusion patients, three were intravenous drug users, and seven were listed as at risk through heterosexual intercourse (the nature of the risk to this latter group was not made clear). Forty of the patients were listed as having no risk identified.

Harris's claim that HIV sceptics had invented wider definitions of Aids to bring in a greater 'catch' of non-HIV Aids cases overlooked the fact that the World Health Organization's own definition for Aids in Africa has had exactly that effect, as revealed in the *Lancet*[11] in October 1992 by Japanese researchers who had for several years been investigating the epidemiology of HIV in Ghana. The group, from the Institute for Virus Research at Kyoto University and the Noguchi Memorial Institute for Medical Research at the University of Ghana, said the revelation of non-HIV Aids cases at the Amsterdam conference 'seems to have provoked dispute about the aetiology of the disease: is Aids truly caused by HIV?' They said that in 1990, blood samples were collected from 227 Ghanaian Aids patients diagnosed by WHO clinical criteria in Africa. Multiple laboratory diagnostic tests showed that 135 of these – 59 per cent – were negative for HIV, leading them to conclude that 'the existence of other agents causing Aids-like syndromes might be possible among these so- called HIV-negative cases'.

Co-factors Come into Fashion

When I next saw Sonnabend, in New York in October 1994, he was a different person from the haunted individual I had met thirty months previously. His days in the wilderness looked as if they might be ending. Gallo was friendly, and had invited Sonnabend to the previous Aids review meeting at the National Institutes of Health. Multifactorial approaches were now officially 'in', though in the context of HIV: witness a recent review article in *Science*[12] by Fauci, entitled 'Multifactorial Nature of Human Immunodeficiency Virus Disease: Implications for Therapy', in which he acknowledged that the disease process is multifactorial, that a 'superantigen' (a protein that stimulates activation of excessive numbers of T-cells) might be involved, not necessarily HIV-related, and that 'repeated or persistent exposure of the immune system to an antigen may ultimately lead to immune system dysfunction and loss of the ability to maintain an adequate immune response to the antigen. Furthermore, the general functional capability of immune competent cells may be impaired if they are maintained in a chronically activated state. In addition, chronic activation of the immune system may induce an abnormal programme of cell death (apoptosis) as well as the secretion of certain cytokines that can induce HIV expression.' It had always been Sonnabend's contention that chronic activation of the immune system, such as he had seen caused by the 'exuberant' gay lifestyle, could in itself eventually cause irreversible loss of immune function.

A further cause for encouragement was that a non-profit, community-based Aids research centre that Sonnabend had founded in New York City, the Community Research Initiative on Aids, was flourishing, though this was partly because it now spoke the language of HIV, declaring itself 'dedicated to the exploration of new methods for treating HIV disease and its associated opportunistic diseases'.

'I'm trying to learn to survive without giving in to the mainstream,' Sonnabend said. 'Things that are threatening don't survive. There is this terrible normalising influence, which means that to get public support you've got to be non-threatening. I think it may be better now; the monolithic Aids establishment is crumbling.

'It took me some years to come to understand the unwillingness of the scientific community to respond to criticism of shoddy science. The reason was that the rush to the single agent was motivated by things other than science. It was obvious to me, and it must have been obvious to anybody trained in microbiology, that the evidence presented in the scientific literature was suspect, but there was just general silence. My trust in the scientific community was shattered because of the way this evolved. We were told at one time that "time is the only co-factor", for example. This was pure science fiction. Why was there no discussion of this among doctors, among academics?

'I'm still puzzled why journalists were so uncritical. When the institutions sent them press kits about HIV and the perils it was supposed to represent, you would have thought they would have gone out and asked, Does everyone agree with you? What is the evidence? Does anyone think differently? But none of that happened. The mainstream journalists received their copy from these institutions and simply reported it as it was given to them. All of the nonsense would have been much more difficult to promote if they had been there to protest.'

When I told Sonnabend that as medical correspondent at the *Sunday Times* during the second half of the 1980s I had played a leading role in promoting the 'deadly new virus' theory, he kindly (though not persuasively) tried to take me off the hook. 'There was a group thing, you were responding to that. But what about the scientists? Why did they let all this happen?'

At the time of writing, Sonnabend has become gloomy again about the prospects of a return to sanity. There has been wide publicity for the theory, extrapolated from the effect on blood T-cell counts of some short-term drug studies, that 'from the first moment of infection HIV may be locked in a titanic struggle with the immune system', with 'more than two billion white blood cells destroyed every 24 hours'.[13] How this squares with the studies of cellular immunity suggesting that thousands or millions of people may be harmlessly infected with HIV, or with the evidence that T-cell decline in HIV-positive haemophiliacs can be reversed by purifying their Factor 8 treatment, is not addressed or explained. It is as though the scientific world is making some final, desperate attempt to rescue the HIV hypothesis. Allied to these face-saving manoeuvres come new calls for ever earlier and more drastic combinations of drugs to try to swing the balance of power in favour of the victims of this 'war of attrition' between the immune system and HIV – even though they might feel themselves to be perfectly healthy, and despite their having – even by conventional thinking – an average life expectancy of ten to fifteen years ahead of them from the time of infection.

Sonnabend feels no bitterness towards Gallo. In fact, he has some sympathy for the US government researcher, who has received much media criticism over his role in promoting as his own discovery the agent originally isolated by Montagnier's group. 'I feel that all the things that unfolded in the early 1980s were done in full public and scientific view, and with the knowledge of his political bosses at NIH. So I feel that by focusing on Bob Gallo, one is simply deflecting attention from the truth about the structure of the whole scientific endeavour in which these things can happen. For that reason I don't see why Bob Gallo should be singled out when the problem belongs to the whole scientific community. He was given permission to do what he did; it was as if wrongdoing is rewarded.'

I asked what lesson Sonnabend had learned from his experience of the scientific world's handling of Aids. 'I'm afraid what I feel I've learned is quite depressing. If you are asking, have I come away with anything constructive and positive, I would have to say no. I have become rather despairing of our ability to approach our problems and questions in a dispassionate way.

'Terrible mistakes happened, and there's no willingness to look back, so they just go on being repeated. We have no idea whether AZT is of any help to people at all, yet it's out there still. When I worked for the MRC, and was part of the antiviral community, the idea of putting a drug that is so evidently a poison as AZT into people for the rest of their lives just wouldn't have been considered. It may be that short-term use in selected people can give some benefit, but the chemical nature of this drug is such that one should be totally frightened of it. The willingness to expose people, including healthy people, to such a drug on a long-term basis is to me remarkable. We are still not looking at whether these agents really work, because we are doing the same poor clinical trials with new agents. I am really quite depressed.'

Based on his clinical and research experience Sonnabend developed the multifactorial theory of Aids causation from which he made several precise predictions. As this chapter has demonstrated, these were mostly confirmed by events, whereas the predictions based on the 'deadly new virus' theory have turned out to be grossly wrong. I suspect that one day his long-neglected contributions to the field of Aids will win him considerable recognition.

He is still predisposed to the view that Aids has multifactorial origins, rather than being caused by a single agent. He considers it likely that HIV is harmless. He says that despite a 'desperate' search for indirect mechanisms whereby HIV could still be held responsible for the death of T-helper lymphocytes, no evidence for this has been observed in infected patients. Although there are well-documented precedents for viral-induced auto-immunity, again, no evidence exists that HIV can do it, whereas there are factors other than HIV that could plausibly explain the auto-immune phenomena seen in Aids.

HIV, he believes, simply became visible because of being introduced into the highly interactive pool of gay men who were caught in a spiral of multiple and repeated immunosuppressive infections and exposures resulting from the promiscuity 'revolution' of the late 1960s, a spiral which meant that by the late 1970s even a casual encounter with a sick, multiply infected man could carry a great risk of disease. 'The essence of this view is that it's not anything new, but that in the current epidemic people are exposed to a new combination and much greater concentration of old immunosuppressive agents. The exercise now should be to try to identify these factors.'

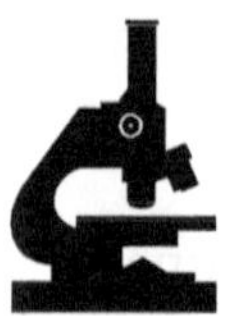

4: DRUGGED

John Lauritsen is a Harvard-educated survey research analyst who began reviewing Aids research in early 1983. Despite being aged around sixty, he could almost pass for a schoolmaster in his late twenties, with tweedy jacket, boyish haircut and large, observant, somewhat doleful eyes. He has lived for nearly thirty years in a flat in St Mark's Place, New York City, at the heart of what was once a gay community in both senses of the word but which he now finds a shadow of its former self. The flat is stacked from floor to ceiling with books and papers. A small corridor between these mounds of documents gives access to a desk by a grubby window. Much of the desk is also piled high with papers, but there is just about room for the computer and keyboard from which the most trenchantly informative, irreverent, funny and tragic writing of the Aids years has emerged. Much of it has appeared in the *New York Native,* often as cover stories presented with enormous panache.

In an introduction to his 1993 book *The Aids War,*[1] Lauritsen has a telling story of how he first became acquainted with the perils of speaking the truth. He was aged six, it was just before Christmas, and he had asked his parents if Santa Claus really existed. They told him, and a few days later he passed the news to his playmates, who had anyway, he says, been at least sceptical. Then the flak began. 'My mother received calls from bitter, sobbing women: *their Christmas had been ruined by me!*' At a family discussion that evening, his father counselled that it was always right to tell the truth – 'but it was also good to be cautious, for others were not so rational as we'.

Lauritsen evidently did not take much notice of his father. Caution is not a word brought to mind by his writing style. Perhaps it might have been better – for him, at least, if not for journalism – if he had been told to try not to be hurtful. But he seems instead to have preferred to be guided by Miss Celestine Brock, who taught him Latin and journalism (she died in 1992 at the age of ninety-nine), and to whom *The Aids War* is dedicated. 'I have not forgotten her disdain for euphemism, sentimentality, and all kinds of phoniness – nor have I forgotten a lecture she gave on the meaning of PROBITAS,' he writes.

There is no euphemism in Lauritsen's descriptions of his views on the 'Aids epidemic' (he often insists on putting 'Aids' in inverted commas, because he considers it a phoney construct). 'It is an epidemic of lies,' he writes, 'through which hundreds of thousands of people have died and are dying unnecessarily, billions of dollars have gone down the drain, the Public Health Service has disgraced itself, and Science has plunged into whoredom. The official Aids paradigm – including the preposterous notion that a biochemically inactive microbe, the so-called "human immunodeficiency virus", causes the (at last count) twenty-nine Aids-indicator diseases – represents the most colossal blunder in medical history... People with "Aids" (PWAs) are not suffering from a deadly new disease; they are people who have become very sick in different ways and for different reasons.'

Lauritsen's journalistic style is unfettered by the conventions of professional detachment. His writings reveal a cool and clear intelligence, however, and I suspect that, ultimately, history will judge his work to have been more valuable than the many skilfully crafted 'objective' reports on HIV and Aids that have appeared in the mainstream media, misleading – as I now believe – readers world-wide.

Unlike Callen and Sonnabend, who took the politically extremely incorrect line that multiple infections arising from gay promiscuity were probably the most important and certainly a much neglected factor in Aids, Lauritsen has targeted the abuse of 'recreational' drugs. There is an overlap, because drugs have been an engine driving gay sex into previously uncharted territory. The *Native's* publisher, Charles Ortleb, who balked at following through the Callen and Berkowitz 'We Know Who We Are' confessions on promiscuity, has given Lauritsen some fine opportunities to air his views, while not necessarily agreeing with them. In years to come, when gay men look back in wonder at the many mistakes surrounding the handling of the Aids epidemic, *Native* readers will have no grounds for saying no one told them there were problems with the conventional approach.

Lauritsen's first shock, and the subject of his first major piece of Aids writing, was the way US government statistics on the syndrome were presented. The assumption that it was an infectious disease spreading primarily among gay or bisexual men was built into the tables from the start. In listing Aids cases by patient characteristics, the Centers for Disease Control under-represented by more than half the role of intravenous drug use. The CDC's 'Patient Characteristics' table of 31 December 1984, for example, listed 73 per cent as gay/bisexual men, and 17 per cent as IV drug abusers. But the latter should really have read *heterosexual* IV drug abusers. Subsequent information suggested that about 25 per cent of the gay men with Aids at that time were also IV drug users — that is, a further 19 per cent of the total Aids cases. Leaving aside sexual orientation, up to a third of total Aids cases through to 28 January 1985 were in IV drug users.

In an article published in the *Philadelphia Gay News* of 14 February 1985 and reprinted in five other papers, Lauritsen wrote about this underplayed drug-Aids connection. 'Why should gay sex make an IV drug abuser cease to be an IV drug abuser?' he asked. He also pointed out that studies on gay men with Aids indicated that most were regular and heavy users of drugs of all kinds, not just those injected intravenously. But the CDC had chosen not to reflect this, either, in its reports. 'Even someone who has taken large quantities of half a dozen different "recreational drugs" every day for years does not qualify as a "drug abuser" in the CDC's epidemiology,' Lauritsen pointed out. That was because, from the beginning, the hypothesis had been that the only way drugs caused Aids was when needles were shared, thereby transmitting an Aids-causing microbe from one person to another. The way the CDC was collecting and presenting its epidemiological evidence was already artificially excluding hypotheses of Aids causation in which drug abuse played a central role.

The CDC had plenty of evidence of the drug-Aids connection. One of its own researchers, Harry Haverkos, conducted a study between September 1981 and October 1982 among eighty-seven homosexual men with Aids. The researchers found that 97 per cent had used nitrite inhalants or 'poppers' (amyl nitrite, butyl nitrite, isobutyl nitrite), drugs that increase the flow of blood by relaxing blood vessel walls. Other drug use levels reported in the study were: 93 per cent marijuana, 68 per cent amphetamines, 66 per cent cocaine, 65 per cent LSD, 59 per cent quaaludes, 48 per cent ethyl chloride, 32 per cent barbiturates, and 12 per cent heroin. Multiple drug use was the rule: 58 per cent of the Aids sufferers used five or more different 'street drugs'. The CDC neither published the study nor cleared it for publication elsewhere, though Haverkos released copies privately.

Every week, the CDC was issuing a table of Aids cases listed according to what was called 'hierarchical presentation', in which the patient characteristics considered predominant in the epidemic were listed first. After that, a patient was included in a subsequent risk group only if he had not already been counted. Since gay/bisexual men were considered the largest category and put at the top of the hierarchy, this was why those who were both gay and IV drug users did not appear in the IV drug abuser category.

Lauritsen pointed out that the effect of this approach was to construe Aids as a venereal disease, rather than a drug-induced condition. To show the distortion produced by this kind of presentation, Lauritsen presented his own table based on the assumption that the CDC had kept records on all drug abusers, intravenous or otherwise, and listed them first instead. In that case, the statistics (Aids cases by patient characteristics to 31 December 1984) read as follows:

	Number of cases	**Per cent of total**
Drug abusers (IV and Non-IV)	7,234	95
Haitians	152	2
Haemophiliacs	76	1
Gay/Bisexual men	75	1
Other	73	1
Total	7,610	

Lauritsen drove home his point: the table was strictly guesswork. No one – including the CDC – had sufficient data to set up a 'hierarchical' table of this kind. 'But before you dismiss this imaginary table based on drug abuse as the primary "patient characteristic", note how dramatically it misrepresents the number of gay/bisexual males with Aids. This element of distortion, inherent in any type of "hierarchical presentation", totally disqualifies the CDC reports as an accurate analysis of the epidemiology of Aids.'

If reliable data on 'drug abusers (IV and non-IV)' did exist, researchers might tend to formulate hypotheses in which drug abuse played a central role in the aetiology of Aids. Lauritsen put forward three such hypotheses:

1. Drugs as primary factor:

Drugs destroy the body's immune system, just as alcohol damages the liver, cigarettes promote lung cancer, and thalidomide causes birth defects.

2. Drug interactions:

Particular combinations of drugs may be injurious to the immune system. By way of analogy, an addict who had built up a tolerance for heroin would find it almost impossible to kill himself with an overdose. Most deaths attributed to 'drug overdose' actually resulted from a combination of two or more different types of drug.

3. Drugs plus bugs:

Microbes which might be harmless in a healthy body become deadly in conjunction with drugs. This hypothesis had been put forward three years previously in a *New England Journal of Medicine* editorial:[2]

Some new factor may have distorted the host-parasite relation. So-called 'recreational' drugs are one possibility. They are widely used in the large cities where most of these cases have occurred, and the only patients in the series reported in this issue who were not homosexual were drug users... Perhaps one or more of these recreational drugs is an immunosuppressive agent. The leading candidates are the nitrites, which are now commonly inhaled to intensify orgasm... Let us postulate that the combined effects of persistent viral infection plus an adjuvant drug cause immunosuppression in some genetically predisposed men.

Lauritsen noted that HTLV-3, the virus isolated (as LAV) by French scientists in 1983 and 'rediscovered' by an American government scientist the following year, was now being 'touted' as the 'Aids virus'. Perhaps it *was* responsible for Aids, but that remained to be proven. It might just be another opportunistic infection. Even if it were the primary factor, mere exposure to it clearly did not suffice to cause Aids.* A necessary precondition might be an already weakened immune system, 'a condition which is a usual and expected consequence of drug abuse'. Much more information was needed, but the evidence strongly implicated drugs in the aetiology of Aids, at the very least as a major co-factor.

The Effects of Poppers

The following year, Lauritsen and Hank Wilson, a long-time gay activist in San Francisco, co-authored a sixty-four-page booklet called *Death Rush: Poppers & Aids,* in which they pulled together scientific evidence of the specific hazards associated with poppers use. In 1981, Wilson had noticed that many of his nitrite-using friends were developing swollen lymph nodes. After reading medical literature on the inhalants, he founded the Committee to Monitor the Cumulative Effects of Poppers, with which Lauritsen began to collaborate in 1983.

From 1981 onwards, Wilson began sending out packets of medical information on poppers to the gay press. For the most part they were ignored. An exception was the *Native,* which in December that year ran an article by Lawrence Mass entitled 'Do Poppers Cause Cancer?' In 1984, Charles Ortleb, the *Native's* publisher, wrote an article 'Poppers May Be Co-factor in Development of KS in Aids Cases', with an editorial in which he called on club owners to discourage the use of poppers on dance floors. (This prompted an attack by the 'health critic' of the *Advocate,* another leading gay publication, who later died of Aids.)

Poppers are usually sold nowadays in small bottles, but they got their name because they were originally made in glass ampoules, enclosed in mesh, as a self-administered emergency treatment for people with heart pain: they

* In the light of the work on cell-mediated immunity to HIV, described in Chapter 3, this statement is even more certain than Lauritsen could have realised a decade ago.

could be 'popped' under the nose and the volatile contents, amyl nitrite, instantly inhaled. The manufacturer in the United States was Burroughs-Wellcome, American arm of the British drug company Wellcome. Amyl nitrite was a controlled drug until 1960, when the prescription requirement was removed by the Food and Drug Administration, and during the 1960s the use of poppers as a sex aid grew among gay men, primarily those involved in sadomasochism. As well as giving the user a rapid 'high', felt as a strong rush of energy that reduced sexual and social inhibitions and intensified and prolonged orgasm, the drug facilitated anal intercourse by relaxing the anal sphincter and deadening the sense of pain in the rectum.

The prescription requirement was reinstated by the FDA in 1969, but from about 1970 onwards commercial brands of butyl and isobutyl nitrite became widely available and, soon, immensely popular in gay sex. A poppers craze was in full swing by 1974, and by 1977 they were in every comer of gay life, marketed under names such as Rush, Ram, Rock Hard, Climax, Thunderbolt, Locker Room and Crypt Tonight. 'At gay discotheques men could be seen shuffling around in a daze, holding popper bottles under the nose,' Lauritsen was to recall in a 1989 *Native* article. 'At gay gathering places – bars, baths, leather clubs – the miasma of volatile nitrites was taken for granted. Some gay men became so addicted to poppers that they were never without their little bottle, from which they snorted nitrite fumes around the clock. For gay men who came out in the 70s, poppers appeared to be as much a part of the gay clone lifestyle as moustaches or flannel shirts. The brilliant red and yellow label of one brand, Rush, was so distinctive that a successful gay political candidate in San Francisco used the colour scheme on his campaign posters.'

Later, again in the *Native,* he wrote that a series of stunning poppers ads that the industry created from the early 1970s through to the late 1980s 'must rank among the most brilliant advertising campaigns in history. Within only a few years, hundreds of thousands of men were persuaded that poppers were an integral part of their own "gender identity". The ads conveyed the message that nothing could be butcher or sexier than to inhale noxious chemical fumes. Bulging muscles were linked to a drug that is indisputably hazardous to the health.' One ad for a brand named 'Discorama' targeted disco dancers. Another, for the poppers brand Rush, focused on the phrase, 'Better Living Through Chemistry'.

The industry became rich and powerful. In 1978, in just one city, an estimated total of $50m a year was being made from sales of more than 100,000 bottles a week. That same year, the *American Journal of Psychiatry* warned that new research 'raises the issue of whether repeated use of these products could increase the risk of developing cancer'. By 1980, sales had reached hundreds of millions of dollars and the National Institute on Drug Abuse reported that more than 5 million people were using poppers more than once a week. Gay men made up virtually the entire market, and many gay organisations depended on a slice of the industry's profits for their existence. Gay publishers carried large ads for the products.

Nitrites do not seem to cause physical dependence, but two separate studies in the 1970s found that some gay men could no longer perform sexually without them. According to *Death Rush,* with regular use they become a sexual crutch, 'and many gay men are incapable of having sex, even solitary masturbation, without the aid of poppers'.

Poppers had become an accepted, even obligatory part of the gay male lifestyle in some cities, but because of that the subject of their use and the dangers associated with them aroused intense emotions. 'Ordinarily rational men become hysterical when it is suggested that the nitrite inhalants are harmful to health and may play a role in causing Aids,' Lauritsen wrote in *Death Rush.* 'This is understandable. Since poppers have become necessary for them to function sexually, giving up poppers would seem, at least in the beginning, like giving up sex itself.'

Less easy to understand was the immunity from controls accorded to the manufacture and sale of poppers. Normally, every drug in the US had to undergo extensive testing before it could be sold legally, but poppers were subject to no testing or quality control whatsoever. Manufacturers had labelled their product a 'room odorizer', and astoundingly, the federal FDA, the California and New York Departments of Health, and other government regulatory agencies had looked the other way. 'If a drug like butyl nitrite can be marketed as a "room odorizer", then anything could be sold as anything,' Lauritsen wrote. 'Heroin could be sold as a mosquito-bite remedy ("for external use only"). Live hand grenades could be sold as "paperweights".'

The problem was made worse by the fact that for several years, government agencies discouraged any approaches to Aids other than the single-infectious-agent hypothesis. 'Researchers who advanced drug abuse or multifactorial hypotheses tended to be ostracised or unfunded. After Robert Gallo's "discovery" of HTLV-3, it became obligatory to regard this as the primary or even sole cause of the syndrome.'

The result of these pressures was that few gay men, physicians or Aids researchers were aware of how extensive and powerful the evidence against poppers was. 'Anyone who has studied even a portion of the medical literature can only shake his head in amazement that this dubious commodity has not been banned,' the booklet said. The only exceptions were Massachusetts, Wisconsin, and, as of June 1985, New York State. In Massachusetts, where poppers had been banned for years, only 378 cases of Aids had been reported as of 31 March 1986. In contrast, there had been 6,265 cases in New York, where poppers had been sold legally in sex shops, baths, discos and even neighbourhood tobacconists.

Death Rush then gave forty-eight pages of abstracts from medical and scientific findings on poppers, summarising hundreds of pages of reports and articles. The drugs had been demonstrated to be mutagenic – causing genes to mutate – and, along with other substances with which they readily combined, carcinogenic. They were directly toxic to blood cells, causing striking deformities as well as decreases in immunological function. Mice exposed to nitrite vapours suffered gross lung damage, weight loss and immunosuppression, with altered T-cell ratios exactly as in Aids. In one study where they were exposed chronically to low dosages of isobutyl nitrite vapours, they developed methemoglobinaemia (a form of anaemia where the blood turns brown and the oxygen supply to critical organs is reduced) and atrophy of the thymus gland, which plays a vital part in programming immune system cells. Destruction of the thymus is a common autopsy finding in Aids patients, and anaemia is typically part of the syndrome.

The study findings included:

- Mice exposed to isobutyl nitrite in a closed environment, 'simulating the practice of the homosexual patient', showed dose-related immune system damage, with decreased lymphocytes and macrophages. They became highly susceptible to disease and death caused by mycobacterial disease, one of the leading killers in Aids.[3] The researchers, at the National Jewish Center for Immunology and

Respiratory Medicine, Denver, concluded: 'We believe our findings establish that inhaling isobutyl nitrite should be considered dangerous to homosexuals and others at high risk for developing Aids.'

- Minute quantities of isobutyl nitrite caused irreversible damage to human immune system cells in laboratory experiments.[4] The researchers concluded: 'These in vitro studies strongly suggest that the inhalant nitrites may indeed be dangerous, and their use should be condemned by those physicians who treat patients who use these drugs regularly.'

- Production and activity of natural killer (NK) cells was suppressed in mice exposed to isobutyl nitrite.[5] The authors of this study suggested that since these cells help protect against tumours as well as various types of infection, poppers use 'could underlie the susceptibility of homosexual men to opportunistic infection and Kaposi's sarcoma'.

- Multivariate analysis of risks among twenty homosexual men with KS, and forty healthy controls, indicated that use of amyl nitrite was an independent and statistically significant risk factor for KS. In the light of their data, the authors considered a tenable hypothesis to be that the drug may have caused KS either by causing immunosuppression, thereby allowing a sexually transmitted cancer-causing virus or other carcinogenic agent to operate, or by acting directly as a carcinogen itself.[6]

- Previous heavy nitrite inhalant use proved the most important factor distinguishing eight patients who developed Aids from thirty-four who did not when forty-two homosexual or bisexual men with persistent swollen lymph glands were followed for thirty months.[7] The link was still statistically significant after adjustment for numbers of sexual contacts, but the same was not true the other way round: in other words, on the basis of this study, nitrite use was implicated more strongly as a factor in causing Aids than promiscuity. A follow-up on this study at four and a half years, when twelve of the men had developed Aids, implicated a previous history of moderate to heavy nitrite use in causing the syndrome, and in particular, Kaposi's sarcoma.

- Inhalation of amyl nitrite for two minutes, five days a week, caused progressive immunosuppression in mice. The trend started after as little as five days' exposure. The authors concluded: 'These data suggest that nitrites may have a primary or contributory role in Aids.'[8]

- Nitrites proved a highly significant risk when lifestyle factors of thirty-one homosexual men with Aids were compared with those of twenty-nine symptom-free homosexual men, only exceeded by frequenting bathhouses. The heavier the nitrite use, the greater the risk of developing Aids. The authors commented that the compounds were among the most highly potent chemical carcinogens for animals; of thirty-nine species tested, none was known to be resistant.[9]

- Mice exposed to amyl nitrite (AN) five days a week for twenty-one weeks showed profound lung damage, and suffered severe loss of helper T-cells, with altered T-helper/suppressor ratio, as occurs in Aids victims. 'It does look, then, that there seems to be a link between AN inhalation and cellular immunity depression.'[10]

- A 1982 editorial from the *Yale Journal of Biology and Medicine*[11] put a strong emphasis on the drug hypothesis, making the point that all the non-homosexual Aids cases identified at that time were drug abusers. The article stressed the likelihood that nitrites were a causative factor, perhaps with an infectious agent. It also referred to studies demonstrating evidence for opiate receptors on lymphocytes, and depression of T-cell numbers and function in opiate addicts.

- Groups of mice exposed to a single capsule of amyl nitrite (Vaporole, 0.3 ml capsule, Burroughs Wellcome) in an eighteen-litre sealed container for four minutes, twice daily, for five consecutive days showed normal antibody responses (to sheep red blood cells) but reductions of 30-45 per cent in cell-mediated immunity.[12]

Dr Sue Watson, co-author of this last study, sent a letter about it to the *Advocate,* the world's largest gay newspaper. She wrote: 'Our studies show that amyl nitrite strongly suppresses the segment of the immune system (cellular immunity) which normally protects individuals against Kaposi's sarcoma, Pneumocystis pneumonia, herpes virus, Candida, amebiasis, and a variety of other opportunistic infections. The upshot of this research is that persons using nitrite inhalants may be at risk for the development of Aids.' The *Advocate* did not see fit to publish the letter, despite carrying pages of articles on Aids at the time. According to Watson, a call to the editor produced the response: 'We're not interested.'

'Garbage In, Garbage Out'

Several key CDC investigators were rooting for the 'lethal new virus' theory from as early as mid-1981, a predisposition that may have helped give rise to some poorly designed studies that appeared to rule out other factors. These studies, however, then became quoted around the world, by commercial interests and others, in support of the 'authorised' version of Aids causation.

A national study of the first fifty gay men with Aids, for example, published in August 1983,[13] was interpreted as finding evidence against the poppers theory, since use of the drug was reported not only by almost all the Aids victims, but by almost all of a group of gay men, used as a control sample, who did *not* have Aids. These 'controls', however, were not representative of healthy gay men. They were selected from venereal disease clinics, and from private practices of doctors specialising in VD. They had various risk factors. Some had immunological abnormalities and swollen lymph glands, and several developed Aids after the study was completed. 'About a third had been "fist-fucked",' Lauritsen says. 'The people in the CDC may be very naive, but in fact it is only a tiny fraction of gay men who have ever been fist-fucked. It's a grotesque and dangerous practice and most gay men would reject the very idea of it. These so-called controls were also heavy, heavy users of recreational drugs. In fact, the majority of gay men across the US are not heavy users of drugs. So this sample was not representative. It could not have been typical in terms of the inferences they drew from the study.'

The researchers had admitted that the study design was biased towards obscuring real risk factors, rather than falsely identifying risk factors that were not real. They stated: 'The expected impact of these potential problems in control selection and classification would be to minimise differences between cases and controls rather than to create false differences.' In the light of such fatal flaws, Lauritsen said, all analyses based on comparison between the Aids patients and the controls would be dismissed by most survey research professionals as 'garbage in, garbage out'. The comparative data were worthless, and should be ignored. The authors of the study did draw comparative conclusions, however, and they were wrong to do so.

For several years, the Committee to Monitor Poppers sent copies of research findings to the CDC and other public health agencies, and on 21 April 1985 Hank Wilson wrote asking Curran, now head of Aids at the Center for Infectious Diseases, for help in alerting gay men to the dangers. He wanted a statement to be issued condemning the use of the inhalants, which, he said, 'continue to be marketed and promoted to the gay male community as if they had no harmful health effects, nor any role in the development of Aids'.

Curran responded evasively. His letter was characterised by phrases such as 'deserving of further attention' and 'warrant further investigation'. He acknowledged that 'it is possible that heavy use of nitrites, or another factor correlated with such use, may contribute in some as yet undefined way to the development of Kaposi's sarcoma in those already infected with HTLV-3 or who have Aids'. He felt the data did not justify 'an absolute "anti-popper" campaign', but said that 'gay men should consider decreasing use of this substance until more data are available to assess those risks that may exist'.

Wilson and Lauritsen deplored this response. They felt there was already ample evidence for banning poppers. 'Gay men should not "consider" anything at this point,' they wrote. 'They should act. And they should *stop* using poppers, not just *decrease* the use of them... Everyone who has studied the issue knows that poppers are dangerous, and almost certainly implicated in the aetiology of Aids. And yet the popper profits continue to roll in, and gay men continue to die. As long as public officials refuse to do their duty, it is up to each of us individually to spread the word about the dangers of using poppers.'

In an appendix to *Death Rush,* Lauritsen pondered on the 'adversary stance' that US government officials had taken against the possibility that toxic agents played a role in causing Aids. 'They have, for example, laid down the line that IV-drug users develop Aids not from the drugs they use, but from allegedly "shared needles", an unproved assumption.' In fact, such epidemiological information as there was seemed more consistent with a toxicological process than with the prevailing microbial model. That included the fact that for five years Aids, unlike a truly communicable disease, had remained compartmentalised. More than nine out of ten Aids cases were either intravenous drug users or homosexual/bisexual men. 'For reasons unknown, the US Public Health Service adheres with military rigidity to the line that Aids *must* be explained in terms of the "Aids virus", and that research efforts must be based solely on this premise. Risk-reduction measures are to be predicated solely on preventing transmission of the putative virus.' That insistence had stifled independent research and thinking, and dangerously missed people as to the risk factors for Aids.

'Intravenous drug users have not been told to quit using drugs, only that they must stop "sharing needles". (Actually, there is no evidence that all, or even most, of the IV-drug users with Aids did "share needles".) Gay men have been told that they must restrict their sexual activities, but not that they ought to stop using cocaine, heroin, quaaludes, amphetamines, ethyl chloride, PCP, marijuana, LSD, barbiturates, poppers, and the other "recreational drugs" (a sick euphemism) that are prominent in the lifestyle of many gay men.'

Why *was* there such readiness to dismiss the nitrite inhalants as central to understanding the epidemic of Kaposi's sarcoma and opportunistic infections in gay men, when it was clear they had immunosuppressive and carcinogenic actions, and when an epidemic of their use among gay men had preceded the arrival of Aids? Even if, one day, a single microbe were proved to be the primary cause of Aids, common sense would dictate that vulnerability to such a germ would be greatly amplified by the widespread phenomenon of chronic and heavy use of nitrite inhalants in gay men. Poppers abuse was an outstanding and novel factor in the lives of the biggest group at risk for Aids. The fact that the new technology of T-cell counting could also demonstrate immune deficiency syndromes in people who abused different drugs – or in babies whose immune systems developed while they were being carried in the womb of such drug abusers – was not an argument for dropping poppers from the picture.

Was there a reluctance to take on the poppers industry? Commercial pressures were certainly present. By default, the industry had become very big and powerful, as regulatory authorities colluded with the absurd fiction that the drugs were being sold as some kind of room fragrance rather than for their pharmacological effects.

On 1 April 1983 a press release was issued by Joseph F. Miller, president of Great Lakes Products, Inc., 'the nation's largest manufacturer of nitrite-based odorants'. It was entitled 'US Government Studies Now Indicate that Nitrite-Odorants Not Related to Aids!' According to Miller, 'the assistant director of the Center for Infectious Diseases (a part of the Centers for Disease Control in Atlanta), Dr James Curran, invited him to Atlanta in late November of last year to discuss the work being done by CDC relative to its Aids investigations'. Miller claimed he had been assured that 'no association exists between nitrite-based odorants and Aids', and that although his company did not advocate the misuse of the 'odorants' as inhalants, it was 'greatly relieved to know that recent Government studies clearly show that such misuse poses no health hazard'.

Miller wrote to the *Advocate* urging them to publicise the press release, adding: 'As the largest advertiser in the Gay press we intend to use the extensive ad space we purchase each month as the vehicle for sending a message of good health and wellness through nutrition and exercise to the North American Gay communities.' The full-page advertisements that followed, promoting 'the world's most refined nitrite-based odorants', were called 'Blueprint for Health'. One of them asked: 'Where are the troublemakers of the gay community that brought Aids into Fantasyland – the wonderful land of drugs, parties and sex? Will this land of enchantment have to be closed for good, or can a few attractions be saved to enjoy on special occasions?' The answer, of course, was that a few health changes (which did not include any mention of nitrite abuse) 'will help keep the gates of Fantasyland open for all to appreciate and enjoy'.

Six months later, on 27 September 1983, Curran complained in a letter to Miller that the press release and advertisements misrepresented the CDC findings. He said that while it was unlikely that nitrites would be implicated as the primary cause of Aids, 'their role as a co-factor in some of the illnesses found in this syndrome has not been ruled out'.

Earlier that same month, however, the CDC had again played directly and damagingly into the hands of the poppers industry with a brief news item in the *Morbidity and Mortality Weekly Report* describing an experiment involving mice and poppers. The mice were exposed to nitrite vapours for time periods ranging from three to eighteen weeks. According to the report, none showed any evidence of a toxic effect on their immune system. On the basis of this study, a 1983 pamphlet published by the CDC, *Gay and Bisexual Men Should Know About Aids,* claimed that there was no relationship between Aids and poppers.

When the study report was published in full – two years later – it became clear that the news item had been grossly misleading. The dosages administered had been very low, 'selected to mimic an occupational exposure setting', a tiny fraction of the doses to which nitrite abusers were exposed when inhaling directly from the bottle (though even at that low level, some of the mice developed thymic atrophy and mild lung damage). One reason why they were so low, as one of the researchers was later to reveal, was that the doses had to be adjusted below the level at which they were 'losing' the mice. The supplier of the animals had subsequently disclosed that they were suffering from a low-grade infection that made them an especially vulnerable batch. But as Lauritsen has pointed out, this means that deaths at the higher doses may well have been due to immunotoxicity – exactly what the study conclusions claimed not to find – rather than the immediate toxic effects of the nitrite fumes. Whatever the explanation, the end result was that the dose was far too low to be meaningful.

By the time the full report appeared, several other studies, using more realistic dosages, had already shown clear evidence of immunotoxicity, and at the end of their published paper the government researchers made a specific disclaimer, that 'this study did not attempt to model the recreational use of these drugs'.[14] But it was too late; the world had wanted a deadly new virus, and it now had one, and for the time being no one wanted to listen any more to alternative theories of Aids causation.

Money *does* make the world go round, and once the megabucks started to flow for HIV research, the virus theory was to prove unstoppable. At the start, however, CDC researchers appear to have attempted to make an honest assessment of what was happening. They put in some hard footwork, interviewing patients, visiting seedy gay bars, sampling bottles of nitrites to check for 'bad lots'. Commercial pressures were almost certainly irrelevant to their assessment, except in so far as the poppers industry was indeed already a force to be reckoned with. So how could they fail to see the evidence that stared Lauritsen and Wilson in the face? Lauritsen rails against their incompetence, but perhaps it goes deeper than that.

'The Sex Got to be Unstoppable'

A deadly new virus was neutral. It avoided those 'twin horns' Randy Shilts had written about as underlying the handling of the epidemic, 'don't offend the gays and don't inflame the homophobes'. It meant neither having to face the ugly homophobia that runs through our excessively machismo western societies, nor the hollow, depersonalised sexual behaviour to which that homophobia had helped give rise. After finding that immune deficiency was also occurring in transfusion recipients, and in 'heavy' drug users such as heroin and cocaine addicts, leading researchers readily came to the unwarranted conclusion that there must be a single cause for this ill-health. 'Somebody who gets a rush from heroin isn't going to toy around with something as lightweight as disco inhalants,' they thought.[15] That was the context in which poppers came to be dismissed as largely an irrelevance.* Then, after a period when neither press nor politicians were showing any interest in a 'gay plague', the politicians started turning up the pressure for a quick fix. Government researchers obliged and HIV took birth as the sole cause of Aids.

There is a late twentieth-century 'scientific' turn of mind, nearuniversal, that shies away from human complexity, particularly anything to do with 'lifestyle' or 'behaviour' or 'morality', and instead looks for single – and simple – external causes and solutions to complex human problems – the

* An exception was Dr Harry Haverkos, who led a 1982 study which concluded that 'using nitrite inhalants may be associated with the occurrence of Kaposi's sarcoma in patients with Aids', and who has persisted ever since in trying to draw attention to the links between KS and Aids.

'pill for every ill' syndrome that has led medicine down many dangerous and damaging paths. It is not truly scientific at all, of course, but it can sometimes give a comforting appearance of being so.

Shilts tells how in mid-1992 Don Francis, the brilliant epidemiologist who was the CDC's leading exponent of the theory that a new sexually transmitted virus was causing the immune deficiencies seen in gay men, asked to see an Aids victim during a visit to the Sloan-Kettering cancer centre.[16] He had gone there with Jim Curran to try to get the hospital's retrovirus laboratory into action on the problem, but felt embarrassed that he had been working on the disease for nearly a year and still had not met a patient. The doctors led him to Brandy Alexander, a thirty-eight-year-old former female impersonator whose flesh was now spotted with purple Kaposi's lesions, and whose once-handsome face was covered with scabs and sores wrought by an uncontrolled herpes virus. He also had an array of the usual opportunistic infections, including severe hepatitis and tuberculosis of the bone marrow.

> Alone, in the room, Brandy talked honestly with Francis about his life. Brandy could tell Francis wasn't particularly shocked at anything he heard.
>
> 'The sex got to be unstoppable,' he said, his eyes wandering around their hollow, gaunt sockets, trying to see the answer. 'I don't know whether it was to be close to another person because I didn't want to be alone. I don't know if I just got bored with normal sex, so I'd try something new. Something more exciting. Fisting. Another rung.'
>
> The monologue was taking Brandy to a conclusion that irked the scientific side of Don Francis's mind. Brandy was trying to find a reason he was lying in pain in that bed in Room 428A about to die. The old moral teachings, Francis thought, die hard.
>
> 'I think this is a communicable disease and you got it,' said Francis, matter-of-factly. 'You're not being punished. A virus made you sick.'

Don Francis used to dream of reaching out for a faint orange light that was suspended in front of him, tantalisingly close, but which drifted farther and farther out of reach. It was The Answer, always there before him, but still beyond his grasp. It wouldn't have occurred to Shilts, who was deeply wedded to the HIV theory, but perhaps, deep in Francis's soul, the orange light represented Brandy. Although the scientist's intellect told him there was no connection between 'unstoppable sex' and this disease, at a deeper level his heart may have known Brandy was right.

In spite of the CDC's premature rejection of nitrites as a prime factor in homosexual Aids, and the poppers industry's forceful marketing tactics, warnings about the dangers of the drugs began to appear in sections of both the gay and the mainstream press during the 1980s. The US Congress, as part of the Anti-Drug Abuse Act of 1986, asked the National Institute on Drug Abuse (NIDA) for up-to-date information on the inhalants, and on 31 March 1987 NIDA sponsored a one-day technical review meeting designed to address questions of usage and health hazards.

The event's main organiser was Harry Haverkos, the former CDC staffer, now chief of the clinical medicine branch at the National Institute on Drug Abuse. In his own presentation, he focused on the suspicion that nitrites could be playing an important part in causing Kaposi's sarcoma. Several epidemiological studies had pointed to a cause-and-effect link. Although other studies had cast doubt on this, their methods had differed and unsuspected bias might have influenced the results.

By this time, it had certainly become clear that among Aids patients, KS was almost exclusively confined to gay men. There was no evidence of a causal agent being either sexually transmitted, or blood-borne. The disease had not been reported in the female partners of bisexual men with KS, nor was there any consistent pattern of KS transmission among clusters of homosexual men linked by sexual contact. Blood donors who had developed KS had apparently transmitted HIV infection to recipients, but those recipients had not developed KS. One study had shown a strong association between risk of KS and increased income, a further pointer to the argument that a drug could be implicated. Common sites for KS in Aids were the chest, mouth and head, including the tip of the nose, all suggestive of nitrite fumes as a cause.

Haverkos called for a multi-agency task force to be set up by the US Public Health Service to resolve the issue, and for more research into the effects of nitrite inhalation in humans, both on their own and in combination with other drugs.

A historical review by Drs Guy Newell and Margaret Spitz of the department of cancer prevention and control, University of Texas, Houston, showed that the production and sales of poppers as 'recreational' drugs first became widespread between 1970 and 1974, preceding the arrival of the Aids epidemic by about seven to ten years, which was consistent with a carcinogenic effect. (Retrospectively, several cases of Aids-type KS, in which the opportunistic infections were also present, had been diagnosed as having occurred in the late 1970s.) Furthermore, the age group in which KS was mainly being seen was consistent with the victims having been first exposed to regular use of the drugs seven to ten years previously. Almost 100 per cent of people with KS had a history of poppers use, and in most cases heavy use was reported. The handful of cases in whom use of the inhalants had not been reported might have been sensitive to passive exposure in the discos or bathhouses, and besides, in any epidemic it was not unusual for some patients not to give a clear history of exposure. The researchers stated: 'We conclude that nitrite use may contribute to the development of Aids-related KS among male homosexuals. Immunosuppression may allow expression of human immunodeficiency virus that was previously suppressed. The interaction of nitrites with other identified risk factors is yet to be elucidated.'

Armed with the report of this review meeting, Congress outlawed poppers in measures passed in 1988 and 1990, citing an 'Aids link'. Their use had in any case declined during the 1980s, as recognition of the hazards began to penetrate the gay community. It has not stopped, however. In 1992 a stand at a gay street fair in Chicago offered iced tea for $1 and poppers for $5. The same year, the manufacturer of Rush poppers sent out a mail order advertisement to 'preferred customers'. The drugs are now being sold as video head cleaner, polish remover, carburettor cleaner and leather stripper ('Not an overpriced "headache in a bottle" like those other brands,' says the advertising copy in a gay magazine), and are on sale openly in Soho, London and other parts of the UK today. According to Hank Wilson, use of poppers is currently increasing again in the big cities across America. Institutional memory in the gay community is short, he told *Spin* magazine in a 1994 interview, and there is concern that young men who have come to the big city in the 1990s will think of poppers as 'the new toy', knowing little of the battles that have been fought for so long.

In May 1994, NIDA held another technical review meeting on the inhalants, once again organised by the patient and persistent Harry Haverkos. And once again, the toxicologists, Aids researchers and others present reached a consensus urging research into the connection between poppers and KS. Fresh evidence included further studies showing immune suppression from nitrite exposure in animals and men; a study showing that nitrite vapour is even more powerfully mutagenic than had previously been thought (in the case of iso-butyl nitrite, the vapour had been shown to be eleven times as mutagenic as when the chemical was in solution); and a demonstration that a decline in nitrite inhalant abuse among gay men from about 1982 to 1988 had been paralleled by a subsequent decline in the proportion of KS cases in homosexual Aids. The meeting also heard that dozens of cases of HIV-negative gay men with KS (sixteen in the practice of one physician alone) have been reported.

The meeting had implications that went beyond the issue of nitrites, as Lauritsen made clear in a brilliant, detailed report in the *Native*.[17] The National Cancer Institute's Robert Gallo was there, as 'unofficial voice of the Aids establishment', and he had disclosed important revisions in the Aids paradigm. 'It is now necessary to consider co-factors,' Lauritsen wrote. 'No longer is HIV believed to cause KS by itself; at most it may aggravate KS after it has been caused by something else.' The meeting indicated a willingness on the part of the Public Health Service to rethink the basic premise of the Aids model that had prevailed since 1984. 'It is high time,' Lauritsen added, 'for the HIV-Aids hypothesis has been a total failure, both in terms of public health benefits and in terms of making accurate predictions.'

Gallo had begun by saying that he had no fixed opinion regarding cofactors for KS, whether chemical, viral, or a combination. He still believed HIV in KS was an 'enormous catalytic factor', but 'there must be something else involved'. He torpedoed the oft-quoted objection to the poppers-KS link – that Africans and others who develop KS are unlikely to have been abusing nitrites – by continuing:

> Do you believe that all Kaposi's is one and the same disease? I don't. Why should we say they are, any more than all leukaemias are the same? Leukaemias don't all have the same pathogenesis. So why should we say a benign disease of old men in East Europe of Mediterranean or Jewish stock is the same disease as a sudden disease in younger people that is far more aggressive? And do we believe that the iatrogenic renal transplant Kaposi's

> associated with therapies and immune suppression is the same disease? I'd at least leave open the possibility that these are quite distinct, even pathogenetically. I know there's a great desire to link the African with the modern or epidemic form of KS, and I can understand that, because they're both aggressive. But they may not be. Therefore, what one tells you may not be good for the other...And when you go to the iatrogenic renal transplant KS, you have to argue that it's a ubiquitous transmitted agent, because all of the people that have it in their kidneys weren't involved in rimming.

Gallo then presented a summary of findings from his laboratory regarding KS.

> The first thing I can tell you is that we've been able to regularly culture from Kaposi's tumours what pathologists say is a tumour cell. We asked: What is the role of HIV in all of this? And we found that inflammatory cytokines [messenger chemicals central to communication between immune system cells] ... were the very likely initiatory events in creating this cell. We said, 'Oh, the role of HIV is likely to be in increasing these inflammatory cytokines.' But we have learned – this should be of interest to everybody that isn't completely married to HIV – that the inflammatory cytokines are reportedly increased in gay men even without HIV infection. Inflammatory cytokines are usually promoted by immune activation, not by immune suppression. So here was a paradox...So the inflammatory cytokines may be increased by HIV, but I wish I knew what else was increasing them before a gay man was ever infected with HIV. Maybe it's nitric oxide [formed during the metabolism of the nitrite inhalants], maybe it's a sexually transmitted virus, maybe it's all of them, maybe it has to do with rimming because it's immune stimulation with non-specific infections...I don't want to get into the semantics. I believe that HIV *obviously* plays a role in this disease. I think the epidemiology is not debatable. But I think that there is more going on. I don't know what that 'more going on' is. For me it's whatever is accounting for the increase in inflammatory cytokines...The nitrites *could* be the primary factor. What if the nitrites had the ability, interacting with endothelial cells, to produce a tremendous amount of 'X', of inflammatory cytokines?

Gallo added:

> I don't know if I made this point clear, but I think that everybody here knows – we never found HIV DNA in the tumour cells of KS...So in other words we've never seen the role of HIV as a transforming virus in any way. The role of HIV has to be indirect.

In the light of Gallo's statements, Lauritsen wrote, 'it is hard not to think of the tens of thousands of gay men with KS who have died, and of the treatments they received. If HIV is not the cause of KS, then how appropriate were the nucleoside analogue drugs like AZT and ddI, whose theoretical basis is the HIV-Aids hypothesis? It may be hoped that this meeting is a signal of greater willingness on the part of the Aids establishment to reconsider the basic Aids paradigm. Kaposi's sarcoma as an Aids phenomenon remains a puzzle, and no hypothesis so far put forward seems fully adequate to explain it. It could be that KS comprises diverse conditions with diverse causes. Having said that, however, the nitrites-KS hypothesis is very much alive, more than a decade after its precipitous rejection by the CDC.'

Nitrites Link Still Unchecked

Writer Tom Bethell, who has recently become a powerful new voice questioning the HIV-Aids hypothesis, quoted Haverkos in a recent *Spin* article on the nitrite controversy as declaring: 'If somebody could find me five white women with Kaposi's who did not use nitrites, between the ages of eighteen and forty-five, sexually linked to a man with Kaposi's – just five couples – that would take me back. But we're thirteen years into this epidemic, and I have not seen such cases reported. If this was a sexually transmitted agent, there ought to be a handful of women like that.' (Twice as many whites as blacks use poppers, and twice as many get KS.)

About 5,000 new cases of Aids-related KS are reported each year in the US, but despite the billions of dollars that have been invested by American taxpayers in Aids research there is still no systematic way of checking the nitrites link, because the forms that doctors fill out lack questions about drug use other than those injected with needles. 'I almost had a question about nitrites put on the CDC surveillance form back in 1984,' Haverkos told Bethell, 'but they had to weed it, make it a little shorter, and that was one of the questions they took off.'

Evidence implicating poppers in Aids has continued to increase, and now includes studies showing that they destroy the capacity of lung cells to protect themselves against the deadly form of pneumonia which, along with KS, originally characterised Aids. But the domination of thinking by the HIV theory has prevented this vital information from reaching doctors, and consequently their patients. The way the 'hidden censor' works was exemplified by the fate of a 1991 study in which the effects of short-term nitrite inhalation were studied experimentally in eighteen healthy male volunteers, who lived as in-patients at NIDA's Addiction Research Centre. The men were given moderate, intermittent doses for up to eighteen days. One class of T-cells fell substantially in number and activity, even during the last two weeks of the study when the men received only two doses a week. There was a gradual increase back to normal levels after inhalation was stopped. There were also 'dramatic' and longer-lasting falls in natural killer cells, which help to protect against cancer, and the authors speculated that this might help to cause KS. The results, they said, while not addressing the possible cumulative effect of long-term inhalation, suggested that chronic exposure, even at relatively infrequent intervals, 'is sufficient to produce sustained alterations to the human immune system'.[18]

When Hank Wilson came across this study, it was listed in the *Index Medicus* under 'amyl nitrite'. There was no reference to it under 'Aids' or 'nitrites'. So on behalf of the Committee to Monitor Poppers he wrote to the National Library of Medicine, which forms part of the US government's National Institutes of Health complex near Washington, to urge that it should be cross-indexed. 'The article is an Aids study and is most relevant to HIV-positive people who continue to use nitrite inhalants or who believe nitrite inhalants to be harmless,' his letter said. 'Unless there is a cross-indexing under "Aids", Aids educators, counsellors and researchers are likely to miss this relevant study.'

The reply that came back demonstrated the compartmentalised thinking that has so bedevilled Aids research from the beginning of the epidemic.

Signed by the head of the index section, bibliographic services division, it affirmed that the article had been indexed correctly, since it was 'about the effects of inhaled *amyl nitrite* on lymphocytes…from human subjects who were, among other criteria, *seronegative* for HIV-1'. The letter added:

> The access points for any given article in *Index Medicus* consist of the central concepts of the article: in this case, the pharmacology of amyl nitrite and the effects of drugs on lymphocytes.
>
> The goal of indexing is to describe, in the most specific terms available, the concepts that are actually discussed in each article. In the article in question, amyl nitrite was the only substance that was administered; for this reason, we did not assign the less specific heading of 'nitrites'. Moreover, the article itself is not *about* acquired immunodeficiency syndrome, no matter how relevant it may be to individuals with an interest in Aids. The 'Aids' heading is reserved for articles that discuss this disease.

Wilson, whose boyfriend, a one-time heavy poppers user, had KS and was soon to die of Aids, did not let the matter rest. He alerted gay health activist contacts around the world to the study, and urged them to write asking the National Library of Medicine to list it in the computerised data source AidsLINE as well as cross-index it under Aids in *Index Medicus*. 'Educational efforts about the hazards of popper use must be increased to counter the promotional efforts of popper sellers,' he said.

He also wrote to Dr William Adler, chief of clinical immunology at the National Institute on Ageing, whose research group had organised the study and who was one of the paper's authors. Adler, whose laboratories also form part of the NIH Washington complex, took the issue up with the medical library. He pointed out that the study had been approved by the Office of Aids Research at NIH, and in fact was the only study supported by the NIH Aids budget 'investigating the effects of illicit drugs on the immune system as they may relate to the establishment and progression of HIV-caused disease'. The reason the subjects had been HIV-negative was to avoid confounding the results, he added. Hank Wilson's efforts were to educate users as well as health professionals as to the effects of drug use 'as they relate to HIV-caused problems'.

New Aids cases in young adults and homosexuals had started to decline. 'The educational programmes are working and should be encouraged. Vaccines are years away and therapy has not resulted in any cures. If the people involved in education feel their efforts could be furthered by a reclassification of this paper I would take their input very seriously.'

On this occasion, Hank Wilson's efforts were successful. The index was changed. But in a way, it was a Pyrrhic victory. Adler knew how to talk the language of HIV; he linked the drug work to 'HIV-caused' disease, to allow the library official to connect a study of drug-induced immunosuppression with Aids, even though the subjects of study were HIV-negative. It wasn't the official's fault that she could not see the connection without having an artificial bridge constructed for her. She was reflecting a decade of brain-washing in favour of the HIV paradigm by scientific authorities, and the powerful apparatus that supported them – the press releases, the science and medical journals, the media correspondents who turned for 'off-the-record' assessments of developments in the field to a small coterie of HIV-predicated Aids barons.

Inertia in the UK

It is not just in the US that the role of drugs (as opposed to needlesharing) in Aids has been so neglected. It has been largely ignored in most parts of the world. As we shall see, the UK Department of Health has had a poor record of equivocation over nitrite inhalants, and even today (1995) is refusing to take action over the drugs, which are freely sold and advertised in Britain. The department's stance on the drug-Aids connection has not just been neutral. It has made no attempt to give a fair assessment of data implicating drugs in Aids. Like its US counterpart, it has been adversarial, citing discredited studies in a one-sided attempt to dismiss evidence that might threaten the HIV paradigm.

The result is that even gay men who have tested HIV-positive are rarely warned about the dangers, and many continue with high levels of drugs use. An idea of the phenomenal extent of this physical abuse in a group of people who, according to the conventional view, are already immunocompromised or dangerously at risk of being so was provided by a paper presented at the 1993 International Aids Conference in Berlin. Out of 200 attenders at an HIV clinic in London, 28 per cent admitted to using poppers during the previous week, 42 per cent during the previous month and 64 per cent during the previous year. There were also high rates of usage of ecstasy, LSD, amphetamines and cocaine.

British gay health activists who have taken up the fight against drugs in the gay community have met a wall of indifference among many doctors and nurses, Aids educators and government advisers, as well as within mainstream gay organisations. It is as though there is a kind of death wish lurking behind superficially expressed concerns to save lives. Worse, those who challenge the HIV hypothesis have been accused of 'blaming the victims', and of various kinds of bigotry including 'homophobia' or 'drugophobia'.

Lauritsen, who is now a full-time Aids researcher and writer, has faced such charges for years, and deals with them effectively. In his 1993 book *The Aids War,* he states:

> I have no desire to point the finger of blame at those who are sick, or to increase their suffering, but I refuse to tell lies under the guise of *sensitivity.* Lives are at stake, and there is no way to formulate rational risk-reduction or treatment guidelines without telling the truth about aetiology. To pretend that the behaviour of PWAs has nothing to do with their being sick, is to kill with a false kindness.

To observers like Lauritsen, the Aids saga is 'an epidemic of lies'. Even worse, in a way, because of the effect on our minds, it is an 'epidemic of information overload':

> Aids technobabble is dumped on us every day by the media: T-cell ratios, CD-4 receptors, DNA, RNA, latency periods, TAT genes, ELISA test, Western Blot test, p-24 antigen test, polymerase chain reaction test, angiogenesis, nucleoside analogues, AZT, ddI, ddC, d4T, macrophages, lentiviruses, reverse transcriptase, apoptosis, and all the rest of it. Over 60,000 papers on Aids have been published to date – untold millions of words. Nearly all

> are the intellectual equivalent of toxic waste, which is to say, both useless and dangerous.[19]

He argues that everything about the HIV paradigm is wrong. The presumed condition of immune deficiency is not present in all 'Aids' patients. The tests used to diagnose immune deficiency are new, highly inaccurate, and without adequate benchmarks; someone's T-cell count can go up or down by several hundred in the course of a day. Many of the diseases held to indicate 'Aids' when found in the presence of antibodies to HIV – the list of these diseases has now grown to twenty-nine – are not even caused by immune deficiency. And in his view, the hypothesised microbial culprit, HIV, is harmless. 'A biochemically inactive microbe cannot cause illness, any more than the reader of this book could rob a bank at the same time he was in a coma.'

Other diseases, such as mumps, measles, polio, chicken pox, rabies, gonorrhoea, malaria, salmonella, the common cold or bubonic plague, could all readily be described and diagnosed. That was not the case with 'Aids', which was defined entirely in terms of *other*, old diseases, in conjunction with dubious test results and even more dubious assumptions. 'Although people are undeniably sick, "Aids" itself does not really exist; it is a phoney construct.' The HIV-Aids hypothesis was foolish from the start. It had persisted for more than eight years 'only owing to the cowardice and stupidity of the media and the ruthlessness of the vested interests that comprise the burgeoning HIV-Aids industry'.

At base, 'Aids' was really very simple. Most, if not necessarily all, gay men who had developed 'Aids' fitted a particular profile, which marked them out from the tens of millions of gay men across America who had had sex with each other, and remained healthy. Lauritsen said he had developed this profile from his own interviews with many dozens of gay men with 'Aids'; from direct observation; from survey research; from interviews with PWA leaders; and from the reminiscences of those who had observed 'the scene'.

In the decade preceding their diagnosis, most of those who developed Aids had contracted venereal diseases many times, treated with ever stronger doses of antibiotics. They had taken antibiotics prophylactically, to avoid getting VD again and again. They drank too much; they used 'recreational' drugs; they smoked heavily; they experienced terror, owing to a war waged against gay men by the Moral Majority (described by Lauritsen as 'an American coalition of fundamentalist Christians'); they experienced loneliness, alienation and depression; they experienced shame and self-hatred, which, in a vicious circle, they acted out in ways that degraded themselves. And as the epidemic developed, they experienced grief: 'they were in perpetual mourning, their hearts broken by the loss of their closest friends'.

Following the gay liberation movement, a gay sex industry mushroomed, bringing with it a lifestyle which many gay men adopted as their own. One might have thought that gay liberation would usher in a new era of sexual freedom and happiness, but according to Lauritsen that did not happen. Sexuality became reduced to frenetic encounters in baths or back rooms.

> Some establishments in New York City and San Francisco provided a Theatre of Depravity, in which the patrons derived erotic satisfaction from psychologically and physically abusing each other. There were commercial sex clubs featuring rooms in which demented beings in bath tubs waited for others to come along and use them as toilets. Some places featured slings, in which people became communal semen receptacles. A 'Black Party' at a popular disco club provided, for entertainment, the spectacle of a young man mutilating himself and of a pig being murdered. It is fair to say that many who died of 'Aids' in the 80s, had died long before that in terms of humanity and self-respect.[20]

Lauritsen argued that the commercial gay milieu was itself extremely unhealthy psychologically – aside from and in addition to the specific health risks (drugs and disease) that existed within it. Inextricably bound up with the physical components of an addictive way of life were the psychological – and foremost was denial: the lies an addict tells himself and others in order to conceal, rationalise, and ultimately sustain his addiction. Here was a root cause of the Aids/HIV mythology: 'Denial of the role of VD and drugs in making gay men sick has insidiously undermined efforts to formulate rational treatment and prevention guidelines.'

The Drug-injured Body

In the past five years, Lauritsen said, he had spoken before hundreds of PWAs. He always asked if there were any to whom his risk-profile did not apply. The overwhelming response had been that the profile was right on target.

> Back in 1983-1984 I had a number of talks with Artie Felson, a founder of People With Aids New York and a member (as I was) of the New York Safer Sex Committee... At that time there were only a few thousands 'Aids' cases, so it was possible for a politically active PWA like Felson to come in contact with a substantial proportion of the PWAs in New York City and around the country. He told me that he had interviewed between 300 and 400 gay men with 'Aids', and had interrogated each of them with regard to sex and drug use. Though none of his respondents were virgins, some of them had not been specially 'promiscuous'. However, they were all drug users. Felson said he had heard stories of drug abuse that would make the hair stand on end. And, without a single exception, they had all used poppers. My conversations with Felson took place before the 'Aids virus' hypothesis had become obligatory Truth, so we were still free to bandy about ideas as to what 'Aids' was and what caused it. Felson adamantly maintained that he himself had become sick as a consequence of drug abuse, and that 'Aids' itself represented drug injuries to the body.[21]

If there was still some room for doubt over which aspects of selfdestructive behaviour contributed most to 'Aids' in gay men, the picture was much clearer in IV drug users, who as of October 1993 represented nearly a third of America's total 'Aids' cases. There were three possible hypotheses on why they were getting sick: one, because of shared needles; two, because of the drugs; or three, because of both. Although the first hypothesis prevailed, it falsely assumed that the drugs themselves were innocuous. Therefore, only the second and third hypotheses were tenable. The toxic consequences of drug abuse had long been common knowledge. For heroin and other opiates, they were listed in one popular home medical guide[22] as including psychological and physical addiction manifested in an intense craving, 'and a host of physical ailments including liver dysfunctions, pneumonia, lung abscesses, and brain disorders'. There were many medical references indicating that addiction to psychoactive drugs leads to immune suppression and clinical abnormalities similar to 'Aids'.

The same point has been made powerfully by Robert Root-Bernstein, associate professor of physiology at Michigan State University, whose 1993 book *Rethinking Aids* contains an enormous and authoritative review of the multiple challenges to the immune system seen in every group at risk of Aids. Root-Bernstein accepts that HIV, when activated, may contribute to immune system decline. But he argues that an important feature of drug abuse that has not been taken into account in defining who is at risk for Aids is 'the possibility that non-intravenous drug abusers who are exposed to HIV or other immunosuppressive agents by sexual routes will be at as great a risk of Aids as are intravenous drug abusers'.[23] This fact, he says, may help to explain why many sexual partners of IV drug abusers – people who are almost all drug users themselves – are developing Aids despite the fact that they do not share needles.

Another explanation of this fact, of course, might be that drugs themselves, independently of the transmission of HIV through shared needles, are the prime cause of Aids in such cases, a possibility that Root-Bernstein half acknowledges in asserting that 'if we are to understand Aids, we must understand the drugs that Aids patients inject, snort, sniff, smoke, skin pop, or otherwise imbibe prior to and during their development of illness. To control Aids we may have to learn how to get millions of addicts off drugs.'

According to Lauritsen, there has never even been a study to determine whether all, or even most, intravenous drug abusers with 'Aids' ever did share needles, although such research would be simple and inexpensive. 'I've spoken to many public health officials who believed that such research existed, but none has ever been able to provide a reference. I have spoken to many IVDUs – some with "Aids" and some not, some still using drugs and some "clean and dry". When I asked them if they had ever shared needles, the overwhelming response has been: "Share needles? Are you crazy? What would I do that for?"' In Italy, IVDUs comprised about 80 per cent of 'Aids' cases, yet needle-sharing was almost unknown as anyone could walk into a drug store and buy one.

Lauritsen quoted from an interview with William Burroughs, author of *The Naked Lunch* and 'a man with many decades of knowledge about drugs', expressing scepticism on the needle-sharing claims:

> They say junkies share needles, and that they can't afford to buy needles. If someone can get up to 50 dollars a day for any sort of habit, he can pay two dollars for needles. For an outfit. Now the outfits, a plastic syringe and needle, are sold right in the drug drop for two dollars. There's no reason for them to share needles — unless some of them are ignorant beyond belief. They know about the danger of serum hepatitis. You can get serum hepatitis, malaria, and syphilis from sharing needles. Serum hepatitis is a very serious condition. So I wonder to what extent they are sharing needles.[24]

To anyone who has eyes to see, Lauritsen says, it is obvious that IVDUs are getting sick now for the same reasons and in the same ways that they were getting sick long before the advent of 'Aids'. Many are dying of lung disease, just as they were thirty, forty or fifty years ago. 'I have lived in New York City's Lower East Side for two and a half decades, and I have observed what drugs do to people. I have seen healthy young guys arrive on the scene in the spring, and then later in the year I have seen the same people standing on the corner and begging – feeble, wizened old men. I have seen dead bodies propped up against walls or sprawled across sidewalks, waiting for emergency service units to haul them away.'

Yet the City Health Department had stated publicly that an IVDU with pneumonia or tuberculosis and HIV antibodies would be counted as an 'Aids' case, under the assumption that HIV was the sole cause, whereas if the same person had pneumonia but no HIV antibodies, it would be assumed that drugs were the cause. He would be just one more junkie with lung disease. 'This kind of logic belongs in *Alice in Wonderland*. The reality is that no one has ever observed the slightest difference in clinical profile between patients with any of the indicator diseases plus HIV and those with the same diseases minus HIV.'

Thousands of Lives Lost

Lauritsen sees the faulty reasoning that divorced understanding of 'Aids' from drugs as having cost the lives of thousands of gay men. He believes the consequences may be even more pernicious in drug users. Large sections of the gay community do at least know of the anti-drugs message, despite the Public Health Service's espousal of the HIV cause. Lauritsen was a member of the New York Safer Sex Committee which in 1984 formulated the first comprehensive safe sex guidelines. 'I had to fight, with the help of Artie Felson and Michael Callen, to get in a section warning about the dangers of drug abuse. We succeeded, with the result that risk-reduction guidelines targeted at gay men included admonitions against drug use, drinking too much, and so on. Our guidelines came right out and said, "Avoid drugs. Shooting up kills…Poppers are also dangerous." Gay men got the message. In addition, the city closed the Mineshaft, the St Mark's Baths, the Saint (disco club) and other establishments which were arenas for truly psychopathic drug abuse. The outlawing of poppers by New York State and Congress also helped.'

In contrast, injecting drug users had been subjected to years of 'safe needle' propaganda: 'Don't share needles, soak your needles in bleach' and so on. 'They received the message that needles were dangerous *but the drugs themselves were safe!* Members of ACT UP went throughout the Lower East Side, giving hypodermic syringes and "clean needle kits" to intravenous drug users. There is no reason to believe that the propaganda was not effective. Many junkies probably did make sure their needles were clean, and then went on shooting up with their usual drugs.'

The consequences could be seen in Aids statistics in New York City. IVDUs now accounted for a much larger proportion of cases – nearly 50 per cent in the twenty-two months to October 1992, compared with less than 30 per cent as of 31 December 1984. Gay men, by contrast, now comprised less than 35 per cent of the cases, compared with more than 55 per cent in 1984.

It is questionable whether that trend will continue. Lauritsen says that in the early 1990s gay men in San Francisco and New York City, two epicentres of the 'Aids epidemic', have gone back to the levels of drug abuse and promiscuity that obtained in the 1970s and early 1980s. A 1991 survey sponsored by the San Francisco Department of Public Health, organised by the Lesbian and Gay Substance Abuse Planning Group, found that almost 40 per cent of gay and bisexual men, and 20 per cent of lesbian and bisexual women, reported substance abuse at levels considered by experts to indicate chemical dependence or addiction.

Many are young men new to the gay scene. On New York City's Fire Island in August 1992, several thousand gay men attended a 'Morning Party', held to benefit Gay Men's Health Crisis (GMHC). One person who was there told Lauritsen that at least 95 per cent of them were in a state of extreme intoxication from such drugs as Ecstasy, poppers and cocaine, as well as alcohol. The playwright Larry Kramer, in an interview published in the *Advocate* headlined 'Kramer vs The World', commented:

> I loathed the Morning Party. The Morning Party sent me into a depression I cannot begin to describe. After twelve years of the plague, I should come back and see the organisation that was started in my living room having a party like that!...There were 4,000 or 5,000 gorgeous young kids on the beach who were drugged out of their minds at high noon, rushing in and out of the Portosans to fuck, all in the name of GMHC.

Writing in late March 1993, having just returned from a trip to the UK, Lauritsen noted that there was an explosion of drug use in the gay scene in London.

> Every Saturday night an estimated 2,000 gay men attend a dance club where drug consumption is the main activity. According to London sources, virtually 100 per cent of the men are on drugs, from 3.00 in the morning, when the club opens, until it closes many hours later. Especially popular is a variety of Ecstasy, whose ingredients are claimed to include heroin... Poppers are sold legally in London. No one seems to think they even count as drugs, as gay physicians, writing in the gay press, have said that poppers are harmless.
>
> None of the major Aids organisations have properly warned about the dangers of drugs. At most, their risk-reduction literature has urged people to use alcohol and drugs in moderation, so as not to affect the

> 'judgement'. Drugs are portrayed as risky only to the extent that they might facilitate a lapse into 'unsafe sex'. Poppers – which cause genes to mutate, which cause severe anaemia, which can kill through heart attacks, which suppress the immune system – are depicted as bad only if they cause someone to forget about condoms.

Lauritsen acknowledges that the thousands who have worked in Aids organisations have included kind and courageous individuals who came to the aid of very sick people at a time of need, demonstrating their basic goodness and decency. For him, however, the bitter reality is that in the Aids war, the mainstream organisations have been in the camp of the enemy. Their leaders were 'not just the passive dupes of the Public Health Service', but actively collaborated in creating the Aids mythologies. They not only endorsed but elaborated and refined on the prevailing paradigm, and never admitted in their literature that anyone had ever doubted HIV, even when scientific controversy was raging.

'Suffice it to say that from the very beginning there were critics of the hypothesis, and that our voices were silenced…Never, indeed, did they admit that the HIV-Aids hypothesis was just that, *a hypothesis*.'

The ethical indictment was not that mistakes were made, though that was nothing to be proud of. 'Rather, their blame consists of having suppressed dialogue. The Aids organisations were rigidly and ruthlessly totalitarian in censoring any viewpoint that did not fit the orthodox dogmas of the moment. They inspired sufficient fear among their employees that none, while still employed, publicly expressed a doubt about the HIV-Aids hypothesis or the benefits of AZT therapy – though some did so after resigning or being fired.' Lauritsen tells of how he has felt the shadow of censorship – 'unofficial, but all-pervasive' – hanging over him in his Aids writings.

The Aids War, which was self-published, is a fearless, passionate work. Lauritsen's consistently informative and challenging reports stand out like a beacon in an ocean of confused thought over Aids. His writing may not seem objective, but in one sense it is, relative to most Aids literature, because he is not looking through the lenses of a compromised orthodoxy. His passion is legitimate because he is extremely well-informed, and on the basis of his knowledge he has concluded that the general state of ignorance is costing thousands of lives, squandering national resources, and destroying 'the good name of Science'. He is surely right, although I believe he may have underestimated the state of our ignorance about what HIV means, and thereby overestimated the culpability of those scientists who promoted it as the cause of Aids. What seems absolutely clear is that it was injudicious to drop drugs from the frame so early on, when they were the common factor among so many people with immune deficiency, and when an explosion in their use, particularly nitrite inhalants, had preceded the arrival of Aids in the gay community.

Lauritsen has shown phenomenal courage in challenging the conventional view of Aids. As well as trying to put across his views through his writings, he has done the same in person at many meetings, and has withstood much abuse as a result. He has been supported by a strong sense of morality. 'Somehow we must return to older and better standards,' he cries. 'This means a return to the authority of intellect and ethics, as opposed to the authority of money and power.'

There is also a certain iciness in his outlook, reminiscent of the six-year-old who could not understand the upset caused when he debunked Santa Claus. Although he accepts that 'in the Aids war, there is a vast army of fools: venal fools and non-venal fools, crooked fools and honest fools, malevolent fools and charitable fools', he also believes there are Aids criminals who, if there were justice in the world, 'would be brought to justice, given fair trials, and executed'.

His view of humanity in general is remarkably detached. This may be one reason why he was able to see so clearly, and from such an early point, the mistakes that were being made, while the rest of the world laboured under so many illusions. He told me: 'Intellectually it is disappointing how far evolution still has to go – the fact that people collectively and individually are so extremely stupid; and also that people have so little in the way of principle. Certainly, the profit motive gone mad is part of it, but a lot of the madness that has taken place is simply mass psychology.

'I think part of it is a question of belief. Part of the anger people feel when you challenge the fantasies they believe in comes from an inability to believe that the Public Health Service of the US would be so dishonest and incompetent. They don't believe that the *New York Times* and other papers would consistently tell them things which were not true. I think it is also in the nature of bureaucracies, the Public Health Service or any other, to be pathologically incapable of ever admitting they have made a mistake; and here, they haven't just made a mistake, they've made the greatest blunder in all medical history, which has killed tens of thousands of people. They can't face up to the enormity of it.

'Then there is the denial on the level of the gay newspapers and gay subculture. These tend to revolve around the gay sex industry, which would include everything from the historic discotheques to the clubs and bars and the poppers industry; and here, it is obviously not in their interests to acknowledge the true cause of Aids. Probably the core phenomenon at these establishments, which made many tens of millions of dollars for their owners, was drug consumption, and in my opinion drug consumption is the main reason these men became sick in ways that are called Aids.

'At the individual level, I can see that as it is now, a gay man diagnosed as having Aids has a certain martyr status, almost like in the old fertility rituals when the sacrificial victims had a great deal of fuss made of them as they were led with chants and flowers in their hair to the sacrificial altar.

'It would be quite different to say that someone with Aids became sick as a consequence of substance abuse. This is not something that would elicit the same type of sympathy, and in fact the response of most ordinary people – the healthy response – would be to say OK, you've made your bed, now you've got to lie on it.'

Thus spake Miss Brock. We may not like the medicine – and a spoonful of sugar would make it a lot easier to swallow. People with Aids should receive as much medical and social support as people with any other life-threatening condition. But in Lauritsen's analysis, thousands have died and are continuing to die because of a phoney construct of Aids causation. If the price to pay for an end to this holocaust were the loss of martyr status of Aids victims, would that really be such a bad exchange?

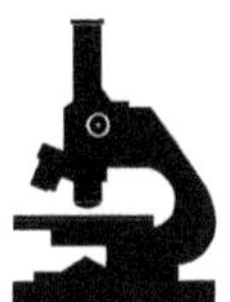

5: A CONSPIRACY OF HUMBUG

When Jim Curran and Don Francis and others in the US Public Health Service came swiftly to the conclusion that a new infectious agent was responsible for Aids, they were acting in line with a tradition that has dominated medical thinking for more than 100 years. The germ theory of disease – the idea that illnesses are caused mainly by transmission of an organism from one host to another – brought so much power to explain and sometimes prevent disease that today it exerts a strong hold over most of us. Yet it has not always seemed so obvious as an adequate description of the disease process.

Although it has no clear point of origin, the essential idea of transmission of specific disease agents grew in strength during the first half of the nineteenth century. It was controversial: most doctors at the time were steeped in the classical tradition in which susceptibility to disease, whether contagious or otherwise, was understood as lying largely in the host. They were resistant to the idea that a living, extrinsic agent was also involved. But the germ theory swept through medical science like a forest fire during the second half of the century, after the French chemist Louis Pasteur and the German bacteriologist Robert Koch triumphantly demonstrated distinct microbial causes of specific syndromes in both animals and humans. At that point, the only opposition came from those who resented changes in established practice, 'or who objected to the sudden burst of incontrovertible facts into sanctuaries of privileged opinion', as the distinguished public health expert Dr Gordon Stewart put it in a *Lancet* article nearly thirty years ago.[1]

At the time, Stewart was professor of epidemiology and pathology at the schools of public health and medicine, University of North Carolina. His five-page article, entitled 'Limitations of the Germ Theory', is strikingly relevant to the difficulties over Aids causation that today's 'sanctuaries of privileged opinion' have encountered.

Stewart accepted the established fact that germs can cause disease. Indeed, he wrote, 'infection without a germ would be as impossible, or miraculous, as conception without a sperm'. But a more balanced view of disease causation was needed. He argued that just as Victorian physicians resented the intrusion of microbiological facts on their practices and views, the same reaction was now operating in favour of, instead of against, the germ theory.

> Medical teaching, diagnosis, and treatment lean heavily upon the prerequisite that, for every disease, there is a single ascertainable cause; the object of most research is to identify this cause, and by prevention or treatment to eliminate it. Thus, our approach to infectious disease is often exclusively germ-oriented, with vaccines and chemotherapy as the principal weapon of attack. The fact that these weapons have been strikingly successful in countless situations supports this attitude but does not necessarily mean that no other attitude is justifiable. The question confronting us is now whether, by accepting the germ theory as the main explanation of infectious disease, we are overlooking other determinants of equal or great importance.

In fact, Stewart argued, the theory supported a grossly oversimplified view of the natural basis of infectious disease. It had become a dogma, neglecting the many other factors which have a part to play in deciding whether the interaction between host, germ and environment is to lead to infection. Such factors include the host's personal susceptibility to infection, for example, which could be increased as a result of travel, changes of diet and antibiotic treatment; social and economic factors such as poverty and over-crowding; behaviour and personality; and genetic constitution. 'It is often easier to use antibiotics or vaccines than to alter human behaviour or the environment, but if a disease is maintained because of attitudes, behaviour, or surroundings, a germ-orientated approach is unlikely to succeed.'

The article, carried by the *Lancet* under its 'Dogma Disputed' slot, included a discussion of the nature of dogmas – 'comfortable things which, like favourite armchairs, increase in appeal as time passes'.

> If accepted uncritically, any theory tends to become a dogma, that is to say, it becomes the captive of its own postulates. The more rigid the postulates, the more complete the captivity ... a theory, to be valid as a continuing vehicle for thought, must provide for exceptions, must convincingly explain anomalies, must have embodied in its fabrication a recognition of its limitation as well as of its extent. A theory lacking in these qualities is vulnerable at any point to disproof; one which seeks to maintain validity in the face of anomalies or in contradiction to new facts, becomes a dogma.

Later, as Mechan professor of public health at Glasgow University in Scotland, Stewart continued to fight the narrowness of outlook that sees illness as dictated by germs alone. He directed a study of hospital admission data which demonstrated that children living in deprived districts in Glasgow were on average nine times more likely to be admitted to hospital for any reason than children in non-deprived districts. When the components of deprivation were tested separately, the factors most strongly linked to admission rates were overcrowding in households, and the parents being out of work. Notably, these factors correlated with admission rates for infectious diseases such as measles and whooping cough much more strongly than did low levels of vaccination in the same districts. Quality of accommodation in terms of physical amenities did not seem to make any difference; there was no excess of admissions in four of five districts in which basic amenities were lacking in up to one fifth of households, and the highest admission rates (100 times greater than the lowest) were found in two districts containing large estates of modern council housing with only a few older properties lacking in amenities. In all, some 55,000 children, about a third of the population studied, were statistically very much more likely to be admitted to hospital than the others.

Stewart and his co-author Dr Alison Maclure concluded in their 1984 report on the study: 'The findings show possibilities of an immense saving in avoidable illness and health service costs by elimination of recognisable disadvantages. But they suggest also the presence of a less recognisable lifestyle factor which may be responsible for a substantial health-damaging effect in some relatively non-deprived environments.'[2]

The study was supported by the European Regional Office of the World Health Organization, with whom Stewart continued as an adviser on his retirement from the Glasgow post in 1983. The following year, he wrote an important report on social and cultural factors in human health, commissioned by WHO, in which he developed further the argument that 'the influence of environment and behaviour upon disease has been consistently forgotten or ignored in the practice of medicine, nowhere more than in the field of communicable diseases'. One reason for this neglect was the maintenance of professional monopoly: since the basic lessons of personal and communal hygiene were simple and unchanging, they could be observed and practised independently of organised medicine, 'which has seldom supported and often resisted or disparaged efforts in public health'.

The 250-page report, completed in 1985, included a chapter on breakdown of immunity to infection in which Stewart set out a case for believing that lifestyle and behaviour factors were probably central to the newly recognised syndrome called Aids, because of the way cases were concentrated among people who had been exposed to some very specific risks. This chapter, Stewart's first written discussion on Aids, still stands today as consistent with most of the evidence that has been accumulated about the condition in the years since. It was well ahead of its time in anticipating problems that were to arise with the HIV theory.

To understand Aids and similar disorders, Stewart wrote, it was necessary to understand the dual nature of the immune response, in which immunity to specific infectious and other foreign agents was enhanced by 'helper' T-cells and inhibited by 'suppressor' T-cells. He quoted the eminent immunologist Sir Macfarlane Burnet on the circumstances necessary to lead to unresponsiveness of the immune system:

> ... for effective inhibition of capacity to respond to a specific antigen, a situation must arise or be contrived by which sufficient antigen can make contact with *all* specifically active immunocytes [lymphocytes] which can have descendants. This means that all cells must either be set into irreversible production or be destroyed...
>
> Since lymphocytes may remain inert but potentially capable of mitosis [division and growth] for long periods (several years in man), this may well

> require that antigen remains present for a long time in order to catch some of the cells in a vulnerable phase.

In other words, if the immune system is challenged by a specific antigen sufficiently strongly and over a long enough period of time, usually several years, a situation may develop in which it will no longer respond to that antigen, and hence no longer be capable of protecting the body against the infectious agent (or other pathogen) involved. This chronic exposure could be brought about by various viruses, but also by 'the insults to immunity conveyed by repeated introductions of infection intravenously in addicts to narcotic drugs'.

Stewart had seen at first hand the devastation wrought on the human body by such mechanisms, having conducted a major study of drug addiction in New York City and New Orleans between 1968 and 1971, while employed as Watkins professor of epidemiology at Tulane University in New Orleans. The study was funded by the National Institute of Mental Health.

In 1967, he recalled, an explosive outbreak in the use of and addiction to narcotic and psychoactive drugs, notably heroin, had begun in the United States and among US soldiers serving in Vietnam. To any doctor working with addicts at that time, it had become obvious within a year or two that a novel range of active, latent and opportunistic infections was being transmitted. This was partly because syringes were often used communally, without sterilisation, and also because it was usual for the heroin or other drug to be diluted with other materials by the pusher or user. The most common infection was hepatitis B, but many other organisms, accompanying increasingly bizarre patterns of injection, became familiar: bacteria, yeasts and fungi, herpes simplex, cytomegalovirus, toxoplasmas, cryptococci, lymph gland infections and multiple abscesses. Many of these infections were chronic or recurring, often unrecognised at first, and difficult to treat. In confirmed addicts who gave themselves intravenous injections with contaminated substances several times a day, multiple infections developed which could not be controlled by medical drugs or by the patient's own overtaxed and diminishing resistance. Many addicts were severely malnourished and already had one or more bisexually or homosexually transmitted diseases.

'The fatality rate was never known but was certainly high. In all but name, the numerous cases – tens of thousands at least – of addicts with incipient or established artificially created infections of this description were clinically very close to the cases subsequently recognised for endpoint diagnosis as Aids.' Yet this went as far back as the late 1960s. It had been said that Aids cases were first seen in the US in 1978 or 1979, at least two years before the first published reports, but the presumption that a new and different disease began then was doubtful. The earlier cases had almost identical histories, habits, symptoms and signs. What was new in 1978 and subsequently was the insight into the immune deficiency, the technical capacity to investigate it, and the recognition in the US of a complex syndrome which was as yet rare in other developed countries.

The question now arising, Stewart wrote, was whether, in addition to the diverse microbial pattern of infection, there was also a single, underlying, transmissible, causal microbe common in all cases.

As far as the cases were concerned, Aids was less a syndrome than a conglomerate of miscellaneous medical data – clinical signs, microbial isolates, lesions with indications of partial or complete exhaustion of the mechanism of immune resistance to various infections, and common factors presumed to predispose the host to the illness. There was also a generalised disorder of the immune and auto-immune mechanisms, and sometimes cancerous changes in the tissues. Most cases were either promiscuous homosexual or bisexual men, and men who took drugs intravenously. The remainder were sexual partners of known or suspected cases, haemophiliacs who had received repeated blood transfusions, and a few infants of mothers who had Aids or whose sexual partners had it. 'There is no evidence of occurrence in other infants nor of transmission on any scale outside the risk groups even among those who in households or hospitals are intimately involved in caring for Aids patients.'

In terms of social evolution, Aids was also new mainly in name. The combination of drug abuse, homosexuality and opportunistic infections had already erupted as a nationwide epidemic in the US as far back as about 1967, and the link between certain viruses, especially those in the herpes group, with lymphocyte disorders and disturbance of cell-mediated immunity was well recognised shortly afterwards. It was also known that these infections were usually associated with malnutrition. There was a strong similarity to the clinical state of the heroin addict, 'wasted by chronic infection and malnutrition'.

What also needed to be explained was the formation of auto-antibodies (in which the immune system begins to attack the body instead of protecting against disease), the extreme exhaustion of immunity, and the cancerous changes in some homosexual men, leading to the development of Kaposi's sarcoma and various lymph gland growths. Here, Stewart favoured the explanation offered by Sonnabend and others, arising from studies of the effects of sperm on the immune system. Repeated exposure, both in experiments with rabbits and in human patients, had been shown to lead to the presence in the blood of antibodies which cross-reacted with components of the immune system. This self-destruct mechanism, along with the fact that the sperm was also often infected with the immunosuppressive herpes virus CMV (cytomegalovirus), allowed other, latent infections to activate and after a certain point meant that responses to any infection would be compromised, as would the body's ability to deal with malignant cells.

All of this, Stewart concluded, 'would appear to provide a remarkably complete behavioural and biological explanation of Aids in the group at highest risk, namely homosexual men with multiple sexual partners'. Since female sexual partners could also – though rarely – develop Aids from bisexual men, and since there were cases in infants and some other low risk groups, Stewart allowed that it remained possible that some other disease agent, such as a retrovirus, could be involved in initiating or maintaining Aids or its component conditions. However, if such an agent existed, it could not be very infectious. That was evident from the extreme rarity of contact cases, even among those who looked after severe and terminal cases of Aids in hospital or at home. It had to be transmissible by blood or blood products, but on the epidemiological evidence it would cause disease only in people whose resistance was compromised by other factors. Presciently, Stewart argued that the new test for antibodies to the retroviruses claimed to be linked to Aids had not yet been shown to be reliable, either as indicators of infection or of Aids. It was particularly important to note that a positive result 'does not indicate past, present or future infectiousness because there is no evidence as yet of transmission of Aids by casual contact'.

The fact that there were far more Aids cases in the US than in the rest of the developed world awaited explanation. 'It has to be remembered,' Stewart wrote, 'that the permissive social climate which fostered widespread use and abuse of psycho-active drugs and perhaps of an extended spectrum of sexual behaviour also began in parts of the USA before becoming apparent in European and Pacific countries. But the change did follow. It might be that Aids will do so too.' Still, on the basis of what had happened so far, the evidence in Europe pointed to a very low level of risk of Aids for the general population.

This authoritative report, by an acknowledged world expert in the field of public health, was treated as an 'inter-office' document by the WHO, and never published. Perhaps it was never even read by those responsible for the fight against Aids. The approach it exemplified has never been reflected by WHO, which instead promoted the HIV theory with great vigour, producing a world-wide pandemic of fear.

Nature Rejects a 'Provocative' Hypothesis

Ten years on, the evidence is still telling us the same as Stewart described, only more strongly than ever: Aids is not behaving as the new, highly infectious disease it has been made out to be, and its spread has remained confined to people facing heavy and persistent challenges to their immune system because of behavioural, medical and lifestyle factors.

Gordon Stewart, however, has still been unable to have his arguments debated, or even published, in any major scientific journal, despite intensive efforts on his part in recent years. A partial exception is the *Lancet*, which has taken a number of letters from him, while turning down his articles. He has become engaged in an extraordinary, unceasing battle with journal editors and professional leaders. He wants them to publish clinical and epidemiological facts in the context of his argument that the data do not fit the 'lethal virus' theory of Aids. To date, they have been unwilling to do this. The *British Medical Journal* has been dismissive. *Nature's* editors have rejected numerous attempts on his part to persuade them to publish his arguments either as a letter or as an article. The Royal Society, Britain's foremost scientific institution, has done the same, even though he has amended his manuscripts many times in response to the demands of referees. His file of correspondence relating to these efforts is very thick. It bears powerful witness to the mental and emotional pathology that has gripped the medical and scientific professions during the Aids era.

After a sensational 'London Declaration on Aids' by official bodies in 1988, Stewart drafted letters with Sir Reginald Murrell, president of the Royal College of Surgeons, objecting to 'alarmist and misleading publicity' being promoted through the media at the time by the government-appointed Health Education Authority. 'Since the journals wouldn't publish anything, we tried to get Sir Douglas Black, president of the Royal College of Physicians, Sir Richard Doll [eminent epidemiologist, and emeritus professor of medicine at Oxford University] and others to join us in a letter to *The Times* but they wouldn't sign,' Stewart says. 'The *Lancet* published an attenuated letter by me in 1989.'

Stewart first tried to persuade *Nature* to allow its readers to learn of 'an alternative hypothesis' on HIV and Aids in March 1990, submitting an abstract and later the full text of a 3,000-word paper questioning the single virus theory. Before submitting the paper, he sent it to Sir David Tyrrell, president of the government's Dangerous Pathogens Committee. He expressed interest, and sent it to the Medical Research Council. 'They denied ever receiving it, and failed to acknowledge a second copy,' Stewart says.

A particular strength in this and in his many other efforts to alert the scientific community to shortcomings in the HIV theory was his familiarity with public health data from New York City (NYC) as well as the UK. Thus, he reported that at the end of 1989, the cumulative total of Aids cases registered in the UK since 1982 was 2,831, about the same as the cumulative total that had been reached in NYC in June 1984. Using this comparison, he was able to show that official predictions in the UK that Aids would soon affect a large proportion of the general population had no support from the US data. By November 1989, the cumulative totals for Aids cases in NYC had risen to 19,476 men and 3,038 women, including a high proportion of injecting drug users. But only thirty-nine of the men, and twenty-one of the women, had no known risk. In the great majority of cases registered reliably in expert Aids centres, the syndrome accompanied risk-prone behaviour, or exposure to toxic and infectious co-factors.

He also demonstrated that the spread of Aids in the UK and US was best predicted by a simple linear model based on time, consistent with the idea that risk-prone lifestyles within finite groups of people are the prime cause. In contrast, greatly exaggerated official predictions had been based on more complicated models that accepted the hypothesis that a new infectious agent was at work, producing exponential growth. These models were constructed on assumptions that drug injectors and bisexual men would infect their women partners, and that all who were infected would spread and develop disease, sooner or later, in all countries in which HIV was detected.

Stewart's alternative hypothesis proposed two primary causes of Aids: anal intercourse, and the sharing of infected injection needles. He argued that either one of these, or both together, was capable of brewing up the cocktail of chronic infections necessary – although not usually sufficient on their own – to cause Aids in the two main risk groups, and that these activities were weakening immunity, impairing healing and nutrition, and causing vitality to be depressed. Drug abuse in general was the main co-factor. Many of the drugs used, including the nitrite inhalants, harmed the immune system. Their cumulative effects, and especially their interactions, were profoundly damaging to vital functions and health generally. Aids in other people, such as the partners of Aids cases who also shared risks, recipients of transfusions, and babies born to at-risk mothers, were secondary consequences of this disease-generating activity in the same communities.

In anal sex, those most at risk were the passive partners, whether male or female. The rectum and its supporting tissues did not favour that kind of activity. When the cell lining was eroded and blood vessels damaged, the tissues and bloodstream were opened to invasion by faecal organisms, by the pathogens of all the sexually transmitted diseases, and many others. The risk of trauma and infections increased greatly with the frequency and violence of the action, and with the multiplicity of partners. Self-treatment of gonorrhoea and other infections with antibiotics was another risk factor, creating microbial mayhem in the intestines, and paving the way for bacterial and fungal super-infections. Semen in the rectum provoked immunological disorder. 'All this, combined with frequent, promiscuous anal and bisexual intercourse with dozens or hundreds of partners had become a way of life amounting to a subculture in the dedicated communities in which Aids was first observed and in those to which it spread. Knowledge of the dangers led to a reduction in risk behaviour but, by this time, various infectious diseases had become inseparable from the way of life.'

Stewart then drew on the experience from his three-year study of drug users in New York and New Orleans, as well as other published studies, to describe how a similarly debilitating, and potentially more widespread, amalgam of diseases had been noted in the late 1960s onwards in young injecting addicts. The drugs themselves were often impure and non-sterile; and needle-sharing, promiscuity and 'general disregard of hygiene – a notorious feature of the drug scene everywhere' – led to the sharing also of whatever infections were around, notably hepatitis, herpes, and cytomegalovirus, which could itself destroy helper T-cells. 'All the psychoactive drugs currently in use in this way, especially heroin and experimental mixtures, are profoundly depressing to appetite, general health and immunity. Alternation of excitement and depression leads quickly to habituation, overdosage and reckless disregard of all the personal and societal consequences of this lifestyle.'

If infection was minimised by using uncontaminated drugs and needles, or especially by opting for oral drugs, many addicts could live equably with their habit for many years. Otherwise, chronic infection, especially with therapy-resistant microbes, led to severe disease in target organs and often to death. 'A pregnant woman can transmit her infections and her drug-toxicity congenitally to her child. An infected donor can transmit latent infections to recipients of blood and blood products.' Most or all of the infections listed as indicators for Aids occurred in people in these categories, together with defects in immunity, before Aids appeared 'almost as a predictable disaster'.

Stewart also summarised weaknesses in the HIV theory itself, including arguments that it was so rarely found in the T-cells that Gallo's original belief, that it destroyed the cells directly, could not possibly be true. Even if HIV were proven to have some kind of priming role in causing Aids, prevention would still require control of the main co-factor, drug abuse; just as trying to manage the illness itself would be useless without dealing independently with the infections that arose.

He accepted Aids as an infectious condition, and fully endorsed the need for precautions against transmission by any route. But he condemned the way the 'monopolistic' HIV theory had led not only to false predictions about spread, but had governed research and control policies. Resources were almost all being directed to a single-factor strategy, aimed at producing an anti-HIV vaccine and anti-HIV drugs. The alternative hypothesis postulated that to prevent and control Aids, the behavioural and existential features of its victims' lifestyles needed to be recognised. Much more effort should be put into researching the risk-prone and health-damaging behaviour present in some adolescent and young adult communities, and into controlling 'the manufacture, distribution and irresponsible use of immunotoxic and psychoactive drugs'.

Nature had thus been presented with a manuscript that would have put before a world scientific and educated lay audience a reasoned alternative to the HIV hypothesis of Aids causation, with extremely important implications for research, prevention and treatment. This was at a time when Aids was generally considered the biggest medical crisis for decades, and when it was already clear that the HIV theory was in trouble. The paper was the work of a senior medical scientist, who had a long background in infectious diseases, who had worked with drug addicts in the US and UK, and who had held consultancies with WHO in this field. He had provided an original analysis and comparison of statistical data from two centres of public health excellence, New York City and the UK. He had studied the issue diligently (the paper had seventy-two references), and had corresponded with and visited or met key persons from various centres in Europe, the US, Africa, South America and Asia. (London was an exception: 'The doors of the Medical Research Council, Department of Health and many important centres of investigation were amazingly closed to any form of inquiry,' he recalls. 'Officials never replied to letters about the erroneous information which they were using for promotional purposes. From late 1987 onward I suggested a closed door, professional seminar with Peter Duesberg but nobody would agree.')

Nature took five months to reach a decision. On 18 June, after several follow-up letters, Stewart was told that the manuscript was receiving the personal attention of John Maddox, the editor. On 8 August, he received a courteous letter from David Concar, assistant editor, apologising for the delay but regretting that the magazine felt unable to publish it. The letter stated:

> Our main concern is the amount of solid epidemiological evidence that exists for your central hypothesis that lifestyle factors such as anal intercourse and IV drug abuse are the primary (but not sufficient) causes of Aids. Given the provocative nature of that hypothesis, we feel that its exposure to a wide general readership such as ours could only be justified in the wake of definitive supporting evidence. As far as we are aware there is no evidence, for example, that the CD4 counts of seropositive individuals who continue to indulge in anal intercourse or IV drug abuse drop any more rapidly than those who don't. At the same time, we are not persuaded that the various manifestations of Aids preclude HIV being its primary cause.
>
> A secondary factor is the manuscript's great length and discursive character. Most of the original scientific papers that *Nature* publishes are written in a highly condensed format, and we seldom publish hypotheses, even when the subject matter is clearly of general interest.
>
> I am sorry that on this occasion we cannot be more positive.

The journal's reference to the 'provocative nature' of Stewart's hypothesis shows clearly that in deciding to reject the paper, the editors had social and political considerations in their minds. The requirement of 'definitive' supporting evidence was an impossible demand, since for years Aids research had been predicated on the HIV theory, and efforts to explore alternative hypotheses had not merely been minimal, but as Sonnabend and others had seen, actively discouraged or prevented.

Even so, the epidemiological evidence linking anal intercourse and IV drug abuse with Aids was clear to all with eyes to see, and there were obvious mechanisms whereby those behaviours could be causing Aids. The main confounding factor was HIV, for which no such mechanisms had been identified. The length of the manuscript was modest for such an important topic, but in any case Stewart had already waited five months for a decision and was not at all averse to having the text edited, provided that its central message could be conveyed.

He wrote back to *Nature* on 16 August, urging that they at least publish an abstract he had freshly prepared on the issue, with a few references, as a short communication or letter. He insisted that his paper was provocative only in so far as it challenged epidemiological assumptions about HIV as the unique cause of Aids. On the basis of those assumptions, predictions had been made about heterosexual spread of Aids in non-risk groups, which clearly did not fit the facts according to the latest statistics. In New York City, out of 21,421 men with Aids as of 2 March 1990 – at least ten years into the epidemic among gay men and drug abusers – the number said to have acquired the disease even after 'sex with women at risk' was only eight. Aids cases in white females (all risks) totalled 501 but only three of those had 'no identified risk'. In the UK, despite an estimated 35,000-100,000 cases of infection with HIV, there were to date only twenty-one Aids cases in which no risk had been identified. 'It is the special duty of epidemiology in a continuing problem of this importance to examine and re-examine all evidence, just as it is surely the duty of Editors to see that statements of verifiable facts and legitimate questions are expressed, not suppressed,' Stewart wrote.

It was to no avail. A cursory note from Maddox, dated 18 September, stated: 'Thank you for your manuscript but sadly we cannot publish it. You will appreciate that the issue with which you deal is of enormous public importance, that the epidemiology of Aids has been much discussed and has become an exceedingly intricate matter and that, as a consequence, it is unlikely that you could convince our readers of the correctness of your conclusion on the basis of such a simple argument.'

Stewart kept fighting. On 27 September, *Nature* published a letter from doctors at two London Aids centres claiming that only subjects infected with HIV developed Aids, and that such data clearly supported a pathogenic role for HIV. In further correspondence with the journal, Stewart tried to press home the point that the correlation between HIV and Aids in high-risk patients was never in doubt; what was at issue was whether or not HIV *caused* Aids and was both necessary and sufficient to explain the disease. 'This is not so,' he wrote on 26 November, 'because Aids is not a single disease. It can occur without HIV, while seropositivity to HIV...is widespread without Aids.' He went on:

> What worries me most is your refusal to allow a reasoned question about the dogma that HIV is the exclusive cause of Aids to be posed in your columns. The matter is of immense importance because it is abundantly clear that, outside the main risk groups of homosexual men, needle-

> sharing drug addicts and their partners, Aids is still a rare disease even in the USA where HIV is very prevalent in both sexes. I have offered you enough verifiable data to justify the question and...I am not dismissing HIV as a factor in the pathogenesis of diseases related to or preceding Aids.
>
> I would suggest that we send our correspondence, dating from last March, to the Press Commission with a copy to the President of the Royal Society, and that you publish the outcome.

In a reply dated 4 December, Dr Maxine Clarke, executive editor, did not respond to Stewart's point about the confusion between correlation and causation. She asserted, however, that after discussing his letter with Maddox, 'it is not our view that *Nature* has not published reasoned debate on the question of HIV and Aids; quite the contrary, in fact'. In his reply on 18 December, Stewart said he could not recall seeing any scientific item questioning the HIV hypothesis in *Nature* except a short letter from Peter Duesberg*, professor of molecular biology at the University of California at Berkeley. 'Please tell me if I am overlooking any other publication,' he wrote.

> Even so, the questions which I have raised in my four submissions to you stand apart from Duesberg's doubts. I suggested that predictions based on the HIV hypothesis are demonstrably wrong and that the epidemiological patterns to date in the UK and USA at least do not support assertions about heterosexual transmission outside risk groups, or an imminent spread to the general population. My message, though no less strict on sexual laxity, is therefore much more optimistic than those from your other contributors and from official quarters. My prediction, made early in 1990 when the paper was sent to you, is right on target and has no caveats, unlike those in the erroneous predictions of mathematical models which you seem to accept...
>
> I have to conclude that you are determined to ignore salient, verifiable facts in contemporary statistical returns and literature, and to reject any communication, however brief, which dares to question the unvalidated hypothesis that HIV is the prime cause of Aids. I can understand that the

* **Duesberg's own battle over HIV and Aids is described in Chapter 6.**

pressures of peer review and consensus politics might discourage you from publishing a controversial paper but, if these are applied also to letters in a journal of your standing, the future for freedom and objectivity of opinion in scientific work is bleak. Except for my short letter in the *Lancet* [1989, volume 1, page 1325] no medical or scientific journal in Britain has seen fit to publish any doubts about HIV. Current research, enormous expenditure and remedial policies generally are therefore subject to the constraints imposed by far-reaching extrapolations of this hypothesis into everyday medical, social and commercial activities. I can think of no situation in peace-time in this country where such censorship – and hence censure – has been applied to informed communication about a serious hazard to the public health.

In response to a letter from Maddox asserting that 'as several of my colleagues have now explained, we do not think your argument is cogent', Stewart replied that 'the fact that you do not accept the cogency of my argument' was not the reason for his intended submission to the Press Complaints Commission, a non-statutory body set up to deal with press grievances in the UK. 'It is that, having given prominence and support to the hypothesis that HIV is causing an unstoppable epidemic of Aids in the general population, you will not publish even a letter raising a question about it.' In fact, he did not follow through with a submission because, on inquiry, he was told that the commission were unsure whether they could handle a scientific issue.

More letters to *Nature* followed. On 25 January 1991, Stewart wrote:

Dear Mr Maddox,

Perhaps you have seen the end-of-1990 figures published by the Aids Surveillance Unit of the PHLS [Public Health Laboratory Service]. They show, in the UK, a cumulative total of 4,098 cases and, in Scotland, 195 cases.

You will perhaps recall, in figure 1 and in the text of the paper written in 1989 which I sent to you early last year and which you rejected after a long delay, my regression lines and equations predicted 3,900 and 200 cases respectively for the end of 1991. These estimates are now confirmed, in contrast to the erroneous higher predictions of the Cox Committee [a Department of Health working group on HIV and Aids that predicted 8,000 cases in the UK by December 1989] and of experts reporting in 1989 to the Meeting on Transmission of HIV and Aids published in the Philosophical Transactions of the Royal Society (325, 37-187). There are even greater contrasts in projections for 1991 and subsequent years, and in breakdown of the data: especially in the absence to date of any evidence of appreciable incidence of Aids in women and infants outside high-risk groups.

My own, more accurate prediction to date is neither clever nor lucky. It is based upon a testable assumption that, in Britain as in the USA, and despite the spread of HIV, Aids is occurring foreseeably as it began, i.e. in subsets of the population whose behaviour or misfortune places them at high risk of exposure to the various infections, drugs, trauma and depletion of immunity which contribute to the variable symptomatology in the complex of diseases registrable as Aids. By the same token, the spread of Aids to the general population and to infants was and is eminently preventable by avoidance of these same risk behaviours which can be summarised in a few plain words for both sexes as promiscuity, anal intercourse, unprotected intercourse with unsafe partners and needle-sharing of drugs.

Might I suggest, finally, that you publish the above as a letter?

It was not published, and nor were letters sent on 16 February, 23 October and 14 November, each written in response to specific new Aids developments. The 14 November letter, addressed to Maxine Clarke, was a response to Maddox's 'Aids Research Turned Upside Down' editorial*, and a subsequent qualifying article. Stewart wrote:

In his Editorial Article of 26 September, Mr Maddox conceded that HIV might not be a sufficient cause of Aids, on the basis of interesting but unconfirmed reports of work in mice and monkeys. In his article, to which

* See Chapter 1

you refer my attention, on 14 November, and obviously under pressure, he qualifies this by saying 'There is no dispute that Aids is triggered by HIV.'

Might I suggest yet again that you and he and, indeed, your entire editorial and reviewing personnel must be well aware that there is a great deal of dispute. You have had visits, data, correspondence and articles from many well-qualified scientists and physicians expressing or conveying doubts about the origins and role of HIV in Aids. The truth is that there is plenty of dispute, for well-stated reasons, but that the editorial staff and advisers of *Nature* are determined to conceal it by rejection and by printing an excess of contrary views.

I have myself submitted and re-submitted to you from 1989 onward, in two articles and three letters, verifiable evidence from epidemiological data in human populations that HIV does not trigger the development of Aids, in the UK and USA at least, unless there is concurrent and continuing risk behaviour, and involvement of cofactors, in well-defined subsets of the population; and that the wider spread of Aids by heterosexual and congenital transmission to the general population, predicted in official forecasts, is not occurring. These findings...are obviously and urgently relevant to the diagnosis and control of Aids, the more so because effective vaccines and drugs based on the HIV hypothesis are not available.

In your issue of 14 November you feature also the fact that the basketball player Hero Johnson is HIV seropositive and use this as an example of transmission of HIV by heterosexual contact to a man whose wife is pregnant and reportedly HIV negative. This is speculative, anecdotal sensationalism at its worst, quite unworthy of a scientific journal. I cannot see how you can justify an editorial policy which accepts articles about mice, monkeys and gossip while rejecting verifiable data from epidemiological surveillance and clinical observations in specified communities affected by Aids.

I am asking you therefore to reconsider the letter already sent to you for Scientific Correspondence, updated by including the enclosed table or rewritten, as you prefer. If you still reject this, will you publish instead the present letter, modified if you wish, as general comment?

Maddox replied:

> I have read your letter to Maxine Clarke responding to an article by me, and I am writing now regretfully to say that we cannot continue our correspondence with you, given that all your earlier manuscripts were assessed at the time.
>
> I am sorry to send you this disappointing news.

Stewart had one more try, in December 1993, when he fired off an angry rebuttal of an editorial stating that 'the evidence that HIV causes Aids is still epidemiological'. That was not so; the epidemiology demonstrated that people's circumstances and behaviour were the primary determinants, not a single germ, though HIV might play some part in the disease, as yet to be determined. Apart from the risk groups in particular locations, Aids was a rare, essentially male disease in the US, Europe and Australasia with a limited spread to women subjected to similar, abnormal risks, to some babies in the womb, and to some people inoculated accidentally with contaminated blood.

> In domestic terms, what this means (and what you and most other editors of professional journals refuse to print) is that the relative risk of Aids to a male aged 20-39 engaging in high-risk behaviours in parts of London is at least 5,000 times that of the general adult population of the UK, and about 50,000 times that of persons who avoid risk-behaviour. In almost all other locations in Britain, Aids is such a rare disease that fewer than 1:100 GPs will see a registrable case in 1994.

Maddox's reply indicated a complete inability to grasp the essence of what Stewart – and the statistics – were saying. He emphasised that the editorial concerned had not represented HIV as the sole cause of Aids, but then showed clearly that his mind was still wedded to the idea that a single infection was the main risk for Aids. 'The "establishment",' he wrote, 'would not be at all put out if, in Britain, the spread of Aids has to be modelled by supposing that there are two distinct sub-groups, male homosexuals and heterosexuals, with bisexuals (and intravenous drug users) serving as the bridge between them.

Nor would it be at odds with the model to suppose that the transmission factor – the chance of infection per act of intercourse with an infected person – differs from one group to the other.' This was why he believed that what Stewart had to say about the relative risks of infection was not relevant to the argument about the HIV hypothesis.

Stewart tried again. Official predictions were wrong conceptually as well as mathematically, he wrote, because they depended on assumptions that all who acquired HIV, by whatever route, would get Aids. If transmission of HIV were the key factor in Aids, 'the huge daily preponderance of heterosexual over homosexual acts of intercourse would already have produced an enormous increase in Aids in females'. But it was no use. After an exchange lasting several more months, Maddox once again refused to publish anything of Stewart's arguments, now accusing him of 'implicitly' misrepresenting the magazine's position on HIV in his latest letter. On 9 May 1994, Stewart replied in his final missive:

> My letter opened with a reference to a statement in your Editorial column of 9 December and to a 'continuing debate' – which is an understatement of your editorial stance in this subject. Am I to take it...that you regard your editorial prerogative as being exempt from correction or even comment? If so, your respected magazine ought to carry a Science Warning to this effect to open a new chapter in the annals of editorial objectivity, and to save you the bother of replying to those who happen to disagree with some of the questionable views that you persist in publishing.

Stewart's frustration was very understandable. As we have seen, he had fought for four years to persuade Britain's leading science journal to accept a communication on a subject that he was eminently well qualified to address, that was of enormous international importance, and on which he had prepared relevant statistical information and analysis that had not been published previously. After all that effort, he had still not been able to persuade the journal to take even a letter.

However, it would be wrong to conclude that the episode demonstrates a special high-handedness, or even obtuseness, on the part of Maddox and his editorial staff. From their perspective, it must also have been frustrating to be dogged so tenaciously by this elderly professor and his 'simple' ideas that could nevertheless not easily be dismissed. The correspondence might have been terminated long previously by an editor with less patience, or less concern for the truth. Indeed, the *British Medical Journal* had rejected a similar, though shorter, article, as had the *Lancet.* The *Journal of Epidemiology and Community Health* also refused to publish Stewart on this subject. *Science* (twice) and the *New England Journal of Medicine* also refused and re-refused to publish anything.

The roots of the problem lay deeper, in the scientific and medical psyche. Maddox had succumbed to a group delusion afflicting the highest levels of the scientific world.

Four-year Battle with Royal Society

In parallel with efforts to persuade *Nature* to give his 'alternative hypothesis' an airing, Stewart was engaged in a similar long-running saga with the Royal Society, the national academy of science for the UK and one of the oldest scientific societies of Europe. This battle concerned a considerably longer document of some 8,000 words, with 160 references, in which he addressed a series of papers published by the society in 1989. Those papers analysed the epidemic and made predictions about future spread. The predictions, like those of the official Cox report of 1988 and other authorities, were mainly wrong, and according to Stewart that was because they rested on two false assumptions. The first was that the essential cause of Aids was HIV; the second was that Aids was already spreading widely beyond the original susceptible groups of homosexual men and drug addicts by heterosexual transmission, and would spread further in that way to cause a pandemic of global dimension in general populations.

The paper was a substantial and clearly argued piece of work, which discussed many detailed aspects of the debate over HIV and Aids, drawing on Stewart's lifetime of work in the field. It was first submitted to the society in September 1990, after prior consultation with them. After several months of assessment, the paper was rejected but according to Stewart the editor of *Philosophical Transactions B,* the learned journal involved, agreed that the reasons given by referees were inadequate. So it was submitted to new referees, including two named by Stewart. 'There was a considerable delay during which the Editor did not conceal his hope that the paper would be published,' Stewart says. 'However, it transpired that the Biological Secretary of the society, a zoologist from Bristol, had "decided" to make the decision himself, and that was to reject the paper.

'When I questioned this violation of editorial prerogative, the Editor agreed because, in fact, three of the second set of referees had favoured publication after minor changes. We were now in 1992, and he invited me to update and resubmit the paper, without promising to publish it but with an understanding that it would not be unreasonably rejected, as previously. Meanwhile, thousands of other papers on Aids had been published, so updating it was difficult.'

Stewart nevertheless rewrote and resubmitted the paper in February 1993. The editor sent him the comments of two anonymous referees on 19 May, asking him to reply. Both were hostile, though neither of them answered his case. In essence, they simply made a series of unreferenced assertions, predicated on the conviction that HIV was responsible for the disease. One of them, moreover, was convinced that everyone who has tested HIV-positive will eventually get Aids, since 'individuals who have become infected with HIV have either developed Aids or are moving towards developing Aids'. At the time, this statement was already demonstrably untrue.

The same reviewer wrote that the number of Aids cases was extremely hard to predict 'because Aids only develops after an extremely long and variable incubation time...The author does not present any data to falsify the assumption that HIV/Aids is spreading in the general population in the United States and the United Kingdom by heterosexual transmission.' But that was exactly what Stewart *had* done, with his demonstration that in both countries Aids was restricted almost exclusively to people facing special risks of immune suppression, regardless of HIV. The reviewer even contradicted himself, writing: 'The extent of spread of HIV in the heterosexual population remains uncertain; if the spread is slow (which current estimates based upon the level of risk behaviour in the general population suggest), then the doubling time of the epidemic will be fairly long and hence it will be extremely hard to detect the initial spread of the epidemic.' In other words, no such spread was yet evident. After at least a decade, it still remained pure speculation that Aids presented a threat to the population at large through heterosexual transmission.

The other reviewer referred to 'errors too numerous to list', and then listed three examples, of which none was an error on Stewart's part. The first was that he had cited a mean incubation time of fifteen years from first testing HIV-positive to developing Aids, whereas the 'generally agreed upon time' was about ten years. In fact, Stewart was right: fifteen years is increasingly commonly cited. The figure, which increases constantly with time, is in any case a meaningless and dangerous generalisation, because many people who test HIV-positive will never develop Aids. Secondly, the referee said it was 'untrue' to state that HIV-negative people could receive an Aids diagnosis. In fact, there were numerous such diagnoses in the US, before the Centers for Disease Control built HIV-positivity into the definition of Aids, and there still are thousands of such cases in Africa.

Thirdly, it was said to be untrue to take the view, as Stewart had done, that the clinical diagnosis of Aids was arbitrary. But this was a matter of opinion, not an 'error'. 'Even in centres of excellence,' Stewart said in his reply, 'like those in which I have habitually worked, clinical diagnosis is sometimes arbitrary. It is very much more so in a condition which can occur independently of infection with HIV and of risk factors for Aids.'

This latter reviewer felt so put out by Stewart's alternative hypothesis as to conclude: 'I do not think that this piece of work should be lent the gravitas of publication by the Royal Society.'

Faced with such negative attitudes and hostile opinion, and after making so much effort to put his analysis before the scientific community, it is surprising that Stewart found the intellectual and emotional stamina to continue. He nevertheless sent back three pages of specific comments on the main points raised by these reviewers. He also wrote a general defence of the paper, summarising its most original and relevant observations, and offered the following general comments:

> This paper has taken nearly four years to write. It is updated and re-submitted at the suggestion of the Editor. It already incorporates suggestions and criticisms by several reviewers. It is relevant to remind assessors that I have a lifetime of professional experience in the diagnosis

and control of infectious diseases, and am on record as being perhaps the first epidemiologist to draw attention, in 1969-72 in the USA, to the unique health hazards of the new wave of drug abuse and sexual experimentation which began then in young adults and adolescents. Having begun work in this field with the support of the National Institute of Mental Health in New Orleans and New York, I continued it during tenure of the Chair of Public Health at the University of Glasgow and then, after retirement in 1983, with the World Health Organization, mainly in Copenhagen. The views expressed in the paper reflect this experience which includes working contact in the UK, USA and elsewhere with patients and drug addicts, as well as with lay and professional personnel in these fields.

The paper is admittedly controversial in that it questions the current hypothesis that HIV is the necessary and sufficient cause of Aids, and that neutralisation or elimination of this virus by vaccination and/or chemotherapy is the essential target and priority for prevention and control of the disease.

Although many experts and almost all authorities regard HIV as the sole cause of Aids, the fact is that this assertion rests upon a hypothesis which is, like any other, open to falsification, and valid and viable only if it resists challenge. If there is no challenge, it becomes a dead letter which, so far from solving the problem, perpetuates it. This has already happened with Aids. Unparalleled efforts and expenditure in biomedical research, prophylactic and therapeutic trials with viricidal agents, and large-scale voluntary participation of asymptomatic persons and patients in extensive trials and experiments have yielded no products of proven value. This alone calls for challenge of the hypothesis. In terms of causal logic, epidemiology and pathogenesis there are several other reasons for challenge. The present paper presents these in a constructive criticism of the hypothesis. It does not reject HIV as a contributor to the development of Aids. But it offers an alternative hypothesis structured on a wider base... This has attracted favourable comment from previous reviewers, and is the main reason for re-submission at the suggestion of the Editor and Biological Secretary of the Society.

Stewart submitted this response on 24 May 1993. Three days later, he received a final rejection from Dr Quentin Bone, the editor involved.

Stewart *still* did not give up. The following March, he wrote to Bone as follows:

> I am writing to suggest that your rejection some months ago of the above paper, originally submitted in 1990, was untimely and inappropriate.
>
> You will be aware that the passage of time has once again demonstrated that the predictions made in 1989 in the paper of the incidence, prevalence and distribution of Aids to date in the UK and through 1992 in New York City were correct to within 10 per cent of actual registrations of cases in specified areas, and within very narrow limits of confidence. This confirms the fact that, in these situations which are representative for developed countries, Aids is a disease which is continuing to spread in specified risk groups. There is no appreciable spread to the general population. The incidence in the female population aged 20-39 is about 1 in 600,000. The risk to the homosexual male population in two postal districts of London is 500,000 times that of couples with stable partnerships. All this, and much more, is verifiable. It is also in sharp contrast to the erroneous predictions and general forecasts published by the Society in 1989/90, and it has enormous implications for the public health, safety and expenditure.
>
> The paper was correct also in predicting the invalidity and failure of the Concorde trial of AZT in babies infected vertically with HIV [this was a mistake – the Concorde trial was in HIV-positive adults], the near-impossibility of preparing a vaccine for general use because of mutation by HIV and for other reasons, the absence in the USA and UK of Aids in infants except those born to mothers engaging in high-risk behaviour, and the uncertainty of Aids in haemophiliacs and their consorts. It drew attention to uncertainties in diagnosis, enumeration and testing in Africa which are obscured by acceptance of unvalidated data. All this points to a need to re-examine the orthodox dogma about the cause and transmission of Aids which the Society, by failing to admit any room for doubt, is sponsoring.
>
> If you review the comments of your anonymous referees and my replies, you will find not only that what I am saying is correct but also that the main reasons given for rejection of the paper were often highly biased,

beside the point or entirely wrong. I find it hard to believe that they would be upheld creditably in open debate, and I would suggest that you might care to review your decision in the light of events.

After the editor asked Dr M. B. Goatly, the Royal Society's head of publishing, to reaffirm the rejection, Stewart wrote to Goatly as follows:

> Obviously I must accept Dr Bone's decision not to publish this oft-amended paper but, for the reasons stated in my letter of 10 March and indeed in correspondence dating from 1990, I am not content to let the matter drop in this way.
>
> It must be obvious to all of you, and I would think that it should be of concern to the Society, that some of the referees whom you consulted were not only wrong in their criticisms but outrageously prejudiced and irresponsible. The passage of time has shown how wrong they were...I cannot believe that the Society would endorse this kind of behaviour as a decent basis for assessing serious work from a medical scientist writing well within his field of expertise, especially when the main arguments are now verified and some main questions explained.

Stewart asked for his paper and all the correspondence to be submitted to the society's council as a matter for complaint 'because it reveals a state of affairs within the Society which is inappropriate to its status and function in the scientific world'. That request was turned down, too, though the file was passed to Sir Francis Graham-Smith, vice-president of the society, who wrote:

> I read the referees' reports and the correspondence. I have to say that I am entirely satisfied that the Editor and the publications staff have behaved completely correctly in the handling of your paper and its refereeing. I have no reason to overturn the Editor's decision in rejecting your paper and conclude that there is no case for any further examination either of the paper or of our editorial procedures.
>
> I hope you can now accept that this must be the end of the matter.

Stewart hopes that it will not be the end of the matter. He considers that a demonstrable error has been made that in other walks of life 'would have been washed out years ago', but which at the time of writing, in mid-1995, medical science has proved incapable of correcting. 'Coming from the top scientific body in the country, if not the world, this is a pretty disgraceful state of affairs,' he says. 'It was the Royal Society that convened the meeting that made the wrong predictions. They are honour-bound to put it right.' He sees the process of peer review, in which specialist referees advise journal editors anonymously on a paper's fitness for publication, as partly to blame. 'If you have a consensus on the part of the leading journals and peer reviewers, nothing gets published.' He feels, however, that 'there is a form of censorship which operates which is not just peer review. There is positive discrimination, which ought to be opposed.'

Inadequacies in the peer review process have long been apparent, with refereeing seen by some as a means of 'settling old scores and burying new research', as a *New Scientist* article put it.[3] Stewart feels that the Royal Society reviewers 'took upon themselves the role of judges rather than referees…they did not answer the points raised, but commented on the way they felt things ought to be. Consensus politics are now becoming obligatory; referees are expecting people to conform. Unless you write in such a way that you do conform with the overall drift of the consensus, your paper will be rejected.'

Ultimately, the value of peer review must surely depend on the quality of editorial judgement, both in the selection of referees and in the decision on whether or not to accept their recommendations. In *Nature's* case, Maddox at least had the courage to take personal responsibility for the rejection of Stewart's work, and to offer some explanations, albeit very limited and inadequate. With the Royal Society, however, at one point a set of favourable comments by referees seems to have been discarded in favour of arbitrary rejection by an official; and then subsequently, two referees chosen whose background was such that they were incapable of addressing Stewart's argument dispassionately. It would appear that the society should indeed look again at its editorial procedures, if it wishes to maintain its reputation as a responsible scientific body.

Dangers of Anal Sex

Apart from their invective and lack of reasoned response to the alternative hypothesis, the quality of the final two referees' reports was such as to give Stewart good factual grounds for complaint. The fatalistic claim that 'individuals who have become infected with HIV have either developed Aids or are moving towards developing Aids' was demonstrably untrue in HIV-positive haemophiliacs, whose immune systems, as Stewart pointed out, had often been seen to stabilise and even recover in strength over a period of years after they were switched to a new treatment that relieved them of having to receive repeated injections of blood concentrates.

A statement by Stewart that individuals who progress to Aids are identifiable in terms of risk-behaviour and exposure to further infection had also been falsely challenged. 'This is untrue,' one referee said. 'Whilst fast and slow progressors have been identified, it has not been possible to identify why there are considerable differences in the disease progression rates of individuals.'

This view, which deprives those diagnosed as HIV-positive of any sense of control over their future, has bedevilled medical handling of the epidemic from the first and caused immeasurable harm around the world. Apart from the dramatic demonstration in HIV-positive haemophiliacs of how improvements in the quality of their blood-clotting treatment can halt immune decline, a major US study, the Multicenter Aids Cohort Study (MACS), has clearly shown that sexual behaviour has a big influence on disease progression in homosexual men.

In one analysis from this study,[4] HIV-positive men who progressed to Aids within five years (group A) were compared with those who did not (group B). It was found that 'receptive anal intercourse both before and after seroconversion with different partners was reported more frequently by men with Aids. The ratio of the differences in this sexual activity between groups A and B was higher at 12 (2.3) and 24 (2.6) months after seroconversion than before seroconversion (2.0).' The study authors concluded that 'sexually transmitted co-factors', acquired both before and after an individual became HIV-positive, 'augment (or determine) the rate of progression to Aids'.

This paper – which also counters Maddox's complaint of a lack of hard evidence supporting Stewart's 'provocative' hypothesis implicating anal intercourse as a main cause of Aids – had been published in 1992. The expert consulted by the Royal Society should surely have been aware of such an important finding.

If it had not been for the total dominance of medical and scientific thought by the HIV paradigm, earlier findings from the same study would also have been seen to give powerful support to the theory that promiscuous, passive anal sex comprised a direct threat to the immune system. As far back as 1987, MACS researchers reported in the *Lancet*[5] a very strong cause-and-effect link between anal sex and HIV-positivity. According to the HIV dogma, this link was interpreted as meaning that anal sex increased the risk of transmission of the virus, rather than being intrinsically dangerous. However, the risk was almost exclusively confined to the receptive partners. Since sexually transmitted infectious agents are bi-directional – they go both ways – the findings suggested that the key factor, while certainly associated with anal sex, was not a single infectious agent, deadly in its own right. Rather, they pointed to semen as being an obvious candidate, along with the general risks of infection with common microbes associated with a microbiologically hazardous act. HIV- positivity then appears as a marker of those who had put themselves at risk in this way.

In that earlier phase of the study, a large number of HIV-negative homosexual men were questioned about their recent sexual activity, and followed for six months, to elucidate risk factors for becoming positive. Of men who did not engage in receptive anal intercourse within six months before the start of the study and during the six-month follow-up, only 0.5 per cent (three out of 646) seroconverted to HIV. By contrast, of men who engaged in receptive anal sex with two or more partners during each of the six-month periods, 10.6 per cent (fifty-eight out of 548) seroconverted. *No* seroconversions were seen in 220 homosexual men who did not practise anal intercourse at all during the twelve months.

The gradient of increased risk of conversion to HIV-positive accelerated in proportion to the number of receptive anal partners, from about threefold for one partner to eighteen-fold for those with five or more partners. Those risk calculations were conservative, the authors wrote, because they were based only on the six-month observation period. Six of nine men who converted to HIV-positive, but who denied passive anal sex during the six-month follow-up, did report having practised that activity within the previous six months.

The authors regarded their most important finding to be much lower rates of seroconversion in men who reduced or stopped receptive anal intercourse (3.2 per cent and 1.8 per cent respectively) compared with 10.6 per cent in men who continued the practice with at least two partners. 'The public health message from these findings is clear. Reduction of this high-risk practice by homosexual men dramatically reduces risk of HIV infection.'

A prudent course would be to stop anal intercourse entirely, they said, since the study showed a three-fold greater risk of seroconversion, in six months, in the men who had passive anal sex even with only one partner. The researchers concluded: 'Avoidance of anal intercourse must be the principal focus of efforts to reduce risk in the male homosexual community. This educational message must be given the highest public health priority.'

It ought also to be a high priority in health education generally. In a survey designed to study heterosexual transmission of HIV, US researchers[6] found that whereas sixty-one out of 307 (20 per cent) of the female partners of HIV-positive men had become positive, there was only one case in which transmission appeared to have happened the other way round, from a woman to a man. This is a further strong indication that whatever is causing people to test HIV-positive, it is not a conventional, bi-directional sexually transmitted infectious agent.

Although the study did not analyse risk factors in relation to becoming HIV-positive, it did show that anal intercourse was common among the couples overall, being reported by 112 of the 307 women (37 per cent) as well as a similar proportion of the men. This is an exceptionally high proportion, probably because the study, based at San Francisco General Hospital, included a large number of bisexual men. However, the Aids years have brought numerous indications that bisexuality, and heterosexual anal intercourse, are much more common than most doctors and researchers realise. As Dr Nancy Padian, who led the San Francisco study, has commented, 'extracting sensitive risk-behaviour information is often difficult for even the most experienced interviewer'.

Men and women in impoverished communities may be particularly at risk. June Dobbs Butts, a black sex therapist in Washington, who is also an assistant professor in psychiatry and behavioural sciences at Mecherry Medical College in Nashville, Tennessee, says that despite the tragedy of a growing Aids death rate in the African-American community, 'people close their eyes to bisexuality. But reality informs me that bisexuality exists all around us.' In a survey, described in a column she wrote for the *Washington Post,* she found that many men who defined themselves as 'gay' actually grew up as bisexual. Conversely, 'many men who defined themselves as "straight" told me that growing up in city slums, same-sex behaviour was *de rigueur.* For them it was devoid of erotic significance or memory and was often associated with alcohol and drug addiction – behaviour they have renounced today, since being in recovery from such addictions.'

A European study[7] has shown that the relative risk to women of becoming HIV-positive through sex with an HIV-positive partner is increased more than five-fold in anal intercourse, compared to vaginal intercourse. Raw data from this study has shown that a massive 46 per cent of women who had anal intercourse with HIV-infected men became HIV-positive. Other risk factors for the women were having sex with a man with full-blown Aids, and a history of sexually transmitted disease in the previous five years. All these factors are consistent with Stewart's hypothesis that a general disease burden on the body arising from risk behaviours, rather than a specific infection, is the real cause of the epidemic of immune deficiency, with accompanying risk of testing HIV-positive and developing Aids.

The one case in which the US researchers presumed female-to-male transmission of HIV, from a wife to her husband, was in any case unique and fully consistent with Stewart's thesis. The couple participated in a 'swinging singles' club and, over the five years before entry to the study, the wife had over 600 male partners, including over 2,000 contacts with a bisexual man, an unidentified number of contacts with an intravenous drug user, and over 1,000 contacts with a person she knew to be HIV-positive. As part of their 'swinging' activity, the woman would often have sex with another partner while her husband first watched and then had intercourse with her himself.

Lack of Spread Outside Risk Groups

In invitations to the 1994 Tenth International Conference on Aids in Japan, the sponsors announced that '60 per cent of the world's population is now being threatened by an explosive growth in HIV infection' and a pandemic of Aids. These are the words, Stewart points out, used by the consensus on HIV in the 1980s about the pandemic of Aids which was said to threaten North America and Europe. But time has made it plain that the long-predicted 'heterosexual onslaught' is not happening. Even in New York City, an epicentre of Aids, the cumulative total of 57,769 adult cases from 1982 to April 1994 includes 54,312 (94 per cent) in the original risk groups.

The picture is similar in Britain, where out of the 8,414 cases reported to April 1994 (70 per cent in two London postal districts), 8,311 (99 per cent) were within the defined risk groups. In most of the countries of Europe and Australasia, Stewart says, Aids is so rare as to be negligible outside those groups. Cases are concentrated in a few cosmopolitan cities, where Aids continues to spread because the behaviours that cause the syndrome are also continuing.

The lack of spread outside risk groups is despite what Stewart interprets as 'a blatant attempt to create a heterosexual epidemic' by the US Centers for Disease Control, who changed the system of classification in 1993 in a way that increased the proportion of women receiving an Aids diagnosis.

The CDC's 1993 annual report on Aids gave the impression of an epidemic out of control. Overall, cases more than doubled on 1992, from 47,572 to 106,949. Those attributed to injecting drug use nearly trebled, from 11,738 to 29,399. Big increases appeared in the 'heterosexual contact' category. For example, 2,833 women and 1,232 men were reported to have caught Aids through having sex with an HIV-infected drug user, compared with 1,428 and 702 the year before. Even more alarmingly, 2,716 women and 1,997 men, a total of 4,713, were said to have got the disease from an HIV-positive partner of the opposite sex who did not fall into any special risk category, compared with totals of 788 and 736 in 1992.

Did that mark the beginning of the long-awaited explosion of heterosexual Aids? Not according to members of a Society of Actuaries task force, set up to examine concerns that Americans – and others – are being misled over the nature and extent of the Aids epidemic. They say the increases are artificial, arising from drawing an ever-widening list of conditions into the Aids net. The society, one of the most conservative and respected professional associations in the US, and which also has an international membership, is concerned at the impact on Aids statistics of several successive changes in the definition of Aids. The original definition was modified in 1985, then in 1987, and again at the beginning of 1993. Each time, more clinical conditions were added to the list of Aids-qualifying diseases, until there are now twenty-nine.

The latest changes have produced the most dramatic impact on Aids numbers. The main reason for this, according to Robert Maver, a member of the task force, is the introduction of an Aids-qualifying condition that does not even require you to be sick. People who test HIV-positive and whose immune system cells fall below a certain level can now be called Aids cases, even though they may feel fine – and even though many different lifestyle factors can affect the T-cell numbers.

Under this new category alone, more than 50,000 cases were added to the 1993 total, including thousands of cases retrospectively diagnosed from previous years. But when these and the other new 'Aids' cases – pulmonary tuberculosis, recurrent pneumonia and cervical cancer – are subtracted from the total, it turns out that the epidemic had levelled off and even probably gone into decline in 1993, the opposite of what the official statistics seemed to show.

The actuarial group, which was set up with the approval of the society's president and board of governors, is tackling two immediate tasks. The first is to quantify the relative risk levels Americans face with regard to Aids, with special emphasis on the risk to heterosexuals. Maver says 'a lot of nonsense' has been written on this subject and the group wants to help set the record straight. The second is to contribute to the debate about the true causes of Aids.

Peter Plumley, who is chairing the task force, says it is now clear that HIV is very hard to transmit to healthy people. He agrees with Stewart that the statistics demonstrate that most Aids victims are homosexual men or drug abusers who have a lifestyle that creates immune system disorders. He accepts that being sexually involved on a long-term basis with anyone in a high-risk group does carry a risk, but since the vast majority of people have neither high-risk behaviour nor a high-risk partner, their risk of HIV infection from normal sexual intercourse is so remote as to be almost non-existent – generally considered less than one chance in a million per episode, about the same as winning a state lottery or being struck by lightning.

For such people, Plumley says, 'using a condom is comparable to wearing a hard hat for a walk down Main Street – it may be theoretically possible that it could save your life, but it really isn't worth the bother and inconvenience' except for contraceptive purposes or as a protection against other sexually transmitted diseases.

Out of the 107,000 new Aids cases registered with the CDC in 1993, 4,713 were reported to have developed as a result of heterosexual contact with an HIV-positive person, with no special risk group specified. Plumley points out, however, that it is an assumption on the CDC's part that these cases came about through heterosexual intercourse, made because there was no other explanation for their illness. Because homosexuals and drug addicts often try to conceal their lifestyles, many cases attributed to 'normal' sex may actually have been linked to known risks such as anal intercourse or drugs.

Nearly all cases of Aids can be *proven* to be associated with significant health problems affecting the immune system other than HIV, Plumley says. 'Many of the cases that cannot be proved to be so associated probably in fact were, if the full facts were known. So while HIV infection may be a factor in the development of clinical Aids, health problems and immune system disorders appear to be at least as closely associated with the disease as is HIV. In view of this fact, from the viewpoint of the actuary, mortality rates would be improved far more if the focus were more on the underlying causes (street drugs, anal sex, other STDs, etc.) of the immune system disorders affecting nearly all those with Aids, rather than merely trying to find a cure for HIV.

'In other words, without HIV, people still would be dying from the many immune system disorders associated with drugs and sexually transmitted diseases. However, if people did not destroy their bodies in those ways, there probably would be few cases of HIV, and little in the way of an Aids epidemic.'

If the Society of Actuaries reaches conclusions similar to those that Stewart delivered to the WHO in 1985, and which he has been trying to persuade the scientific world to publish since 1990, perhaps he will at last win some recognition for his tireless efforts. For most of these years he has been almost alone among doctors in attempting to challenge conventional thinking on Aids.

Occasionally, another voice has been raised. As far back as February 1987, for example, Dr Brian Evans, a London genito-urinary specialist, warned that the British government's Aids education leaflets could be exaggerating the dangers of heterosexual intercourse (a message also contained in a book[8] published that year by Dr Michael Fitzpatrick, an east London family doctor). With colleagues from the Central Public Health Laboratory, Evans had found in a study of 300 gay men that passive anal sex was the only risk factor for becoming HIV-positive, with homosexual activity for more than five years the strongest predictor for seropositivity. A screening study of 200 female clinic attendees found none was HIV-positive. His findings were published in *Genitourinary Medicine,* but made no impact.

Similarly, a *Lancet* letter citing evidence of the dangers of anal sex, whether homosexual or heterosexual, was a voice in the wilderness at the time of publication (14 May 1988). Dr Victor Lorian, of the department of epidemiology and infection control, Bronx Lebanon Hospital Center, New York, wrote: 'It is unfortunate that anal sex has not been considered separately from other practices as the main mode of HIV transmission, regardless of the gender of the partners. Calls for abstinence and warnings that all forms of heterosexual activity are equally dangerous are invalid. Warnings that anal intercourse is dangerous are valid, can be understood by most lay people, and could save many lives.'

The reason that these facts were ignored was that they did not fit the theory. Since the world had been persuaded that HIV was the cause of Aids, it followed that HIV was *bound* to put the sexually active population at risk, sooner or later. If it did not happen in five years, then maybe in ten, or twenty. Besides, the HIV protagonists said, look at what is happening in Africa, where equal numbers of men and women were thought to be HIV-infected. That was said to be the future for millions of others elsewhere, even though Stewart, and a few others, insisted that the situation in Africa was far from clear. In the third world, it was very difficult and in some situations impossible to disentangle Aids from malnutrition, and from epidemics of sexually transmitted diseases and other infections in what were often chronically diseased populations. Stewart was also concerned that HIV testing, whose reliability was particularly questionable in third world conditions, might itself be causing widespread loss of life, apart from enormous unwarranted distress.

In some African countries, the stigma attached to a positive test result was so great that victims were at risk of losing their jobs, of being denied hospital treatment, and even, in the case of some mothers and children, of being thrown out of their homes.

Stewart is also distressed over the waste of time and money caused by the medical establishment's acquiescence in 'this fiction' that Aids is a threat to everyone, and that all HIV-positive people will eventually develop the syndrome. In 1993 he co-authored a paper[9] showing that the earmarking by the government of huge sums of cash for Aids prevention and treatment had caused many UK health regions to have considerably more Aids workers than patients. In an analysis of data provided by thirteen health regions in England, researchers found there were 3,400 staff overall (including the full-time equivalent of part-timers) dedicated to Aids work, and 1,800 Aids patients, an average of two to one. Separate research showed an even higher ratio in Scotland, with 550 Aids workers employed by health boards who between them had only a total of 164 Aids patients. Orkney and Outer Hebrides had three full-time staff, costing £70,000 a year, despite having no cases at all of either HIV or Aids. Another health district spent an estimated £100,000 on a counselling and testing programme that identified two people as HIV-positive.

If staff employed by local authorities, charities, research councils and industry were added, the ratio of employees to patients was higher still, the report said. 'In no other area of health service medicine is there so high a ratio of health workers to patients. Aids has provided levels of employment unprecedented in medical history in many medical and non-medical fields.'

Adoption of the deadly virus idea created an atmosphere of crisis in which resource decisions were rushed through, on the basis that regardless of actual cases, health authorities needed to prepare for and try to reduce the impact of the forthcoming disaster. But the threat was unreal in the UK. 'There is not an epidemic of either Aids cases or HIV...the projected epidemic in the general population is not occurring,' the report said. Despite continuing expert claims to the contrary, it was obvious from the distribution of Aids both in Britain and the US that lifestyle and personal behaviour were the main causes. Health campaigns should therefore be directed towards those at risk, and concentrate on preventing high-risk activities such as drug consumption and certain types of sexual behaviour. 'A number of people who are not at risk have been scared out of their wits by being told that they are, and the people who really are at risk are not receiving the attention they need,' Stewart commented.

The report acknowledged that some of the cash contributed to the fight against Aids had probably saved lives when directed to the right targets. The Mersey regional health authority, for example, despite finding itself awash with money because of a very small number of Aids cases, had directed much of this cash to combating Aids risks involved in drug misuse. But often, the special status granted to Aids had prevented surplus funds from being allocated elsewhere. It provided numerous permanent jobs, including non-medical ones like Aids education officers, counsellors, prevention coordinators, social workers and psychologists. It also created special interest groups likely to resist any cutbacks.

Barry Craven, of the University of Northumbria Business School, the paper's main author, said that for each Aids death, health authorities were spending thousands of times more on HIV prevention and research than for heart disease or cancer. It was averaging £290,000 for each person who died of Aids, compared with £50 for each death from heart disease. 'Coming fresh to the issue as an economist,' he said, 'I am surprised by the anomalous way the Department of Health and their medical advisers have arranged their priorities. I feel sure time will show it to have been the biggest misallocation of resources in the history of medicine.'

In 1994 the British government eased the strict 'ring-fencing' of Aids funds, but was still spending over £200m a year, grossly disproportionate for a syndrome producing about 1,500 cases a year. Reallocation of resources continued in 1995 as it began to become apparent to politicians and others that at the very least, the heterosexual risk had been enormously exaggerated. The medical and scientific professions had still not publicly acknowledged, debated or come to terms with the significance of such developments, however, a failure which Stewart describes as 'an absolutely monstrous deceit'. Thus, when Luc Montagnier told a British newspaper in June 1995 that there was no 'explosion' of Aids in Northern Europe and that it was wrong to frighten the public into thinking there was a high risk of catching the disease, the Aids industry was said to be in turmoil over the claims. It is essential that alternative ways of thinking about the entire Aids story should now be admitted, Stewart says.

Why, at the time of writing, are scientific leaders still refusing to comply with that call? One stated reason is concern for the sensibilities of gay men: linking Aids to sex and drugs is considered 'provocative'. Stewart regards such explanations as humbug. Thousands of gay men and drug abusers around the world are still dying because of a condition in which their immune system goes into steep decline. If this tragedy is being perpetuated, as he believes, because science – and most of the rest of us – went down the wrong road in 1984, genuine compassion would demand that a change of direction should at least be considered. Besides, the whole of the homosexual community, as well as millions of people worldwide who have tested HIV-positive, have been tainted with the HIV theory. If a mistake has been made, the longer it is perpetuated, the greater the harm. 'The immediate and knock-on effects of doubts and mistakes about aetiology, testing, diagnosis, transmission, contacts and misunderstandings generally are enormous,' Stewart says.

It seems more likely that at this point, an important component of what we are seeing is a less creditable reaction than compassion, but nonetheless still very human: the fear of being found out. None of us likes to make mistakes, but it is already clear that much is wrong with the HIV paradigm, and it may turn out to be so flawed as to present a substantial challenge to the high regard in which science and scientists are held. So the sensibilities are on the part of the scientific mainstream, as it seeks to defend an indefensible theory.

In a letter to a fellow 'dissident' scientist in the US in November 1991, Stewart wrote of his sense of a decline of integrity in scientific debate:

> We have ample proof now of unreasonable and perhaps organised resistance to the publication, not only of relevant data but also of even the simplest of questions about the HIV dogma; and we have evidence from our correspondents that the same is happening in other fields. It is time to draw attention to the wider implications of this. The whole show from Socrates onward – Magna Carta, Bill of Rights, American Constitution, UN Charter – depends upon the need no less than the right to give and take criticism. Given this, any amount of cheating in politics and public affairs can be somehow resolved. But if taboos are placed upon any criticism

> which conflicts with beliefs and opinions in official or influential quarters, we shall instantly go back to a darker age. Until now, despite efforts by almost every tyranny in history, Science has stood out as an activity characterised by and deeply respected for freedom of expression and critical debate in its efforts in any field of inquiry to get as close as possible to the truth. What we are seeing, amazingly, in our dealings with scientific journals and respected colleagues, is the reverse of this...None of us wants to be sanctimonious but I fear that the moral aspect of our experience is becoming imperative.

The ultimate lessons of the Aids years may lie in what they can teach us not just about the limitations of the germ theory, but about the limitations of science itself.

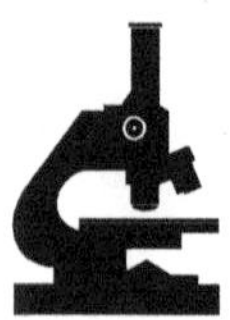

6: A CHALLENGE FROM WITHIN

We have seen how two scientists, both with much to contribute to an understanding of Aids, were easily marginalised by the Procrustean dynamics of the HIV story. Joe Sonnabend started out in a strong position to influence debate, but his multifactorial thinking suited neither the gay nor the scientific community, and, sadly, he was rapidly outmanoeuvred. Gordon Stewart's persistence, integrity and long years of experience were not enough to compensate for the fact that from the start, as a retired professor, he had no power base from which to fight. The strength of his argument meant he could not instantly be dismissed, but he was still fobbed off, albeit in a long-drawn-out process.

Peter Duesberg has created considerably more discomfort for those resting on the HIV bed. As a world expert on retroviruses, elected in 1986 to the American National Academy of Sciences for his outstanding work in that field, he proved impossible to ignore for long when he persisted in questioning the ability of HIV to do the damage attributed to it. At first the scientific mainstream made no response. Then, as Duesberg found his way into various sections of the scientific and lay press, he was gradually marginalised, and eventually ridiculed. Many leading figures in the worlds of science and medicine repeatedly insisted that there was no serious debate on Aids causation, and that it was 'stupid' to think otherwise. They implied that anyone who questioned the HIV theory must *ipso facto* have something wrong with them. When ridicule still failed to silence Duesberg, he was subjected to financial privations. He has not allowed any of these barriers to stop him. Although at the time of writing he sits disconsolate and secretary-less, stripped of a research empire that used to be funded by a $350,000 'outstanding investigator' award from the National Institutes of Health, the reality is that his persistent challenge has resulted in what is probably the mortal wounding of the HIV paradigm.

A prominent factor has been his ability to win the support of a handful of determined and effective journalistic allies. For the most part, these have not been employed by the major news media. Key allies have been John Lauritsen, of the *Native,* Celia Farber, a writer with the rock magazine *Spin,* and Joan Shenton and Jad Adams, two London television journalists working on medical and scientific programmes. Between them, these writers and documentary-makers bypassed the mental blocks that had afflicted the normal channels of scientific communication and kept dissent alive. Courage and sacrifice were also required on their part. Sometimes, they were unkindly treated not only by scientific and medical leaders, but by professional associates too.

Duesberg, who trained in chemistry, was brought from Germany's Max Planck Institute in 1964 to join the virus laboratory at the University of California at Berkeley as a young researcher. By 1970 he had become an assistant professor in molecular biology, and in that same year he and virologist Peter Vogt earned acclaim for resolving a long-standing mystery concerning a chicken tumour agent called the Rous Sarcoma Virus.

Since its discovery half a century earlier, there had been debate over the nature of this agent, which did not behave like a conventional virus. Eventually it was found that rather than killing cells, it seemed to become part of the infected cell, permanently incorporating itself into the genetic material in the nucleus. Studies at the University of Wisconsin by the late Howard Temin, who had previously worked in the virus laboratory at Berkeley, showed that in its free form the Rous agent was a small segment of genetic information encoded as RNA (ribonucleic acid) instead of the DNA (deoxyribonucleic acid) of normal viruses. This was a novel idea for molecular biologists, who previously had known RNA only as an intermediary in the process whereby genetic information stored in the nucleus of a cell is decoded in order to make the proteins the body needs. (The RNA reads off strips of information encoded in the cells as DNA.) Temin proposed that in the case of the Rous agent, and other examples of what came to be called retroviruses, the RNA worked the other way round, copying its small slug of genetic information into DNA, which then became incorporated in the host cell's DNA. He met disbelief at first, but won recognition for this theory in 1970 after isolating an enzyme, 'reverse transcriptase', that catalyses the process.

During the 1970s, Duesberg was among the first scientists to map the genetic structure of retroviruses, and describe their structural proteins. But the breakthrough that particularly excited fellow virologists, also in 1970, was to show how the Rous agent was connected to the development of cancer. This had been a profound mystery, since chickens carried many other similar agents that were entirely harmless. It turned out that the Rous agent was an aberration: it had picked up an extra gene that gave it a cancer-causing potential. When this gene was removed, the retrovirus no longer had the same ability to transform cells into a state of uncontrolled growth.

Along with Temin's discovery, this finding helped trigger an avalanche of interest – and funding – for work on retroviruses. If one of these newly characterised agents could cause cancer in chickens, it was felt, there might be others that did the same in people. Retrovirus research became a prime beneficiary of President Richard Nixon's ill-fated but hugely expensive 'war on cancer' that ran throughout the 1970s.

Much false hope and many premature claims were engendered by scientists who chose to interpret signs of the presence in cancer cells of retroviruses, or of retrovirus activity, as evidence of a viral cause for specific human cancers such as breast cancer and leukaemia. To date, most if not all such claims have proved unfounded. It is uncertain whether *any* of these agents cause disease in humans ('agent' is in some ways a better term than 'retrovirus', since the latter carries unproven connotations of disease-inducing infectiousness). The vast majority of those that have been identified in animals are also harmless. Even when they have been shown to be associated with cancer, as with the Rous agent, some scientists question whether they should really be considered infectious pathogens. Rather, they seem to appear in conditions of chronic distress in specially vulnerable animal strains, often derived from long-term animal breeding. Even though they sometimes have a gene capable of transforming normal cells into cancerous ones, those genes have been shown to originate in the DNA of *normal* cells.

It is true that as with the Rous agent, a mutated gene or collection of genes can cause cancer when injected into another animal or when brought into contact with healthy cells in the laboratory. But it now seems that the appearance of such a pathogenic 'package' of genes, and its transfer from one animal to another in such a way as to cause disease, is exceptional. Activation of these gene packages, and their release from cells in the form of the particles that have come to be known as retroviruses, may be a natural response of the cell to certain types of chronic stress, rather than signifying the presence of an unwanted invader. The connection with cancer probably comes about because chronically stressed cells are driven into increased rates of genetic activity, putting them at higher risk of developing mutations or other genetic faults.

In other words, what scientists have been calling 'retroviruses' may in reality be a part of the body's normal genetic machinery, rather than an aberration; an endogenous activity, related to multiplying the production by stressed cells of certain protein products, rather than an invasion from without.

This way of thinking is unfamiliar to those brought up with earlier ideas of genes, and the DNA of which they are made, as fixed mechanisms of inheritance, but it is in keeping with a much more dynamic model emerging from current research. 'DNA isn't this inert thing encased in Lucite, sending out instructions,' Jeffrey Pollard, a developmental biologist at Albert Einstein College of Medicine, told *Scientific American* in a 1993 review article.[1] 'It's part of the cell, and it's responding to what's happening around it.'

One of the first scientists to appreciate this dynamism was the American geneticist Barbara McClintock, who put forward the idea of transposable genetic elements, also known as transposons or 'jumping genes', as far back as 1947. She developed the theory as a result of observations made during breeding experiments on maize at Cold Spring Harbor Laboratory, when odd patterns appeared in the inheritance of pigments that conventional genetics could not explain. McClintock concluded that a few of the genes did not have fixed locations on a chromosome, but rather, they seemed to leap from one spot to another between parent and progeny. Environmental stress such as heat increased the rate at which such genes transposed. The idea of 'movable DNA' was a heresy at the time and McClintock's insights were neglected for decades, but she was awarded the Nobel Prize in 1983 for her discoveries.

It is now known that within the human genome – the totality of genes in the cell – about 10 per cent is comprised of transposons,[2] genes that can move both from one part of a chromosome to another, and from one chromosome to another. Some move around the cell in the form of an RNA intermediate, just like retroviruses, and use reverse transcriptase to integrate themselves as DNA at their new site. So-called retroviruses differ from transposons in that they have a protein coat to allow them to leave the cell and travel elsewhere in the body, but the coat is not foreign to the cell; it is made from proteins in the cell wall. There is no reason to think of these processes as necessarily abnormal or harmful, though they may well signify a genetic response to abnormal circumstances. Some scientists believe that within these mechanisms, we may be looking at ways whereby the body adjusts to environmental stresses; and even more heretically, that the mechanisms may facilitate and even direct evolutionary change, since the fruits of the alterations can sometimes be passed on to subsequent generations.

Duesberg's 1970 breakthrough earned him acclaim among fellow virologists, particularly those within the powerful retrovirology 'club'. However, he subsequently made himself very unpopular by questioning aspects of the theory of cancer-causing genes. Some genes have the job of promoting cell growth, while others have products that restrict cell growth, and an imbalance between these two, sometimes resulting from a mutation, can certainly lead to cancer. But Duesberg wanted to challenge the simplistic conclusion that because a particular gene could be shown to be associated with cancer, it was therefore 'cancer-causing'.

His perception of the need for caution in that area both stemmed from and spilled over into his doubts about some of the claims for cancer-causing retroviruses. Thus, he was sceptical when in 1980 the National Cancer Institute's Robert Gallo said he had identified a human retrovirus that was a cause of leukaemia. The scientific community has accepted this claim, despite its being unproven, and certainly unproductive in terms of prevention or treatment.

Bryan Ellison explains some of the reasons for scepticism in his self-published 1994 book *Why We Will Never Win the War on Aids.*[3] Ellison is a young biologist who spent nearly five years in various research laboratories at the University of California at Berkeley, including Duesberg's, and the book draws substantially on Duesberg's research. Ellison also investigated the recent history of science and his book holds authoritative information concerning the shaky foundations of many of the claims of the modern 'virus hunters'.

The ground for many false claims was prepared through the development of conceptual tools by which innocent viruses became implicated as causes of disease. These misconceptions then became hidden behind 'a torrent of useless and misinterpreted data', as Ellison puts it, driven by vast infusions of federal money and by the huge profits to be obtained from the test kits and vaccine funding that accompany the creation of virus scares. The biomedical research establishment had itself grown into an enormous and powerful bureaucracy, 'that amplifies obvious mistakes while stifling dissent'. Individual researchers who played along saw their careers advance, while those who raised questions became objects of derision. The public, meanwhile, 'has no choice but to take the momentary "consensus" of expert opinion at face value'.

Ellison sees these processes as having reduced opportunities for self-correction through internal challenge and debate, so that what is left cannot really be called science. With team cooperation and technical skills having replaced independent thinking, virus-hunting disasters became inevitable. In this way of thinking, the most spectacular disaster of all, the false implication of HIV in Aids, is simply the culmination of such trends.

After an embarrassing 1975 incident in which Gallo's laboratory claimed to have isolated the first human retrovirus from leukaemic cells – subsequent tests showed a contaminating mixture of retroviruses from monkeys, apes and baboons – Gallo persisted with leukaemic cells and in 1980 announced the discovery of what he called the Human T-cell Leukaemia Virus, or HTLV. This time, he found the scientific community ready to accept the idea, although some members of the retrovirology 'club', including Duesberg, had their doubts. The cells had been grown for a long time in the laboratory, and had also had to be stimulated with potent chemicals, before they began producing the package of genetic material that Gallo had interpreted as causing the leukaemia.

Still, something had emerged, and the next step was to see if leukaemia could be linked epidemiologically to the presence of antibodies indicating exposure to this agent. Ellison writes:

> With the help of other scientific teams, Gallo soon found HTLV concentrated among residents of the Japanese island of Kyushu, as well as in certain parts of Africa and among Caribbean people. Among these peoples

> also happened to exist one type of leukaemia, a disease since dubbed Adult T-cell Leukaemia (ATL). Having found an overlap between his virus and a cancer, Gallo swung the weight of scientific consensus behind his hypothesis, which now ranks among the most popular virus-cancer programmes. Even standard biology textbooks now discuss Gallo's hypothesis as unquestioned fact.
>
> But no one should worry about catching this leukaemia. By testing the blood supply, the Red Cross counted some 65,000 Americans as having been infected by HTLV, of whom about 90, or one out of every thousand, have contracted the cancer. Kyushu natives fare little worse, with only one per cent of infected people developing the leukaemia ever in their lives. For that matter, not a single American infected by HTLV through a blood transfusion has ever developed the disease. Conversely, quite a number of people worldwide have this cancer without HTLV infection.

The scientists first assumed that 'HTLV' was spread between adults, and calculated a 'latent period' between infection and disease of five years. As they found increasing numbers of healthy people with antibodies to the supposed virus, they extended the latency to ten and then to thirty years. According to Ellison, 'Once they decided the virus is transmitted sexually, while the leukaemia strikes roughly at age sixty, they subtracted twenty from sixty to generate a forty-year latent period. Then, upon realising that the virus is actually transmitted from mother to child around birth, the latent period grew to an official fifty-five years.'

There is no proof that the 'virus', even if it exists as such, is causing this disease, or a brain disorder also now attributed to it.[4] The appearance of 'HTLV' antibodies in the blood of some leukaemia victims may be a consequence rather than a cause of their condition. Nevertheless, since 1989, the American Association of Blood Banks has required a test for these antibodies to be performed on each of the 12 million blood donations handled every year, at a cost of between five and eleven dollars per test. As Ellison remarks, for scientists holding interests in the biotechnology companies producing these tests, the income is enormous.

Gallo claimed to have isolated a second human retrovirus in 1982, from a patient with a different type of leukaemia. He called it HTLV-2. Although antibodies relating to this agent have only been reported found in two patients with that form of leukaemia – and in many others who do *not* have leukaemia – the fact that a second human retrovirus was now recorded in the scientific literature lent credence to the concept that these were genuine human pathogens.

Thus, by 1984, when the Public Health Service, politicians, gay leaders, government scientists and the virological community in general were all strongly predisposed to finding a viral explanation for Aids, the ground had been prepared for ready acceptance of Gallo's claim – first at a press conference, and then through the papers published in *Science* – that what he called HTLV-3, later to be known as HIV, was the culprit.

'Seek, and Ye Shall Find a Retrovirus'

At this time, Gallo and Duesberg were still friends, fellow barons of retroviral research. Duesberg appreciated Gallo's warm-heartedness, and the political and leadership skills he had brought to bear on the research field. Gallo enjoyed Duesberg's incisive intellect and wit. Introducing him to a scientific audience in 1984, he said that he 'is a man of extraordinary energy, unusual honesty, enormous sense of humour and a rare critical sense. This critical sense often makes us look twice, then a third time, at a conclusion many of us believed to be foregone.' Gallo was also grateful to Duesberg for his work on animal retroviruses. Without the genetic map Duesberg had established for these agents, Gallo would have lacked a framework with which to make his claims for having isolated the HTLVs.

Duesberg, however, had been puzzled from the start by Gallo's claims for HIV. He knew that if you look hard enough, 'when you're in the retrovirus business you can detect a retrovirus'. He wondered what was so special about this new one that could make it the cause of such a devastating and varied disease syndrome as Aids. Checking the literature on HIV to see if there were some aspect he could investigate at Berkeley, he concluded that although an association had been shown between the virus and the disease, there was no evidence demonstrating it to be the cause.

He found that no one had been able to show appreciable levels of active virus in patients, even those with full-blown Aids. In fact, in many, the only evidence of infection was the presence of antibodies, usually a sign of the body having mounted a successful immune defence against a microbe. Furthermore, HIV antibodies were not present in all Aids patients (until later, when the CDC made their presence a condition of an Aids diagnosis). The HIV genes did appear to be present in some Aids patients, but only in a latent form, quiescent inside the cells. And they stayed that way: the idea that, like the herpes virus, HIV was waiting to strike when immunity was lowered, also did not fit. When herpes became active, antibodies increased to contain the attack, then fell. In Aids patients the virus remained dormant, even when patients were dying. 'There is no report in the literature describing the virus ever to be active in a patient, only in cell culture,' Duesberg said.

In 1986, he had taken leave from Berkeley to work for some months at a retrovirus facility in the NIH complex near Washington, which happened to be housed in the same building as Gallo's laboratory. Unknown to Gallo, Duesberg was by this time deeply involved in preparing a fundamental critique of current ideas concerning cancer genes and the role of animal and human retroviruses in the disease. He wanted to question some of the assumptions underlying much of the work on retroviruses, arguing that they were essentially harmless. He had been asked to write a major review article on this topic by the editor of *Cancer Research,* the top journal in the cancer field.

While at the NIH, Duesberg took the opportunity to test his growing conviction that HIV could not be the cause of Aids. One day, as an invited speaker at one of Gallo's regular lab seminars, after questioning the importance of cancer genes, Duesberg mentioned some of his doubts about the HIV-Aids hypothesis. Gallo took it lightly, but over following weeks became increasingly sensitive to Duesberg's questions, and resistant to talking about HIV, on one occasion storming out of a lift on the wrong floor. It became clear to Duesberg that neither Gallo nor others in his laboratory had any answers to the problem of not finding HIV active in the body, though several researchers privately admitted to Duesberg that they recognised it was an enormous difficulty.

Duesberg's article, 'Retroviruses as Carcinogens and Pathogens: Expectation and Reality', was published in the March 1987 issue of *Cancer*

Research. It was twenty-one pages long, and referenced 278 papers, many of them concerning Aids – Duesberg reckoned he had read every major paper on HIV to date. He pointed out that although it was postulated that HIV killed the T-cells which were deficient in Aids patients, there was no evidence that it did so, or even any idea of how it could do so. Besides, it appeared to be active in so few of them that even if it were to kill them all, every twenty-four or forty-eight hours, the body's ability to regenerate T-cells would far exceed the losses. Even in patients who had developed Aids, cells had to be propagated for several weeks in culture, away from the host's immune system, before evidence of either spontaneous or chemically induced virus expression occurred*. He pointed out the apparent paradox that people with a high level of antibodies to HIV, making them positive on the HIV test but also effectively preventing virus spread and expression, are considered to be those most at risk of being killed by the same virus. He questioned why in some parts of the world there were huge numbers of people testing positive, but relatively very few actual Aids cases. He asked why research among Venezuelan Indians, for example, showed that while up to 13 per cent tested HIV-positive, *none* had Aids.

Duesberg also took up the issue of Koch's postulates (first raised in relation to HIV a year previously by John Lauritsen in an appendix to *Death Rush*). These classic principles for ascertaining whether a micro-organism detected in a patient actually causes a disease were drawn up in the last century by the German bacteriologist Robert Koch. They gave no support to the HIV hypothesis.

The first, that the organism must be found in all cases of the disease, was fulfilled neither in the letter nor in the spirit. HIV was not found in all Aids patients, but that might be accounted for by deficiencies in detection techniques. More importantly, Koch's explicit expectation that a causal germ would be found in high quantities in the patient, and distributed in diseased tissues in such a way as to account for symptoms, was in no way fulfilled by HIV. It had even proved impossible to find HIV in cells from the lesions of Kaposi's sarcoma, one of the original and most obvious of the Aids-defining diseases.

* Some scientists were later to go further than Duesberg, questioning whether even after this long process there really was a virus present at all.

Duesberg accepted that Koch's second principle, that the microbe must be isolated from the host and grown in culture, had technically been fulfilled, although other scientists have since challenged this belief. As with HTLV-1, the procedure for coaxing HIV into activity is long and arduous. Active virus is not normally freely available in a patient, so instead the genetic machinery of the cell has to be driven into expression in highly artificial ways. Millions of white blood cells are taken from an Aids patient, mixed with cells taken from a patient with leukaemia (as these are cancer cells, they keep the culture going), grown in the laboratory for weeks, and subjected to chemical stimulants. Eventually a single 'virus' is released by a cell, which only then starts benignly stimulating other cells to do the same. As we shall see later, a good case can be made for questioning whether the results of a procedure of this kind can truly be considered evidence for the presence of an infectious disease agent in any conventional sense, let alone anything causally related to Aids.

The third and fourth principles, that the microbe must reproduce the original disease when introduced into a susceptible host, and be found present in the experimental host so infected, has found no support from animal experiments. When chimpanzees and other animals used as models for many human diseases are injected either with fluid from Aids patients, or with purified HIV antigens, none has developed symptoms of Aids, although they do become HIV-positive within about a month of inoculation. Not one of 150 chimpanzees inoculated with HIV since 1983 has developed Aids. There have been no documented case reports of medical workers developing Aids after accidental infection by HIV, despite more than 300,000 Aids patients being treated in the US over the past ten years by a system employing 5 million medical workers and Aids researchers. Furthermore, HIV does not kill T-cells in culture, which is another reason why it has been able to grow endlessly since 1984 in the leukaemia cell line used by Gallo.

Duesberg concluded in the *Cancer Research* paper that HIV was not sufficient to cause Aids, and that there was no evidence, besides its presence in a latent form, that it was necessary to the development of the syndrome. It seemed likely that it was just the most common among the many viral infections that had been picked up by Aids patients, and by those at risk for Aids, rather than the cause. 'The disease would then be caused by an as yet unidentified agent which may not even be a virus.'

At the start of the paper, Duesberg quoted Sherlock Holmes: 'How often have I said to you, that when you have eliminated the impossible, whatever remains, however improbable, must be the truth.' The improbable, as Jad Adams noted in an account of this early challenge to HIV,[5] was that scientists had chased after a microbe that was no more than a harmless passenger, simply because it was new and present in many Aids patients. The impossible was that it could cause a disease as serious as Aids.

The response to Duesberg's paper brought another Holmes passage to Adams's mind:

> 'Is there any other point to which you would wish to draw my attention?'
>
> 'To the curious incident of the dog in the night-time.'
>
> 'The dog did nothing in the night-time.'
>
> 'That was the curious incident,' remarked Sherlock Holmes.

Privately, some of Duesberg's colleagues admitted that they found the paper shocking, but not one came forward to *Cancer Research* with even so much as a letter in response. Peter McGee, the journal's editor, told Adams in January 1988: 'Peter Duesberg is a distinguished scientist. He is a member of the National Academy of Sciences. I knew he had these views so I asked him to contribute. There was no response at all. I was surprised, I would have thought someone like Duesberg would have elicited a response from all the big names. I would have thought people involved in retrovirology would have leapt upon it.'

Duesberg said at the time that when supporters of the HIV hypothesis were asked to comment on the paper, none wanted to reply on the record. Instead, they told reporters how terrible it was to question the hypothesis, because of the public health implications – a form of blackmail that has been used to stifle debate ever since. 'I'm convinced now they don't have the answers,' he said. 'They have made all the claims and the vested interests are so great they can't go back now. I have never seen a situation like this before. I know all the people involved here, I have known them fifteen or twenty years. We have been in the same retrovirus club. When there was a challenge to anyone's hypothesis they would strike back right away if they could. If they couldn't, they had lost the argument.'[6]

Bryan Ellison comments:

> Traditionally, such deafening silence has always been universally interpreted as a victory for the author, indicating the arguments to be irrefutable. However, despite being unable to find any flaws in the article, no researcher could afford to take on the powerful HIV-Aids establishment. Unwilling to risk status and career by challenging the growing Aids research structure, but having no arguments to defend the virus hypothesis, scientists chose the safety of quietly studying HIV. Most even rationalised their stand, convincing themselves they were actually producing beneficial 'spin-off' research by studying an 'interesting' virus, or that they were furthering science in some vague, undefined way. These researchers became quite sensitive about the virus hypothesis, reacting in anger to any criticisms.[7]

Word about the Duesberg critique nevertheless began to spread. Chuck Ortleb, the *Native's* editor, reviewed the *Cancer Research* paper favourably in June 1987, and a month later ran an interview with Duesberg, the first ever, by John Lauritsen. The following February, Lauritsen wrote a follow-up article for the *Native* on the lack of reasoned response to what he called Duesberg's 'devastating refutation' of the prevailing HIV hypothesis on Aids. No scientist in the world had attempted to refute Duesberg, nor had any scientist come forward to defend the hypothesis that HIV was the cause. 'For that matter, no paper has ever been published that systematically presented the evidence that HIV should be considered the cause of Aids.'

For months, Lauritsen had tried without success to get any of the leading government 'Aids experts' to discuss the question, 'What is the proof that HIV is the cause of Aids?' He had not been allowed to speak to them. At the National Cancer Institute (NCI), officials told him repeatedly that none of their scientists was 'interested' in discussing the aetiology of Aids. It was therefore infuriating to read Dr Anthony Fauci, director of the National Institute of Allergy and Infectious Diseases (NIAID), quoted in the *New York Times* as declaring that 'the evidence that HIV causes Aids is so overwhelming that it almost doesn't deserve discussion any more'. Lauritsen commented:

> As a member of the press, I believe I should be allowed to speak to Fauci, so that he can give me just one or two little bits of 'overwhelming evidence'

> that HIV is the cause. Or is the evidence so very overwhelming by now, that no one should even be allowed to discuss the matter? What exactly is Fauci trying to say? Does he believe that he and his colleagues have an obligation to reply to Duesberg, or is the public supposed to accept the 'Aids virus' theory as matter of faith, or perhaps as a matter of patriotism?

The *New York Times* article, published on 12 January 1988, acknowledged that 'no scientist working on Aids has published a detailed response to Dr Duesberg' and that 'scientists acknowledge that there is much they do not understand about HIV'. Its tone was generally dismissive, however, with Duesberg portrayed as a 'solitary dissenter' whose 'paper sank without a ripple in the scientific world, winning few if any converts'.

That approach, said Lauritsen, followed the tack of the NCI, whose press officers had attempted to give the impression that Duesberg's ideas were too 'off the wall' or 'insignificant' for their busy scientists to respond. But that was misleading. Rather than advancing any new theories, what Duesberg had done was put the prevailing hypothesis to the test. 'It is the HIV hypothesis that needs to be defended, not any supposedly novel ideas of Peter Duesberg.' Eventually, the NCI press office produced a statement by their chief epidemiologist, William Blattner, to the effect that 'the weight of epidemiological evidence' was against Duesberg's arguments against HIV. There were no data, no references to published material, and no attempts to address the points Duesberg had raised. In short, Lauritsen felt, it was nothing more than a stalling tactic, designed to fend off questions which the NCI was unable and unwilling to answer.

That assessment was spot on, as internal documents released to Duesberg and Ellison later revealed. On 28 April 1987, less than two months after publication of Duesberg's *Cancer Research* paper, a memo was sent from the office of the Secretary of Health and Human Services (HHS) headed MEDIA ALERT. Copies were addressed to the Secretary, Under Secretary and Assistant Secretary of HHS, and to the 'Assistant Secretary for Public Affairs', the 'Chief of Staff', the Surgeon General and 'The White House'. The memo described the situation created by Duesberg's paper, noting that 'The article apparently went through the normal prepublication process and should have been flagged at NIH.' It went on:

> This obviously has the potential to raise a lot of controversy (If this isn't the virus, how do we know the blood supply is safe? How do we know anything about transmission? How could you all be so stupid and why should we ever believe you again?) and we need to be prepared to respond. I have already asked NIH public affairs to start digging into this.

On the same day, Florence Karlsberg, an NCI public relations officer to whom Lauritsen had spoken before going to see Duesberg, sent a memo to top NIH officials reporting several inquiries about the *Cancer Research* paper, and emphasising that the Department of Health and Human Services 'is quite anxious and awaiting feedback re NIH/NCI response to and strategy for this provocative situation'. The memo added that 'Bob Gallo and others have tried to educate Peter [Duesberg] re HTLV-3 and Aids – but it's hopeless.' Karlsberg recommended forming a response team comprising Blattner, Dani Bolognesi, Anthony Fauci and Robert Gallo. 'Perhaps the epidemiologic approach might be more productive in countering Peter's assertions,' she said.

Blattner drafted a memo that went through several drafts as a potential press release, but it was never issued to the public. In another memo, dated 30 December, Karlsberg wrote that the Blattner memo 'was not pursued in June because Paul [an NIH staff member] suggested at that time that this project be put aside temporarily – at least until necessary. Alas – in the past few months, inquiries have been mounting…The calls and interest are mounting. Perhaps it's time to review and activate the attached statement.' A handwritten response on the bottom, initialled 'PVN', confirmed: 'I guess it is time to get off the dime. This isn't going away.'

Indeed it wasn't. In November 1987, the journal *Bio/Technology* published an editorial by Duesberg at the invitation of its research editor, Dr Harvey Bialy, a graduate of Berkeley and an associate professor at the University of Miami. Again, there was no answer to it, but Bialy had been struck by the logic of Duesberg's original critique and has since become a formidable proponent of the need for a reappraisal of the HIV hypothesis. He came to Duesberg's defence after an attack by *Science* a few months later, demanding fairer coverage. *Science* responded by publishing a brief written debate, with some comments from Duesberg on the one side, and from Blattner, Gallo and Howard Temin on the other. Thereafter, however, for several years, this leading science journal refused to publish anything but the occasional letter, seemingly regarding the issue as a mildly embarrassing irrelevance.

But the cat was out of the bag. In the UK, even before the *Cancer Research* article, Meditel's Joan Shenton and Jad Adams had been alerted to problems with the HIV hypothesis by researcher Michael Verney-Elliott, who was subsequently to become a linchpin of resistance to the theory, immeasurably generous to inquirers with his time and information as well as with his humour (he once summed the story up by saying, 'From the people who didn't bring you the virus which causes cancer, it's the virus that doesn't cause Aids'). Meditel interviewed Duesberg in the summer of 1987 and a film featuring his critique, *Aids: The Unheard Voices,* received the Royal Television Society Award for the best international current affairs documentary for that year, although there was little in the way of recognition or debate outside television circles; the film went out into 'a pool of silence', as Joan Shenton later described it.

In January 1988, *Spin* magazine became the first general circulation publication to put Duesberg's case before the public, with a column and interview by Celia Farber. The introduction went straight to the point:

> The HIV virus is thought to be the cause of Aids, but there's strong evidence that it isn't. The frightening truth is that no one knows for sure, and few scientists are admitting it. Are precious time, money, and lives being lost while we fight a harmless virus?

As well as setting out the essence of Duesberg's scientific case, Farber asked him how his theory had been received by the scientific community. Duesberg replied:

> Those who are really direct targets of this – who are working closely with it and making these major claims that HIV is what causes Aids – have not responded at all directly. And indirectly, well, I know them. Like Bob Gallo, for instance, we are old friends. I spoke to him two weeks ago, and he said, 'With friends like you, who needs enemies?' And he literally runs away from me. Usually when you challenge a major hypothesis, you get a rebuttal, but here it's total avoidance. They don't want to talk, they don't want to be

> seen by me. A few examples: I was at the NIH two months ago, in the same building where Gallo works. We went to the movies, and I said, 'Look, Bob, I really don't believe these claims. I am really convinced now that it can't be so. You have to find another explanation.' He's certainly not a shy person, but ever since, he just doesn't want to be seen arguing or talking about it with me, not even at a party. There was a party with mutual friends of ours who invited us because they wanted to see us debate it, and he refused to come. We were both invited to a memorial meeting for a colleague. Gallo said, 'Is Peter Duesberg coming? Because if he comes, I don't want to come on the same day.' It's very strange.

Asked how it was possible for the entire scientific community, in the face of a serious epidemic, to turn their backs on scientific method and accept, without scrutiny, that this was the Aids virus, Duesberg commented:

> It gives a lot of comfort to say here's the virus and this is the cause. If you say who's done it you'll feel much better, even if it's a monster.

He also spoke of how 'the veterans of the virus cancer programme' – including himself – who had made names and careers for themselves, and developed tremendous skills, were looking for a cause. 'So you show us a new windmill, and we are marching.' Money was a very real contributing factor. Scientists researching Aids were much less inclined to ask scrutinising questions about the cause of Aids when they had invested huge sums in companies whose future rested on the HIV theory. Two of the top five Aids researchers in the country had millions in stocks in a company they founded that had developed Aids kits to test for HIV. And entire reputations depended on the virus.

> The stakes are too high now. Ten years ago, when they were lower, theories could be exchanged and examined more rationally. This cannot be done now. Gallo's lab works so closely with the news media. Every progress report from their laboratories is discussed by Dan Rather and Barbara Walters, *Newsweek*, and *Time* magazine. Every little observation

is in all newspapers. To say that now, maybe, the antibody wasn't worth committing suicide for or burning houses for, would be very embarrassing.

SPIN: Obviously, you must consider the mass testing for HIV antibodies to be an absolute farce.

DUESBERG: Oh yes, of course. The whole thing is a hoax.

Duesberg also gave *Spin* the beginnings of an alternative theory on the cause of Aids. He doubted that it was any kind of a contagious agent – a germ – since casual contact was not enough to cause it, and there was an absolute preference for males. 'There is no such thing as a germ that would prefer Rock Hudson over Cheryl Tiegs.' To get Aids, you needed intimate contact, involving the exchange of human cells. But a virus, by definition, was a 'cell-free infection', something that could be transmitted without transmitting cells – from sneezing or towels or whatever.

Lifestyle probably had a lot to do with it. The 'acquired' in Aids didn't mean it must be a virus or bacterium. 'You can acquire lung cancer from smoking cigarettes, and a number of diseases, as well as immune deficiencies, from shooting up heroin, and even from anal intercourse. It's not great for your health to do that every day.'

Gallo did not respond to repeated attempts by *Spin* to reach him before Farber's article was published. The following month, however, the magazine published a telephone interview obtained by reporter Anthony Liversidge, who had persisted in dialling Gallo's number dozens of times until one night the lab chief picked up the phone himself. His hurt and upset were evident. 'The whole world...everyone is working on the problem of this virus causing Aids,' he said. 'Every virologist on earth will tell you the same thing... Everyone knows this is the cause of Aids. Except maybe two people. There is no debate. Call 5,000 scientists and ask.'

On the question of low virus titre, he said: 'Hasn't Duesberg ever understood indirect mechanisms in cell killing? There are immune responses to the virus that destroy the proliferation of the T-cell. That's crystal-clear now. It is not just a matter of the virus going in and killing the cell directly. Does that take a genius?' He added that HIV 'kills like a truck', as every thinking scientist in the world knew. 'HIV would cause Aids in Clark Kent, given the right dose and the right strain of the virus. Given the right dose and the right route of administration and the right time in someone's life. Alone and of itself. No doubt in my mind. However, that doesn't mean co-factors can't make things more likely.'

Spin was to return to the controversy repeatedly over subsequent years, keeping the issue alive when it had all but died elsewhere. But the major media in the US have so far proved unable to explore the arguments in any depth. According to Ellison,[8] several prospective TV interviews with Duesberg were cancelled at the last minute as a result of behind-the-scenes manoeuvring by NIH chiefs. The *New York Times* had mentioned Duesberg only four times in seven years, every time attacking him. The *Washington Post* had done likewise, with one hostile article and one small, neutral piece.

Duesberg even began to be excluded from scientific gatherings, after Gallo, Fauci and others refused to attend conferences if Duesberg was to be allowed to make a presentation. As a result, many of the invitations stopped. Publication of papers also became difficult, even in the *Proceedings of the National Academy of Sciences*, where members such as Duesberg have a right to appear without the standard peer review.

Duesberg's Case Against HIV

Nevertheless, the *Proceedings* have twice given Duesberg a chance to set out his case in detail. The first paper, submitted in June 1988 and originally rejected, was published in February 1989 after a change of editor and nine months of hurdles posed by hostile reviewers and disputed points. It was nearly 10,000 words long, with 200 references, and represented a huge amount of work.

Duesberg began by acknowledging that the basis for the HIV hypothesis was a correlation between risk of Aids and the appearance of HIV antibodies detected by the 'Aids test', and then set out to show that this did not mean HIV was the cause of the syndrome. In a style which has often been enormously irritating to his opponents, he argued that premature acceptance of the hypothesis had given rise to several 'surprising' paradoxes (references excluded):

> The early adoption of the virus-Aids hypothesis by the US Department of Health and Human Services and by retrovirologists is the probable reason that the hypothesis was generally accepted without scrutiny. For instance, the virus is typically referred to as deadly by the popular press, and public enemy number one by the DHHS. In view of this, it is surprising that the virus has yet to cause the first Aids case among hundreds of unvaccinated scientists who have propagated it for the past five years at titres that exceed those in Aids patients by up to six orders of magnitude with no more containment than is required for marginally pathogenic animal viruses. It is also surprising that despite 2,000 recorded (and probably many more unrecorded) parenteral [needlestick] exposures to HIV-infected materials, unvaccinated health care workers have exactly the same incidence of Aids as the rest of the US labour force. Further, it is difficult to believe that a sexually transmitted virus would not have caused more than 1,649 sex-linked Aids cases among the 125 million American women in eight years — and this number is not even corrected for the antibody-negative women who might have developed such diseases over an eight-year period. Moreover, it is paradoxical for a supposedly new viral epidemic that the estimates of infected persons in the US have remained constant at 0.5 to 1.5 million or even declined to less than 1 million since the 'Aids test' became available in 1985.

He then set out in detail the evidence that active HIV is so hard to find that it cannot account for the loss of T-cells and the clinical course of Aids, a case that even Gallo had already implicitly acknowledged by his invocation of 'indirect mechanisms in cell killing'.

He also discussed the difficulty of isolating the virus, and the fact that even when inoculated into either animals or humans, HIV does not lead on to Aids. Four women who received HIV-positive semen during fertility treatment in 1984 had developed antibody to HIV, but none had developed Aids, nor had they transmitted the virus to their husbands. Three of the women had become pregnant, and their babies were healthy. Furthermore, in fifteen to twenty cases of accidental infection of health care workers, or scientists propagating HIV, during the last four years, in which infection was identified on the basis of antiviral antibodies, none had developed Aids. There was just one case cited in which an HIV-positive health care worker was said to have developed Aids, reportedly after occupational exposure. But there were no data on gender, latent period or symptoms. Besides, a subsequent study that included this case described only transient, fever-like symptoms, but not one Aids case among occupationally infected health workers.

Blood transfusions were another source of documented cases of HIV infection, but transfusion-related Aids cases occurred mainly in people with other health risks, such as haemophilia, and there were no controlled studies, comparing like with like, to show that HIV-positive transfusion recipients had more of the diseases now called Aids than those without antibody to HIV.

The idea that HIV caused Aids after progressively destroying the immune system for two years in the case of children, and an average of eight years in adults (now increased to ten-to-fifteen years or more), was bizarre. After twenty-four years working with retroviruses, Duesberg knew of no example of any other virus capable of such a feat. Although the retroviruses and herpes viruses could persist in the body, it was normally only as truly latent infections. That is, while the immune system remained strong, they did no damage. When symptoms recurred, because of a decline in immunity caused by something else, it was because the virus had become reactivated; but that was not the case in Aids, because no free HIV could be found.

Duesberg cited numerous other biochemical, genetic and epidemiological reasons for his central conclusion, that HIV is like some 50-100 other harmless, idle retroviruses that sit in the human genome, and has nothing to do with the multiplicity of Aids diseases, which are caused by a multiplicity of risk factors. The sophistication of modern molecular biology meant that 'we can now…detect latent viruses or microbes at concentrations that are far below those required for clinical detectability and relevance'. That was why it was necessary to re-examine the claims that HIV is the cause of Aids.

Recognition of the fact that HIV was for the most part inactive in the body had led to a variety of theories as to how it might cause Aids indirectly. One was that it might work in some way similar to the hepatitis virus, which is believed to be able to cause cancer many years after infection. But what happened in such cases was not at all comparable with Aids. The hepatitis virus was thought able to integrate a gene or genes at a specific site in the cell's genome, in such a way that a normal gene became a cancer gene. That cell would then grow out of control and become a tumour. But that was a rare event, and a single event, and there were no grounds for believing that any such interaction could cause the loss of billions of cells during a degenerative disease like Aids.

It was also hard to accept that HIV could cause Aids through an autoimmune process, partly because there was so little of it. In addition, although it was true that auto-immune processes could occasionally be triggered by viruses, it was only the very rare patient in whom that happened, whereas HIV was thought to cause Aids in 50-100 per cent of those infected.

Duesberg accepted that in the US and Europe, antibody to HIV might serve as a surrogate marker for the risk of Aids. Because HIV was so difficult to transmit, it specifically identified those who habitually received transfusions, or intravenous drugs, or who were promiscuous. Indeed, there was a well-established direct correlation between the probability of being antibody-positive and *frequency* of drug use, transfusions and male homosexual activity. Once picked up by such patients, HIV could persist as a minimally active virus in a small number of cells, just enough to provoke the immune system into maintaining antibodies to it. Chronic exposure to such lifestyle risks appeared to provide a biochemically more tangible and plausible basis for Aids than an 'idle' retrovirus, as did the well-documented immunosuppressive effects of malnutrition and parasitic infections in developing countries. The doses of Factor 8 received by haemophiliacs were directly proportional to subsequent immune deficiencies. Epstein-Barr virus, cytomegalovirus, herpes simplex virus, and administration of blood components and Factor 8 had all been shown to cause immune deficiency not only in HIV-positive haemophiliacs, but in those who tested HIV-negative as well.

Duesberg mentioned for the first time in this paper his opposition to the use of anti-HIV drugs such as AZT, later to become one of his central concerns. Since there was no proven mechanism whereby HIV could cause Aids, he argued, the use of these drugs had no rational basis. Since AZT, originally developed as cancer chemotherapy, killed dividing blood cells and other cells, it was directly immunosuppressive.

In response to arguments that Aids was new, whereas the lifestyle factors were old, Duesberg argued that the major risk groups, homosexuals and drug-takers, had only become visible and acceptable in the US and Europe during the previous ten to fifteen years, about the same time that Aids became visible. That change had facilitated risky behaviour, and the particular permissiveness seen in some metropolitan centres had encouraged the clustering of cases that made it easy to detect Aids.

This analysis, Duesberg concluded, offered several benefits, one of which was that it ended the fear of infection by HIV because it proved that HIV could not cause Aids on its own, although it remained to be seen whether it played any part in the syndrome. Studies were now needed to see whether people with antibodies to HIV really did become ill more often than HIV-negative people who had exactly the same level of risk behaviours in their lives.

In August 1990, Duesberg submitted another paper to the *Proceedings*, this time concentrating on the epidemiology, arguing that the evidence pointed much more strongly to drug use as the main cause of Aids, rather than to HIV. The paper was rejected. Duesberg then resubmitted the first part of the paper, concentrating on the challenge to HIV, and that was eventually published in February 1991. In it, he reiterated the argument which Sonnabend and Callen had propounded, that pathogens linked to abnormal lifestyles may be the real causes of Aids. The statistics strongly supported this: 97 per cent of American Aids patients were from groups in which special health risks had been identified, either to do with lifestyle, as with sex and drugs, or clinical treatment, as with the transfusion of blood and blood products.

But what about people who became sick with Aids who had none of the risk factors in their lives? Duesberg pointed out that to date, those comprised a total of 3,900 cases in the US, accumulated over the past nine years, and covering twenty-five Aids-defining diseases which in themselves were not new. To determine whether those illnesses were really caused by HIV, their incidence should be compared with that in the normal, HIV-free population. However, that had not been done, because the diseases were only reportable and recorded by the CDC as Aids if HIV was present.

Surprisingly, in view of the many claims that HIV causes Aids in haemophiliacs, there was not one controlled study that had found HIV to be a health risk. There was a low annual incidence of Aids-like diseases in haemophiliacs, but that was likely to reflect illness related to the inherited condition itself and its treatment, rather than HIV. Severe immunodeficiency had been reported in HIV-negative haemophiliacs. The greater the amount of Factor 8 clotting factor they had received, the greater the deficiency.

The theory that blood transfusions contaminated with HIV caused Aids in other patients was entirely uncontrolled: that is, no one had checked to see whether people with matching conditions, who had received the same amount of blood but who did NOT become HIV-positive, had any less risk of immune deficiency and disease. In fact, there was good evidence that taken as a whole, patients receiving transfusions were a very high-risk group. In one US study, half of a group of patients who received a blood transfusion were dead within a year, and another showed that more than 60 per cent were dead within three years. In other words, people in need of transfusions were often very sick anyway, regardless of HIV, and there was no reason to blame their subsequent illness on HIV just because sophisticated tests were now available to detect antibodies to the virus.

Other risk groups also had conditions indicative of Aids without HIV. Kaposi's sarcoma, and various immunodeficiencies, were seen in HIV-negative gay men, for example. And in a group of twenty-one heroin addicts, of whom only two were HIV-positive, the ratio of helper to suppressor T-cells was found to decline within thirteen years to the level typical of Aids. Among intravenous drug users in New York representing 'a spectrum of HIV-related diseases', HIV was not observed in twenty-six of fifty pneumonia deaths, fifteen of twenty-two endocarditis deaths, and five of sixteen tuberculosis deaths.

Duesberg reiterated that since HIV became detectable with the 'Aids test' in 1985, the number of infected Americans had remained at around a million, or 0.4 per cent of the population. Likewise, the percentage of HIV-positive US Army recruits had stayed at around 0.03 per cent for five years, although more than 70 per cent of seventeen- to nineteen-year-olds were sexually active. 'The strikingly constant incidence of HIV indicates that it is epidemiologically not new in the US and thus not a plausible cause for the new epidemic Aids.'

In fact, because of HIV's chronic latency, it could hardly ever be found either in semen or in T-cells, which meant it was very hard to transmit sexually. That was in keeping with what was known about retroviruses from both animal and human studies: since the virus was normally locked up in the cells, they depended almost exclusively on 'vertical' transmission, down the generations from mother to child, rather than on 'horizontal', person-to-person spread. Practices involving the exchange of cells, such as unsterile drug use, multiple transfusions and promiscuous anal sex, could also transmit the virus, but in Duesberg's view it was just as harmless in those circumstances as when transmitted perinatally.

Among children with Aids, 95 per cent in the US were subject to disease-causing conditions regardless of HIV, caused either by the mother's drug addiction or by deficiencies of their own that required blood transfusions. The few remaining cases probably reflected the normal background incidence of childhood disease, called Aids because the mother, though healthy, had passed on HIV perinatally.

The Drug-Aids Hypothesis

Duesberg had been repeatedly asked, 'If it isn't HIV, what is it?' This is a natural question, even though it might be illogical to expect a world expert on retroviruses to answer it, just because he felt he had demonstrated it was not HIV. The argument that there were probably different explanations for different cases, falsely unified by the newly available techniques for counting T-cells and for detecting retroviral antibodies, was somehow less satisfying than the virus theory.

Perhaps partly in response to such pressures, from 1990 onwards Duesberg was to put increasing emphasis on what he called the 'drug- Aids hypothesis', in which he identified an explosion of drug use as the main cause of the epidemic of Aids in America. He gave a brief summary of this hypothesis in the final paragraph of his truncated *Proceedings* paper, but all efforts to persuade the editor to take the other half of the paper, arguing the detailed case, came to nothing, making him the second member in the 128-year history of the academy to have a paper rejected from its journal (the first, apparently, was Linus Pauling, who had argued that vitamin C might prevent cancer). Duesberg had taken advice from several scientific colleagues in writing it, but it was sent out to three anonymous referees by the editor, two of whom voted to block it. One called any questioning of the HIV hypothesis 'extreme and highly dubious' and warned that the drug-Aids hypothesis 'has a potential for being harmful to the HIV-infected segment of the population'. A similar comment came from one of four new reviewers to whom the paper was sent after a further change of editor at the *Proceedings*. If it was published, he wrote, 'one is further tempted to blame the victim'. All four recommended against publication. So did a further three anonymous reviewers who were asked for an assessment by the new editor, after it was resubmitted by another academy member with favourable comment from four other scientists.

Shortcomings of the peer-review process are evident in these events. The reference to 'the HIV-infected segment of the population' makes it clear that for that reviewer at least, there was no room for doubt about HIV as the cause of Aids; and hence to allow public questioning of the theory would of course be an irresponsible act. Worse still, Duesberg was now including ill-effects from AZT – by this time adopted by the medical profession as the mainstay of Aids treatment – as a major risk factor for Aids, allegedly extending and amplifying the epidemic. He was even discouraging HIV-positive people and Aids patients from taking AZT. For the medical profession, with its firm belief that HIV-positivity represented a deadly infection, this public challenge was the biggest sin imaginable, not least because of the damaging effect on physician-patient relationships. The referees who voted down Duesberg's paper would have done so in the belief that they were protecting the public from dangerous nonsense.

Such *beliefs* did not address the logic of Duesberg's case. Furthermore, the human mind is very clever at finding justification for manoeuvres that are essentially self-protective as being in the interests of others. The drug-Aids theory confronted doctors treating Aids patients with some unimaginably awful possibilities concerning their professional competence and role. There was particular hurt among Aids doctors at having their authority challenged by a 'chemist', as Duesberg's opponents liked to call him.

However, whereas an embarrassed silence, followed by a grudging, gradual and limited acceptance, followed Duesberg's retrovirology-based strictures over the 'lethal virus' theory, he was now moving into a position in which he became vulnerable to direct counter-attack. By focusing on a narrow group of risks, the drug-Aids hypothesis had the advantage both of being more easily testable, in a scientific sense, and more easily understood as an alternative to HIV than the multifactorial approaches favoured by Sonnabend and Stewart. But because it excluded other risks, it had the disadvantage of presenting a clear-cut target through which Duesberg's many opponents could hit back at him, in an area where relatively little research had been performed by anyone, let alone by Duesberg himself.

The idea that the explosion of drug-taking seen during recent decades was a primary factor in Aids was not at all unreasonable. It was a hypothesis considered at the outset, albeit very briefly, by the CDC, and although long propounded by John Lauritsen, it had never been properly investigated.

An enormous escalation of drug-taking started in the US after the Vietnam War, with cocaine seizures rising from about 500 kilograms in 1980 to 100,000 kilograms in 1990. The number of dosage units of domestic stimulants confiscated, such as amphetamines, rose from 2 million in 1981 to 97 million in 1989. These seizures reflected increased consumption, not just better drug control, as was witnessed by a twenty-four-fold increase in cocaine-related hospital emergencies – from 3,296 to 80,355, and with deaths up from 195 to 2,483 – between 1981 and 1990.

There was evidence that long before 1980, injecting drug users died of the diseases that later came to be called Aids. But they became more visible as victims of immune deficiency from 1980 onwards, partly because their numbers increased as a result of the drug epidemic, but more importantly because from 1980 onwards, techniques for counting T-cells became routine.

It was that same T-cell counting technology that highlighted the immune deficiency 'acquired' by haemophiliacs after many years of treatment with the blood concentrates developed during the 1960s and 1970s. Many also tested HIV-positive, because a high rate of infection resulted from pooling blood from large numbers of donors, but there was no evidence that HIV caused their immune deficiency, nor that their condition was infectious. The deficiency came about because of the repeated assault on the immune system arising from having other people's blood proteins injected into them.

Further, the recreational use of psychoactive and aphrodisiac nitrite inhalants had begun in the 1960s and reached epidemic proportions in the mid-1970s, a few years before Aids appeared. According to the National

Institute on Drug Abuse (NIDA), in 1979-80 over 5 million people used nitrite inhalants in the US at least once a week.

Numerous correlations linked Aids with drug consumption, and with the malnutrition that often accompanied heavy and addictive drug use. The syndrome appeared in the groups in whom drug-taking had increased, but not elsewhere. Those in the gay community who were getting Aids had been heavy drug users almost without exception, and usually for many years. A French study among homosexual men who had all inhaled nitrites found that those with Aids were significantly older – approximately ten years – than those without Aids. Other researchers had pointed to a time lag of seven to ten years between onset of chronic drug use and the development of Kaposi's sarcoma. A German study saw Kaposi's sarcoma in an HIV-negative man after he had inhaled nitrites for ten years. Female prostitutes only developed Aids when they were drug abusers.

Most babies with Aids were born to drug-abusing mothers. When they died, there was no need to invoke HIV as the cause. Many studies showed physiological and neurological deficiencies, including mental retardation, in children born to mothers addicted to cocaine and other narcotics, regardless of HIV. In one example, ten HIV-negative infants born to mothers who were addicted to taking drugs intravenously had diseases that would have been called Aids if they had tested positive, including failure to thrive, persistent generalised swollen lymph glands, persistent oral Candida and developmental delay. Another study found that one HIV-positive and eighteen HIV-negative babies born to drug-addicted mothers had only half as many white blood cells as normal babies. At twelve months after birth, the capacity of the cells to proliferate was 50-70 per cent lower than normal. In 1991, a European collaborative study of children born to HIV-positive mothers reported that those with drug withdrawal symptoms were most likely to develop diseases, those with no withdrawal symptoms but whose mothers had used recreational drugs in the final six months of pregnancy were intermediate on all indices, while children of former drug users did not differ significantly from those born to women who had no history of intravenous drug abuse.

Also in 1991, a review article[9] entitled 'Aids, Drugs of Abuse and the Immune System: A Complex Immunotoxicological Network' concluded that there was overwhelming evidence, both circumstantial and direct, of a possible role for drug-induced immunosuppression. 'What is required now is better and more accurate detection of substance abuse, a direct elucidation of the immune and related mechanisms involved, and appropriate techniques to analyse it.' Nearly three-quarters of all American Aids patients were men aged twenty to forty-four, and NIDA surveys showed that men in that same age group accounted for a similar proportion of 'hard' drug-taking.

Aids was new because the drug epidemic was new, according to Duesberg, whereas HIV was a long-established, perinatally transmitted retrovirus, probably 'as old as America', which only appeared new because, being chronically latent, it only became detectable with recently developed technology. This was why, contrary to predictions, Aids did not explode into the general population.

The drugs hypothesis of American Aids also resolved the long-standing paradox that 'Aids' in Africa had a completely different time course, involving mostly different diseases, compared with Aids in the US and Europe: it had different causes. Because of the HIV-based Aids definition, a new drug epidemic in America and an epidemic of old Africa-specific diseases like fever, diarrhoea and tuberculosis were both called Aids when HIV became detectable. But they were not the same disease syndrome.

'Aids by Prescription'

As a central part of his drug-Aids theory, Duesberg also took up and developed a critique of the anti-HIV drug AZT. He argued that the mode of action of this drug was such that it must eventually *cause* Aids when given to people who had tested HIV-positive, but were otherwise healthy. Because it blocked DNA synthesis, it killed dividing cells anywhere in the body, causing ulceration, haemorrhaging, damage to hair and skin, wasting away of muscles, and destruction of the immune system and other blood cells. Uncritical acceptance of the HIV story had in any case been a disaster for those who tested antibody-positive. They had been given to understand that they were the doomed victims of a freak biological event, and that there was nothing they could do to alter their fate – a prophecy that could so easily become self-fulfilling. Giving them AZT amounted to 'Aids by prescription'; yet belief in AZT had also become a part of Aids ideology.

Much groundwork on AZT had been covered by John Lauritsen, who in a long series of articles published in the *Native*, and in *Poison by Prescription: The AZT Story*, had analysed the studies that allegedly demonstrated the drug's effectiveness, and concluded that there was no scientifically credible evidence that it had benefits of any kind. Although individual doctors insisted the drug did appear capable of producing short-term relief in patients whose immune systems had collapsed, those benefits – if indeed attributable to the drug itself, as opposed to a 'placebo' effect arising from the patient's hope in the drug – were rapidly outweighed by AZT's toxicity. There was no scientific case whatsoever for taking such an unquestionably toxic substance for such paltry returns, in fact every reason not to do so. According to some doctors, at least the same level of relief, without the devastating ill-effects, could be achieved by using well-established anti-microbial drugs to counter the specific diseases afflicting patients.

Documents obtained from the Food and Drug Administration through the Freedom of Information Act showed that the main trial of AZT, on the basis of which the drug received its licence, was invalid, because many of the rules for the conduct of such studies had been broken. It became apparent at an early stage, to both patients and doctors, who was receiving active drug and who was on the placebo (the dummy pill). The death rate among the placebo patients was far higher during the few weeks of the trial than ever seen before or since among Aids patients, suggesting either that a disproportionate number were at death's door before the trial began, or that their deaths were accelerated because of their being deprived of conventional treatment for their infections during the course of the trial. Nearly half the patients on AZT, by contrast, were kept alive with blood transfusions, needed to overcome the anaemia caused by the treatment. Deaths in the AZT group accelerated after the trial was prematurely ended.

Most of these shortcomings had become apparent before the drug was given its licence, and they were the subject of extensive discussions. But the concerns were put on one side after intervention by a senior official of the FDA, which was under immense public and political pressure to fast-track an Aids drug on to the market.

Although taken off the shelf (as a failed anti-cancer drug) and investigated for its anti-viral potential by Burroughs Wellcome, the American arm of the British-based drug company Wellcome, AZT was hugely important to the two key US government institutions involved in the Aids fight, the NCI and the NIAID. Both were intimately involved in its testing and promotion, and key officials, particularly Dr Sam Broder, the NCI's clinical director, had worked extremely hard to get it to market. Burroughs Wellcome acknowledged this with a $55,000 donation, in 1985, in support of work on Aids at Broder's laboratory, and a further $25,000 the following year. That did not prevent Broder (later to become director of the NCI) from becoming furious with David Barry, the company's vice-president of research, for making out at a 1987 inquiry into AZT's $10,000-a-year price tag that the drug was developed within the company with hardly any help from others. 'I view AZT as the battle of El Alamein,' Broder was to declare later. 'It is symbolic that we can do something against the virus that causes Aids; that we can make progress; that those who preached that it was inherently untreatable were wrong.'

In effect, AZT became an official government drug, a kind of talisman for HIV. Despite Lauritsen's dismissiveness of all the research surrounding it, some severely ill Aids patients did improve in the short term, and there were laboratory indications of potential benefit. Nevertheless, there has been a totalitarianism about its marketing – not just in the US, but in the UK and elsewhere – that has been truly shameful and frightening. The hundreds of millions of dollars that it earned, along with the fact that it held a flagship role in the fight against HIV, helped generate a climate of opinion in scientific, medical and political circles that was fiercely intolerant of any alternative approaches to Aids. Left-wing author Martin Walker performed a monumental research effort in documenting these abuses of power, which included putting enormous pressure on Aids patients to take the drug, in his 1993 book *Dirty Medicine*.[10]

The Department of Health and Human Services, which had launched HIV to the world in 1984, did the same with a press conference for AZT in September 1986. It also issued press releases in August 1989, again on the basis of a prematurely terminated study, claiming that AZT 'delays progression of disease in certain HIV-infected persons who have not yet developed symptoms'. DHHS secretary Dr Louis Sullivan said the finding was a milestone in the battle to change Aids from a fatal disease to a treatable one. 'These results provide real hope for the millions of people worldwide who are infected with HIV.'

The announcement sent sales of AZT soaring over the next few years, with 'early treatment' becoming the new hope for effectiveness, until a much longer, more carefully conducted study involving Britain's Medical Research Council and French government scientists (the 'Concorde' trial) demonstrated that the drug proved worse than useless in the HIV-positive people who took part. Side-effects were considerable, though not as devastating – in the controlled circumstances of a major trial – as some of AZT's opponents had feared. Over the three years of the trial there were seventy-nine Aids-related deaths in the AZT group, compared with sixty-seven in the 'deferred treatment' group, a difference which, although declared statistically insignificant, was certainly pointing in the wrong direction. Further, there were nearly twice as many 'non-HIV-related' deaths in the AZT group over the period of the study – sixteen, compared with nine. So in all, ninety-five of the patients on 'early treatment' died, compared with seventy-six whose treatment was deferred. The gap might have been even larger if those 'deferred treatment' patients had been spared AZT completely. Findings pointing in a similar direction had been made public in 1991 from a US study headed by Dr John Hamilton, but largely ignored.

To people like Lauritsen, who knew the data and its deficiencies inside out, and Duesberg, whose conviction that HIV was harmless rendered the entire AZT exercise a cruel deception from the start, the persistence with which Burroughs Wellcome, the NIH and the medical profession promoted AZT was unforgivable. Lauritsen, who first used the phrase 'iatrogenic genocide' for the mass prescription of the drug to gay men, wrote in the *Native* in January 1991:

> Those who have eyes to see are witnessing genocide – the genocide of gay men. Millions of dollars are now being spent on an international advertising campaign, 'Living With HIV', in which gay men and other members of 'risk groups' are being told: Get tested for antibodies to HIV – if you 'test positive' you need 'medical intervention' which could 'put time on your side'. The 'medical intervention' is AZT (also known as Retrovir and zidovudine), and

the campaign is paid for, directly and indirectly, by Burroughs Wellcome, the manufacturer of AZT.

The campaign consists of a phoney diagnosis followed by a lethal treatment. Already tens of thousands of objectively healthy gay men have been scared and bullied and bamboozled into taking AZT, allegedly in order to 'slow the progression to Aids'. Optimism regarding their prognosis would be foolish. Except for the lucky few who stop 'treatment' in time, they will die. Death is the inevitable biochemical consequence of taking AZT, for the fundamental action of the drug is to terminate DNA synthesis, the very life process itself.

The only explanations Lauritsen could find for such behaviour were homophobia, and profit. Bruce Nussbaum, in *Good Intentions,*[11] a remarkable account of the mishandling of Aids research during the 1980s, offered a more sophisticated but no less chilling description of what he found during hundreds of hours of interviews with the leading players. Despite his twenty years as a journalist, he wrote, much of it covering business and finance for *Business Week,* he was not prepared for the behind-the-scenes realities of big-time medical research.

On Wall Street, the financial crooks, the insider traders, knew for the most part that they were cheating, breaking the law. The games they played were new...but the corruption itself was as old-fashioned as embezzlement.

Nothing of the sort exists in medical science. In that arena, people have good intentions. They believe they are doing good works for the general health of the nation. Indeed, personal corruption is still rare, although faking experimental data appears to be on the rise. The corruption in medical science goes much deeper. It derives from the very way the Food and Drug Administration, the National Institutes of Health, and the dozen or so elite academic biomedical research centres work with private drug companies. An old-boy network of powerful medical researchers dominates in every disease field, from Aids to Alzheimer's. They control the major committees, they run the most important trials, they determine what gets published and who gets promoted. They are accountable to no one. Despite the billions of taxpayer dollars that go to them every year,

> there is no public oversight. Medical scientists have convinced society that only they can police themselves. Yet behind the closed doors of 'peer review', conflicts of interest abound. These are not perceived as conflicts of interest by the scientists themselves. The researchers are convinced that they have only good intentions.

AZT, Nussbaum found, had been taken up by the NIH, and its network of well-funded trial investigators at major medical institutions around the country, to the exclusion of almost all other therapeutic approaches to Aids. Inquiries by the Aids activist group ACT UP had shown that by early 1988, practically 80 per cent of the patient slots in the NIAID's Aids clinical trials group were for AZT trials. 'ACT UP basically discovered that the entire government clinical testing system was testing one drug – AZT,' Nussbaum wrote.

> Within science, AZT joined the Aids virus in a medical mantra that was repeated over and over again: 'There is one cause of Aids: the Aids virus, or Human Immunodeficiency Virus – HIV. There is one treatment for Aids: AZT'.
>
> AZT both reflected and reinforced the basic paradigm within which almost all Aids research was to take place. The hot fields in virology in the eighties were molecular biology and protein biochemistry. The biggest players were in those fields. Molecular biology focuses on nucleic acids, DNA and RNA, hence the focus on nucleoside compounds such as AZT.
>
> It was simple, it was elegant. That's where the grant money flowed, that's where the articles being published in the best journals originated, that's where the awards for brilliance were. The HIV-AZT litany became dogma. As one scientist prominent in Aids put it: 'If you don't swallow the dogma and repeat it word for word, to everybody around you, in your hospital, in your institution, you get cut off. It's very, very difficult to continue doing research unless you have private funds.'

In a foreword to Jad Adams's 1989 book, Duesberg said he was often asked why it was just himself and a handful of others who questioned the virus-Aids hypothesis. Why didn't a young, ambitious scientist make a name for himself by questioning it? The answer lay in the strong conformist pressures on scientists, particularly young, untenured scientists, in the age of biotechnology. 'Their conceptual obedience to the establishment is maintained by controlled access to research grants, journals and positions, and rewarded by conference engagements, personal prizes, consultantships, stocks and co-ownership in companies.' A dissenter would have to be truly independent and prepared for a variety of sanctions. 'I, for instance, was sarcastically called a "brilliant chemist", but labelled a bigot for considering daily administration of psychoactive and immunosuppressive chemicals more likely to be the cause of Aids than a chronically dormant and chemically almost undetectable retrovirus. Invitations were issued only on the condition that I did not debate the "control" of Aids with the Aids test or the DNA-inhibitor AZT, both of which are based exclusively on the virus-Aids hypothesis.'

Ill-effects of Conventional View

Duesberg became increasingly virulent in his criticisms of the conventional view of Aids. The HIV theory, he claimed, had not saved a single life. Screening blood for antibodies to HIV was superfluous, and probably harmful in view of the anxiety a positive test generated. For him, since HIV could not be the cause, the public health and educational campaigns launched world-wide on the basis of the HIV alert were also tragically and damagingly misplaced, and probably costing thousands of lives. He became passionate about propounding this view, considering it his responsibility to do so. Indeed, he dedicated one of his major articles[12] to 'all intravenous drug users, oral users of recreational drugs and AZT recipients who were never told that drugs cause Aids diseases', and to 'all "antibody-positives" who were never told that the virus-Aids hypothesis is unproven'.

By accepting and promoting his own hypothesis as fact, Duesberg was falling into the same trap as HIV's advocates. For a variety of reasons, none of them having anything to do with science, HIV had been adopted as the cause of Aids when, by any reckoning, the case for it was far from complete. But even if Duesberg felt entitled, on the basis of his expertise in molecular biology, to dismiss HIV from the picture, his drug-Aids theory was only one of a number of alternative hypotheses.

With the perspective he now held, however, he was understandably distressed at the profound ill-effects he saw being generated by the HIV description of Aids. One was that it broke the connection in people's minds between behaviour and consequences – between cause and effect. You were just as liable to die of Aids if you picked up HIV in a single casual encounter as you were if you had thousands of partners, in an orgy of drug-driven sex. Thus, the message behind the public health campaigns had been a pusillanimous one: anything goes, as long as it doesn't transmit HIV. While comforting to those addicted to heavy drug use and heavy sex, it was unquestionably a weak and dangerous position to take.

The long 'latent periods' between the gratification provided by recreational drugs such as cocaine and nitrite inhalants – as also by alcohol and tobacco – and their potentially irreversible health effects, gave credence to the perilous message that drugs were safe but bugs were not. It led to injecting drug users being subjected to years of 'safe needle' propaganda in which the hidden message was that while needles could be hazardous when shared or inadequately sterilised, the drugs themselves were safe. Yet in one rare, controlled study among 300 HIV-positive intravenous drug abusers, the risk of developing Aids over sixteen months was three times higher in those who persisted than in those who stopped injecting drugs.[13]

The 'anything goes' message was not confined to the US. It had gone out internationally, as part of the HIV ideology. Sometimes there was even explicit encouragement of promiscuity, as in a pornographically illustrated leaflet entitled 'Tie Him Down', distributed by the Terrence Higgins Trust, the UK's largest Aids charity. There was nothing wrong in being picked up at a club by a stranger, and bound and gagged on a bondage frame, the storyline indicated, as long as you checked he was into safer sex first. As one outraged young gay man noted, this was at a time when a serial killer was on the loose who throttled homosexual men after tying them up! The Trust helped organise an army of volunteers to ease the plight of Aids victims, priceless work that has continued throughout the Aids years, but it has seemed to lack effective leadership on a number of key issues, perhaps demonstrating the mind-numbing effect of HIV's dominance of thinking. At one time – in common with many other Aids organisations – the Trust entered into an over-close relationship with Wellcome, AZT's manufacturer, promoting the drug through some of its literature. It also took a very liberal line on recreational drugs, ignoring the pleas of gay health activists to highlight the hazards of poppers and other destructive chemicals. One of its senior officials is on record as calling poppers 'a harmless bit of fun' – the kind of thinking which, as Lauritsen had discovered during a trip to London, led some Aids patients to keep bottles of nitrite inhalants at their hospital bedside. When Cass Mann, of the British Aids organisation Positively Healthy, described the toxicities of poppers to the nurses, they said they had been given orders 'not to interfere with the pleasures of the patients'.

Even the British government's Health Department was taking an uncharacteristically permissive line on poppers, becoming dismissive and obstructive of efforts to highlight the dangers of the drugs. In common with the Aids charities and the medical and scientific bodies involved in the fight against Aids, officials felt nothing should dilute the message about the dangers posed by the virus. But this was an irrational stand that owed more to the shaky foundations of the HIV-AZT ideology than to science. The mantra of belief was chanted almost as strongly in Britain as in the US.

On 13 June 1990, a second documentary featuring Duesberg, *The Aids Catch,* appeared on British television. Produced and directed by Joan Shenton with Michael Verney-Elliott as reporter, and shown in the 'Dispatches' series on Channel 4, it developed further the story told in *Aids: The Unheard Voices* not only by questioning whether HIV caused Aids, but by reporting Duesberg's drug-Aids hypothesis, and the startling corollary that Aids was not even an infectious condition. The film included an interview with HIV's discoverer, Luc Montagnier, in which he spoke of his doubts over whether the virus could kill immune system cells on its own. He had found that when cultures of HIV and human cells were treated with the antibiotic tetracycline, the cells stopped dying. His theory, to be spelled out at the Sixth International Aids Conference in San Francisco later that month, was that HIV might have to interact with a co-factor before it could cause Aids. In other words, it might be harmless on its own.

The programme struck home. It was well received by television writers, and for the first time in HIV's six-year history there was the beginnings of a debate over its role in Aids. In a preview entitled 'The Real Facts About

Aids', the *Independent* summarised the message as: 'Understanding the effects of designer-drug abuse (in the West) and malnutrition (in the Third World) may be more important in isolating the factors leading to Aids than sexual behaviour.' The *Guardian's* reviewer noted the film's argument 'that excessive drug use may be one of the activities which precipitates a systematic breakdown of the immune system. Will time and money be wasted on researching the wrath-of-God scenario, when further inquiries on these lines might do more good?'

In the *Financial Times*, Chris Dunkley described the documentary as an outstanding piece of 'Sez who?' journalism. 'That bright, clear-thinking producer/director Joan Shenton looks at the panic-mongering and special pleading which has characterised so much of the previous material about Aids amongst broadcasters...takes that sort of journalism by the neck, shakes it vigorously, and sets off to see what the calm thinkers outside the multi-million dollar research lobby are saying. The result is eye-opening.' The programme was the 'Pick of the Day' choice in the *Daily Mail,* where Elizabeth Cowley wrote: 'Why, after so long in its shadow, can't the medical profession get it right about Aids?' *Today*'s critic, Pam Francis, said the programme left viewers with the thought 'that if HIV has nothing to do with Aids, and Aids is not infectious, we must be living with one of the biggest scientific errors in history'.

In a media column in *The Times,* Jad Adams wrote that the view expressed in the programme appeared particularly startling because it seemed to have sprung from nowhere. In fact, there had been robust criticisms of the HIV theory for years, but they had not been generally reported. 'Why are medical journalists apparently so reluctant to cover dissent? They seem to have a consensus that if the Government's chief medical officer makes a statement, they must print it as fact*.' After the *Independent on Sunday* ran a story by their medical correspondent headlined 'Careless Aids talk costs lives', in which Aids doctors complained about the programme, Adams responded that he found this 'less than amusing'.

* This question is examined further in the next chapter.

> Having failed to rise to the challenge to their orthodoxy in the scientific papers, they are now complaining that criticism of the HIV theory has been presented to the public. If they are so sure of their position, why have their voices not been raised to justify the HIV theory in *Proceedings of the National Academy of Sciences* or *Cancer Research,* both of which have carried very detailed criticism of the theory? Why protest only now?
>
> The reason is probably the one given at the Channel 4 press conference to launch this programme: many of the people from the Aids world present accepted that there had long been doubts about HIV as the cause of Aids but felt that this was not something which should be known to the public as it might undermine preventive measures designed to stop the transmission of HIV. This was admitting doubts about the theory but calling upon the uncertainties to be suppressed so the public would act as if the HIV theory were an incontrovertible fact. Thus doubt is placed in the service of certainty in the public interest.
>
> When the whole story finally emerges, I would suggest the principal victim will be public confidence in scientists.

No longer able to ignore Duesberg's challenge, the Aids 'establishment' hit back. The programme brought a strong protest from Lord Kilmarnock, chairman of the All-party Parliamentary Group on Aids, and eighteen other senior figures in the fight against Aids in the UK. In a letter to the *Independent* they said the public health effects of such a programme were a source of grave concern for anyone involved in health education and the prevention of the spread of HIV, and it should not have been transmitted as it stood. It was irresponsible to push the idea that 'Aids is not and cannot be an infectious disease' without giving other scientists the opportunity to challenge it directly.

Pointing out that Aids was a disease syndrome rather than an infectious disease, they went on to assert that 'HIV is the infection and the transmissible aetiological agent'. In response to remarks in the programme about the ever-extending supposed time lag between infection and disease, they commented that there were a significant number of other infectious diseases with a long incubation period, such as chronic hepatitis, herpes and tuberculosis. 'The vast majority of Aids researchers believe that Aids is a further example.'

It was understood that co-factors such as the presence of other infections, malnutrition, drug abuse and perhaps stress might influence the speed with which signs of immunodeficiency developed following infection with HIV. But without any of these, HIV remained a very serious threat to health. Best available data suggested that by ten years after infection, 50 per cent of patients had developed Aids.

The letter prompted a reply from David Lloyd, the Channel 4 editor who commissioned the two 'Dispatches' programmes. Apart from these two forty-minute reports, he said, in the thousands of hours of broadcast reporting predicated on the HIV hypothesis, there had not been a mention of dissenting opinion. 'A lack of balance? When those programmes that identify themselves with mainstream opinion are prepared to grant the minority a voice, then *Dispatches* will be guilty of imbalance in not seeking out replies from the majority.'

The *Independent* also published a reply from Duesberg, Shenton and Verney-Elliott, in which they countered the analogy between HIV and other infections. Unlike HIV in Aids, which infected only an insignificant fraction of T-cells, hepatitis virus remained chronically active in large numbers of liver cells and this progressively caused disease in about 5 per cent of those infected. It was true that herpes virus could cause disease after a long latency, but when it did so it was because it became reactivated in many target cells. That was not the case with HIV. Similarly, the only possible condition in which the TB bacillus could cause the progressive symptoms of the disease was when it was very active.

Their letter added that it was not irresponsible to question 'an unproven and unsuccessful hypothesis, particularly if it affects the lives of so many. The virus-Aids hypothesis has yet to save the first Aids patient, and has yet to stop the spread of Aids despite enormous research efforts that have cost more than the battles against all viruses in history combined'.

One scientist came to the programme's defence. Professor P. D. Wall, of the department of anatomy and developmental biology at the Middlesex School of Medicine in London, and a Fellow of the Royal Society, wrote:

> I detect excessive reaction in the cries of 'irresponsibility' directed at Channel 4 and the participants in the Aids programme. For the person at

> risk of developing this terrible disease there is no practical difference in the advice given by the two groups. Both insist that we should all avoid 'like the plague' any action that will insert mucky foreign protein into the bloodstream. There is a genuine difference of opinion between scientists as to the precise nature of the muck in the protein. A very vocal majority is convinced that it is precisely and uniquely the HIV virus. A smaller group thinks that generalised abuse of the body opens the way to any number of opportunistic infections, including HIV.
>
> The eventual prevention and cure of Aids will require a resolution of this issue. Whichever side is correct, we still need cures for the bizarre spectrum of bacterial and virus infections that cause the prolonged misery of the Aids patients. In the meantime, while such cures are being developed, both sides insist on the same cautions and precautions.

Nevertheless, for their troubles, the programme makers were taken to the Broadcasting Complaints Commission (BCC) by Wellcome and the Terrence Higgins Trust. After nine months, two hearings and 'mountains of paperwork', as Shenton put it, that a tiny company like Meditel could ill afford, the Commission partially upheld the complaints. It found the programme to have been unfair in its 'treatment of the subject of Aids' and 'likely to have confused many viewers about the risk of HIV infection', despite ruling that it could not go into the scientific arguments. The decision hurt Shenton and the team who had worked for months on the documentary. It was some compensation that the Independent Television Commission stood by the programme and its methods, and Channel 4 itself declared that on this issue the BCC had 'strayed beyond its normal area of competence into one in which it is extremely difficult for it to be seen to adjudicate fairly'. That did not, however, stop Wellcome from refusing to participate in a subsequent Meditel documentary, *AZT: Cause for Concern,* on grounds that 'we did not believe [Shenton] to be willing to make a balanced and accurate programme on this subject'.

From their perspective, they were no doubt right. This was why John Robb, Wellcome's chief executive, felt entitled to protest about the AZT programme to Michael Grade, chief executive of Channel 4, in terms that made it clear he would like Shenton stopped. 'We feel that it is questionable to commission a programme from a producer who has already proved unable to tolerate authoritative public criticism and we are therefore surprised that your Channel should have commissioned a further programme on a very similar topic from such a source,' he wrote.

> As a manufacturer of prescription pharmaceutical products, we are acutely aware of the importance of providing people with medicines of the highest quality, and of making claims for those medicines which in no way build false hopes in the minds of people who may be suffering the psychological strains of coming to terms with life-threatening diseases. We find it deplorable that your company does not seem willing to apply similarly high standards of quality control when entering the public arena on these highly emotive issues.

Wellcome's American arm demonstrated their own ideas of balance in a 1990 video, *The Psychology of Treating Patients with HIV Disease,* sent to doctors treating Aids patients. The basic premises of the video were that 'HIV disease' was coming to be seen as a chronic infection, for many 'the first intimate realisation of death and disease'. Patients needed to be 'motivated' towards early medical intervention with AZT, and helped to realise that their fears of side-effects were unfounded. Doctors were warned that some patients had complained about side-effects which, 'once they've talked about it with their counsellors, were determined to be more related to their anxiety about being on the drug, than to the drug itself'. Patients should be encouraged to 'handle attribution' of symptoms accurately, 'to ally with the drug against the disease' – that is, to blame sideeffects on HIV rather than the drug. A New York physician smilingly declared that the AZT pill 'should be an absolute symbol of life... The whole issue of empowerment here, of people taking charge of their own lives, is involved with this decision-making, to take this drug'.

John Lauritsen, who described the video in a *Native* article entitled 'HIV Voodoo From Burroughs Wellcome', said its whole thrust was to downplay AZT's side-effects. 'Doctors are to dismiss their patients' objections to AZT therapy as "psychological", as short-term depression or anxiety... The hidden message to gay men is this: "You are doomed. Be brave, willing sacrificial victims. Do not listen to the messages of your body."'

'Dr Duesberg Has Become Sidetracked'

For several years, almost single-handed, Duesberg had run into the might not just of a very powerful multinational company, but of the medical and scientific establishment world-wide. In effect, he was challenging the credibility of the hottest fields in scientific research, molecular biology and protein biochemistry, which between them fund most of the advertisements in journals such as *Science* and *Nature*. He had laid down the gauntlet against HIV, now the basis of an enormous research industry; against the 'Aids test', which was the means whereby a sense of political and public alarm over HIV could be maintained; and against AZT, which headed the medical profession's fight against Aids. The health bureaucracy and Aids charities, counsellors and educationists were also understandably upset over his implied – and sometimes explicit – attacks on 'safer sex', the mainstay of their efforts to counter the threatened epidemic. If he was right, and Aids was non-infectious – a possibility few found it possible to contemplate – much of their work might have been misplaced. On the other hand, if, as they believed, he was wrong, it was a disaster to put doubts in the public's mind.

Perhaps because of a siege mentality induced by this near-universal hostility, Duesberg had become increasingly outspoken in favour of his drug-Aids hypothesis, and against the 'safer sex' and condom campaigns that meant so much to so many, particularly in the gay community. In doing this, he achieved some wider publicity for his views, but he weakened his scientific position.

For one thing, he might have been wrong about HIV. The correlation between testing HIV-positive and risk of Aids was real, and as yet inadequately explained. Duesberg's original view had been that the virus always remained inactive, even in Aids itself, and that the presence of antibodies meant nothing more than a successful immune response. That did not fit with Gene Shearer's work, suggesting that the primary response to HIV, perhaps mounted successfully by millions of people, was an immune mechanism mediated by whole cells, with antibodies appearing only as a second line of defence. Later, Duesberg seemed to be taking a position closer to Sonnabend's, that the virus did become active in immunocompromised people, but that the appearance of HIV antibodies was an effect rather than a cause of their immune deficiency.

Even if Duesberg was right, and HIV was harmless, there were other non-HIV theories of Aids causation, such as Sonnabend's ideas involving multiple infections and the immunosuppressive effects of semen from many partners, which remained to be examined, and in which 'safer sex' practices were still highly relevant. Kilmarnock, and the Terrence Higgins Trust, did have grounds for complaint in this respect, although it was true that they were themselves culpable in having failed – along with just about every other institution and organisation claiming responsibility in the field – to face and examine the fundamentals of the case Duesberg made against the idea that HIV had been proved to be the cause of Aids.

As the retrovirologist who had been able to see through some of the web of illusion surrounding HIV, Duesberg's criticisms had a force and a logic that made him an embarrassment and threat. Now those criticisms could be side-stepped. He had alienated some potential supporters, and made it easier for those who did not share his views to dismiss them.

The Aids Catch succeeded in flushing out a response from *Nature*, the first time the journal had given Duesberg's challenge any serious attention. But it was an emotive 'commentary' rather than a scientific rebuttal. Appearing in the issue of 21 June 1990, the two-page article by Robin Weiss, the virologist and cancer researcher who developed Britain's first HIV test for Wellcome, and Harold Jaffe, the former head of the CDC's Aids task force now on sabbatical leave in London, began by declaring that Duesberg's proposition – 'that HIV is not the cause of Aids at all' – was as absurd as theories that HIV originated from outer space. It went on to say that the authors regarded critics such as Duesberg as '"flat-earthers" bogged down in molecular minutiae and miasmal theories of disease, while HIV continues to spread'. It concluded that 'if he and his supporters belittle "safe sex", would have us abandon HIV screening of blood donations, and curtail research into anti-HIV drugs and vaccines, then their message is perilous'.

Gallo took a similar line on Duesberg in his book *Virus Hunting*.[14] He wrote that when asked to explain why such critics 'do not accept the scientific results we have achieved with HIV', he replies that 'there actually are people (I hope not many scientists) who do not believe the United States placed a man on the moon. There is also, I am told, a Flat Earth Society, which has evolved a complex rationale to explain away all the evidence that the earth is round'.

For twenty years, Duesberg had received federal funding for his research. In 1985 the NCI had awarded him an 'outstanding investigator' grant (OIG), a special seven-year award, worth $350,000, designed to give top scientists freedom to explore new research ideas. Four months after the *Nature* commentary, a committee reviewing Duesberg's application for renewal of this grant gave him such a low rating as to guarantee that it would be discontinued. In their resume, the committee stated:

> Dr Peter H. Duesberg, a senior investigator with a distinguished past in molecular virology, requests continued support for studies to pursue his hypotheses regarding the genetics and role of oncogenes and the genetics of viral leukaemia and Aids. Despite the applicant's eminent track record, the relatively low past productivity, the logically and functionally flawed rationale, and the poor prospect of the proposed study for advancing knowledge in important areas greatly weakens the overall merit of this application.

In their report, the committee concluded that a 'lack of substantive productivity during the tenure of this award and the absence of convincing evidence in the current application that this trend will be corrected indicates that Dr Duesberg can no longer be considered at the forefront of his field'. This was 'highly disappointing', considering his strong record of accomplishment up to his receipt of the OIG, but perhaps reflected 'a dilution of his efforts with non-scientific issues'. Though describing him as 'one of the pioneers of modern retrovirology', the reviewers complained that 'Dr Duesberg has become sidetracked'. Much of his time and effort had been occupied by theoretical issues, with many of his publications taking the form of letters on various subjects 'but principally reflecting commentaries on Aids'.

The committee had ten members, but Duesberg found later that three did not participate in the review, and one did so only informally over the phone (with a favourable recommendation). He regarded several of the other members as incapable of giving an unbiased opinion. These included Gallo's close friends Dani Bolognesi, whose Duke University laboratory had originally tested AZT for Burroughs Wellcome (and who took over as editor of the revamped *Aids Research* journal when Sonnabend was fired), and Flossie Wong-Staal, now a professor of medicine at the University of California at San Diego, both of whom, in Duesberg's words, had 'built their careers almost exclusively on the Virus-Aids hypothesis'.

Duesberg fought for the next two years to save his funding, but in vain; and since then, every one of his peer-reviewed grant applications to other federal, state or private agencies has been turned down. He has also suffered discrimination from antagonistic fellow professors at Berkeley. While other faculty members regulate teaching policies, speaker invitations, appointments and similar weighty matters, Duesberg has been placed in charge of the annual picnic committee.

Gordon Stewart says of Duesberg: 'He is now ostracised in scientific circles and deprived of all his research grants. The main reason is that his work lacks scientific support, but this in turn is because the main journals repeatedly refuse to publish details of independent work which falsifies predictions of heterosexual spread of Aids in general populations and questions other assertions in the consensus about HIV. This would be disgraceful in any situation. In the world of science, where over 80,000 papers on Aids have been published, it is utterly indefensible.'

Duesberg has not gone out of his way to win friends among his colleagues. Not content with disparaging the virus-cancer theory, and then the whole of the current scientific enterprise surrounding Aids, in December 1990 he extended his critique to the whole of virology. In a letter to his division head at Berkeley, he declined to teach virology because 'there is no significant clinical frontier in viral pathogenesis since the polio epidemic was ended in the '50s, and thus viruses have become mostly an academic issue'.

According to a report in *Science* headed 'Virology Dead, Says Duesberg', his concern was that so often, viruses were being blamed for illnesses when there was far too little present to cause disease. He favoured the 'innocent until proven guilty' approach over what *Science* described as the usual scientific method, in which a hypothesis remained a candidate until it was disproven. He told the journal that he could not teach about viruses 'because I don't believe in them enough', provoking the comment: 'Perhaps this stand will exempt him from teaching any course that relies on the scientific method.'

That brought a response which summed up this brilliant but deeply disillusioned scientist's view of the field in which he had laboured for thirty years. After remarking that *Science's* suggestion was 'perhaps the most honourable discharge I have earned so far', he wrote:

> Unfortunately, the view that according to 'the usual scientific method ... a hypothesis remains a candidate until it is disproven' can have serious consequences, in particular, if it is a candidate for a way to confront disease.
>
> Take the currently popular virus-Aids hypothesis. The virus remains to be proven guilty. But the hypothesis is currently the only candidate for a way to confront Aids. This confrontation has produced no cure, no vaccine, a highly toxic anti-viral medicine, and an infectious syndrome that does not spread from behavioural or clinical risk groups [the United States has now lifted its ban on visitors who test positive for the human immunodeficiency virus (HIV)], and all that for about $3 billion a year. Lately it looks as if there is even disagreement about how to prove HIV guilty, in particular, about what kind of microbial allies are needed to cause Aids. In view of the emerging HIV schism, I wonder which candidate hypothesis professors should be 'exempt' from teaching. Other examples demonstrate that the ever-popular germ theory has at times 'remained a candidate' far too long, until finally disproved at great cost to the affected people. In the United States tens of thousands died unnecessarily in the 1920s because pellagra was considered infectious by the US Public Health Service, until Joseph Goldberger proved it to be a non-infectious vitamin B deficiency. Indeed, the disease was said to be transmitted by 'poor hygiene' among corn farmers in the South – the primary risk group for pellagra. In Japan, at least 10,000 suffered in the 1960s and 1970s from a drug-induced neuropathy, including blindness, that had been misdiagnosed as a viral disease for more than ten years. The pursuit of oncogenic viruses as the cause of cancer by me and by many of my learned retrovirology colleagues provides another example. Although it has generated such academic triumphs as viral oncogenes and reverse transcriptase, it has been a total failure in terms of clinical relevance to cancer, primarily because, with a very few exceptions, cancers are not infectious. Perhaps professors should not be exempt from questioning clinically unproductive hypotheses from a generation of virus hunters who have never seen a frontier outside the laboratory.

Can one quarrel with that? Duesberg may be annoying, he may play games with people's feelings, he may dance around lesser intellects like a picador baiting a bull, and he may sometimes have overstated his case. But one does not need to be a molecular biologist, nor pass any final judgement on his ideas at this point, to know that much is wrong with the HIV hypothesis, and that Duesberg is no fool. Nor does one need to be a psychologist to see that he cares about truth, and falsehood, as they relate to human suffering, and has made many sacrifices in defence of the facts as he sees them.

Duesberg's 'rush to the media' has been condemned by Gallo and others. 'His voice has diminished confidence in science and scientists, medicine, physicians, and health care workers,' Gallo writes. 'Undermining confidence in the only people working on Aids is not likely to help unify our efforts to conquer it. Instead, it breeds distrust and perhaps frank hostility, often turning researchers into convenient targets for those whose business it is to attack government institutions and people... Irresponsible rantings against HIV as a cause of Aids may lead some infected people to forgo anti-HIV therapy or, worse, not to care about whom they might infect.'[15]

Surely, the irresponsibility that undermines confidence has been on the part of those who ignored, suppressed and ridiculed information they did not want to hear. One can only feel grateful that science has at least been kept alive, albeit by a thread, through the arguments of experts like Sonnabend, Stewart and Duesberg, and the passion and persistence exemplified by Callen, Lauritsen and the Meditel team.

Nature's introduction to the Weiss-Jaffe commentary on Duesberg's views stated: 'Last century there was a sharp difference of opinion between those, such as Koch and Pasteur, who proposed that disease could be caused by invisible microbes, and others who held that epidemics are the result of evil vapours (mal'aria). Arguments that Aids does not have an infectious basis are as quaint as those of the miasmalists.' It was a dereliction of duty on the part of this leading journal that it should present such a travesty of Duesberg's case, but the article had the desired effect; for a further two years, the controversy was to continue to stay almost entirely out of public view. Then in April 1992, the London *Sunday Times* blasted forth with a two-page article which marked the beginning of a genuine scientific reappraisal of the HIV theory.

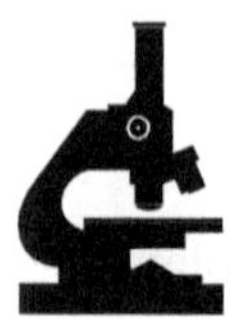

7: AIDS: CAN WE BE POSITIVE?

I remember my sense of dismay and scepticism when in 1984 I heard that a new virus had been named as the cause of Aids. I was editing an avant-garde (and ill-fated) health magazine, which put a big emphasis on the role of attitudes and feelings, and in particular our ability to find and give happiness in life, in determining behaviour and consequent health. This outlook led me to believe that the explanation for the sudden appearance of Aids would more likely be found in the dynamics of the victims' lives than in a new microbe, so my heart sank at the announcement. Instinctively, I felt that doctors and scientists had adopted this microbial explanation not because the facts demanded that they should, but as a means of trying to take control over a worrying situation.

The following year, however, that gut reaction was soon forgotten after I became exposed to the full range of Aids literature and scientific concern on joining the *Sunday Times* as medical correspondent, a job I was to hold until the end of the decade. I quite soon became a convert to the HIV cause, writing of how the growth in confirmed victims of Aids, both in deaths and in full-blown disease, had been exponential both in Britain and in the United States, doubling every nine months to a year, though with Britain lagging behind the US by about four years. This was a typical pattern for a new infectious agent, and it meant that the world did indeed face a new medical emergency.

In November 1986 the *Sunday Times* showed a picture of an ordinary-looking couple with three children, under the headline 'At Risk'. The caption stated:

> A British family out for a walk: father (39), mother (35), two teenage children and a baby. They look happy and healthy. But from what we now know

> about the way the Aids epidemic is developing, all are potential victims. The father could be infected by a prostitute or by a homosexual relationship; his wife through an affair with a casual stranger – or from her husband. And the boy and girl, if they have a drugs problem, could pick it up from an infected hypodermic needle. Even the baby could be infected, if either parent was a carrier. Many like these may soon be under threat.

The article, which was greeted as being 'very helpful' by the UK's Health Department, did contain some worthwhile information and comment. It told of how all over the US, HIV infection, and the paranoia generated by it, was wrecking careers, blighting lives, and inspiring irrational behaviour. The previous week, in Birmingham, Alabama, the local newspaper insisted that all future recruits must take the HIV test as a condition of employment. Twenty-nine Californian telephone workers walked off the job when an afflicted mate returned to work after winning a nine-month legal fight for reinstatement. A virus-carrying construction worker in Indianapolis was forbidden by a judge from seeing his two-year-old daughter, although he had no actual disease. As a British Aids counsellor, Father Bill Kirkpatrick, had said on returning from a recent US visit: 'There is a new disease in America, which ought to be called Afraids.'

By contrast, we said, the attitude in Britain might be too relaxed. Only now were the public and health authorities beginning to realise the novel and horrific dangers presented by the virus, with its long time-lag between infection and disease. Although the Health Minister had described Aids as 'the biggest medical threat of our time', the actual amount of money addressed to the problem had been minute – perhaps £lm for research, and £2.5m for what had so far been a low-key publicity campaign. We reported that there were calls for widespread screening, to establish exactly how far and fast the virus was spreading – but also a great need to maintain anonymity, in view of the terrible psychological consequences of a positive test result. Dr John Galwey, of the Oxford Health Authority, who had seen a brilliant academic kill himself in such circumstances, summarised the meaning of a positive test result as it was understood at that time.

> If you tell somebody they are positive for Aids antibodies, what you are doing is saying that they are infectious and will remain so for a long time, probably for life; that over the next six or seven years they have a chance of at least 30 per cent of developing an illness for which we have no treatment and from which they will almost certainly die; that even if they don't get this disease they may well develop the Aids-related complex, a degree of illness often severe enough to prevent them from leading a normal life; and that if they don't develop Aids they may well become demented.

The *Sunday Times* continued to reflect the uncertainty that prevailed. In January 1987 we reported on a big contrast between Aids cases, which were mostly confined to London, and reported cases of HIV positivity, which were much more widely distributed across the country. We interpreted this (wrongly, because of the false identification between HIV-positivity and Aids) as 'illustrating dramatically how the epidemic is spreading across Britain'. In fact, there was no evidence of HIV spreading, as nationwide anonymous screening was to confirm five years later. We did report in March 1987 that a dramatic rise in the number of people tested in the wake of a big government publicity campaign had failed to reveal any appreciable increase in cases. Thousands who went to their doctor or clinic fearing that recent affairs might have put them at risk had been reassured that they were free of the virus, which remained confined almost exclusively to high-risk groups such as male homosexuals and intravenous drug users.

By June that year, however, I returned from the third international conference on Aids in Washington as a fully-fledged Aids alarmist. The event had been almost like a religious rally, with a total consensus in the idea that a new and deadly virus was sweeping the world. I remember being particularly impressed by assurances from a British haemophilia centre director that his HIV-positive patients were indeed showing signs of continuous decline in their immune system, even though they did not yet have Aids. Their experience seemed to confirm the theory that the virus was a slow but sure killer. I was also struck by a graph presented to the conference by a US Army researcher showing how levels of viral protein in the blood of HIV-infected people changed over time. The graph purported to show a short peak soon after infection, followed by a lull lasting anything from two to ten years, then a gradual rise as Aids developed. The alarming implication was that after some years of carrying HIV relatively harmlessly, there would be a surge of infectiousness in HIV-positive people, providing yet another reason for concern about future spread. It was only years later that it was pointed out to me that the graph had no units, and was not based on any published data; it was worthless, as John Lauritsen put it, except as a simple illustration of belief.

A week mingling among the 6,000 delegates was capped by a visit to the White House, where I met Gary Bauer, President Reagan's domestic policy adviser, a genial man who told me that Reagan had decided to let 'his own good common sense' and long experience overrule the advice of public health officials in announcing a tougher line on Aids testing that week. His stand reflected his concern that the epidemic was set to 'decimate' the American people, and their allies in Europe, unless more positive action was taken to stop it. Bauer urged Britain and Europe to learn from America's tragic mistakes and not delay facing the tough issues posed by the virus.

Reagan's proposals, to screen immigrants and prisoners, and to start routine testing in hospitals and clinics, drew boos and hisses at the conference, where the health care community showed itself deeply divided on the testing issue. The atmosphere there, I reported, was more like a football match than a learned gathering, in which there were clearly two teams at work. The main concern of one team was to help those who already had the virus, while the other was more worried about its spread. But there was at least agreement on the scale of the threat: one American adult in ten could become infected by 1994, according to a computer model prepared at the Los Alamos National Laboratory, although researchers admitted that was based on inadequate information. This was the year that Oprah Winfrey opened her show with the words: 'Hello everybody. Aids has both sexes running scared. Research studies now project that one in five – listen to me, hard to believe – one in five heterosexuals could be dead of Aids in the next three years.'

At about this same time, Andrew Neil, editor of the *Sunday Times*, devoted a whole issue of the newspaper's magazine to Aids and the threat posed by HIV. Neil was always somewhat sceptical, however, about claims of heterosexual spread. Over the next couple of years, in response to memos demanding to know what had happened to the promised epidemic, I re-emphasised the conventional view about the long time-lag between infection and illness. The 'slow virus' idea was of course a marvellous way of allowing us to believe what our eyes could not see. But as the years went by, with Aids cases remaining stubbornly confined to the original risk groups, and no evidence of HIV spreading either, it became increasingly difficult to maintain the line that Aids was a danger to us all. Whereas in 1985 the Royal College of Nursing had predicted that 1 million people in Britain – one in fifty – 'will have Aids in six years unless the killer disease is checked', the actual cumulative total of Aids cases by 1990 was still below 5,000.

The first person to make a real dent in the belief that everyone was at risk was Michael Fumento, a young lawyer who had worked as an Aids analyst for the US government's Commission on Human Rights. In 1988, after he wrote an article for the *New Republic* magazine attacking Aids lobbyists and health educators for exaggerating the risks – and arguing that conservatives were using the epidemic to further political ends such as chastity (as opposed to sex) education, and anti-homosexual legislation – he was effectively sacked. But he went on to produce *The Myth of Heterosexual Aids*,[1] demonstrating that the heterosexual break-out widely predicted in the 1980s had not happened, and was not likely to, although he accepted that heterosexual transmission of HIV and Aids did occur. 'Among what is known as the general population... there is no epidemic,' he wrote. He also argued that inappropriate Aids funding had such detrimental effects on care provision for people with other health problems that it had probably cost more lives than it would save. Gay rights groups feared that his words would spark an anti-gay backlash and campaigned against the book, which sold only 12,000 copies in the US, despite extensive controversy over its message. It failed to find a publisher in Britain, although it was serialised in the *Sunday Times*.

In 1990 I had left my job for a junior executive role at the *Sunday Express*, still covering health and medicine but with commissioning and editing as well as writing forming a part of my brief, and with a greater emphasis on health stories than on medical science. I was no longer in such close contact with day-to-day developments in Aids. In June that year, however, Joan Shenton called me about *The Aids Catch*, her second film for Channel 4 featuring Peter Duesberg's ideas. From all I had seen and heard over the past few years, the theory seemed highly unlikely, but I spoke to Duesberg to try to get a taste of his viewpoint. I seem to remember him producing a stream of ideas and arguments that left me intrigued, though unconvinced.

It so happened that during that same week I received a report from Britain's Medical Research Council on its current Aids research, in which there was a description of findings from a unique group of haemophiliac patients in Edinburgh. Whereas most haemophiliacs treated with commercial Factor 8 concentrate were believed to have been infected with HIV between 1979 and 1983, those in Scotland received 'cleaner' transfusions, locally collected, and tests on their stored blood samples indicated that they remained negative for HIV-antibodies until 1984. In that year, eighteen out of thirty-two, all of whom were treated from the same batch, became positive. Now, ten of those had 'CDC Group IV' disease (symptoms of immune deficiency), whereas the remaining fourteen who stayed HIV-negative were well. This looked like just the sort of proof Duesberg had been arguing was needed before HIV could be accepted as causing Aids, and I said as much in a short comment column in the *Express* headed 'TV professor's Aids theory fails the test'.

> Aids doctors busy trying to persuade people to have 'safe sex' to avoid risking exposure to the virus will not be well pleased by a Channel 4 programme to be screened on Wednesday. Dispatches argues that Aids is just a hotchpotch of old diseases that have become more apparent through the damaging effects on the immune system of abuse of drugs in the West, and of malnutrition in Africa.
>
> The programme is based on the ideas of Professor Peter Duesberg, a molecular biologist at the University of California, Berkeley, who says: 'I believe that Aids is not and cannot even be an infectious disease. We are told you get sick ten years after infection. That is not how viruses or bacteria ever work.' When I asked Dr Duesberg last week about illnesses such as hepatitis, syphilis and TB – which can break out years after the initial infection – he back-pedalled immediately, saying he had been talking about 'the general rule'. But that was not what he said on the programme. And if some old-established microbes can break the rule, why not Aids?
>
> He claims that people with haemophilia carrying the human immunodeficiency virus are made ill by their inherited illness, not by HIV.
>
> A useful study, he told a newspaper recently, would be to compare a group of haemophiliacs with antibodies to the virus with a similar group

> without antibody, follow them for a year and see what happened. If the HIV-positive ones became ill and the others stayed well, that would be evidence that the virus was to blame.
>
> That has been done in Edinburgh, where thirty-two haemophiliacs known to have been exposed to a single batch of HIV-infected blood concentrate in 1984 are being studied in a Medical Research Council project.
>
> Only eighteen developed antibodies to HIV, and ten of those now have Aids-type diseases. But the remaining fourteen who did not become infected are all well.

For the time being, I could continue to rest secure in the comforting certainty of the HIV theory.

The *Sunday Times* Puts Down the Questions

In late 1991 I returned to the *Sunday Times,* this time in the role of science correspondent. Soon afterwards, I was visiting Meditel's offices when Joan Shenton said: 'You know, Neville, you were wrong to dismiss Duesberg's ideas on the basis of the Edinburgh study. It did not compare like with like. The haemophiliacs who became unwell differed in a number of ways from those who did not, regardless of HIV.' I was concerned to hear this, but when I checked the scientific literature to which she referred me, I found it was true: even *before* they developed antibodies to HIV, the HIV-positive haemophiliac patients showed evidence of immune system disorders, and they differed from the others in that their immune systems were more hyper-reactive. After they had seroconverted, there was still a very clear correlation between markers of immune system activation and progression towards disease. These patients had also received more Factor 8 than those who stayed HIV-negative.

Why, then, had the scientists concluded HIV was responsible for the immune system deficiency in these patients? The latest report on the Edinburgh study, published in November 1991,[2] tried to address that question (perhaps in response to Duesberg's critique). The authors acknowledged that many haemophilia patients 'show some degree of immunological abnormalities' even in the absence of HIV infection, probably as a consequence of repeated infusions of foreign protein and/or of infection with hepatitis viruses. They went on:

> However, these can be no more than contributory factors to the gross and progressive changes seen especially in the symptomatic members of the Edinburgh cohort, since the patient subgroups were comparable in terms of age, severity of haemophilia, and degree of liver damage. Past infection with hepatitis B was universal... All patients were infected with hepatitis C virus and had abnormal liver function.
>
> Although we have previously reported that Factor 8 requirements throughout 1984 were significantly higher for the seropositive than the seronegative patients, this difference was not detectable before infection.

In fact, there *was* a difference in Factor 8 usage in 1983 as well as 1984, although it was regarded as statistically insignificant. The mean figure for patients later to be deemed symptomatic for 'HIV disease' was 46,300 units of concentrate (ranging from 0 to 99,000) in 1983, compared with 38,000 in the HIV-negative group. The range among the latter went from 0 to a massive 133,700, which may well have artificially inflated the mean figure for the group.

Furthermore, a 1985 report[3] on the same group of patients had found that T-cell numbers and ratios did not change after infection, a fact which, as the authors said, 'supports our previous conclusion that the abnormal T-lymphocyte subsets are a result of the intravenous infusion of Factor 8 concentrates per se, not HTLV-3 [HIV] infection'. Several other studies showed that the length of time patients had been receiving the transfusions was their biggest risk factor for developing immune disorders.

The latest study also demonstrated differences in immune responsiveness between the patients, probably genetically determined, that were linked to the speed with which they developed disease. Those with a tendency to mount a prolonged and intense antibody response to many antigens went downhill faster than those who were less reactive. This led the authors to conclude that hyper-reactivity to HIV was the cause of their speedier decline, but it would have been at least as plausible to argue that hyper-reactivity to other people's blood proteins was the real reason – and probably more plausible, in view of the known mechanisms of antigenic stimulation associated with repeated transfusions. A further complication was that some of the HIV-positive patients were being treated with AZT, which according to critics like Duesberg could only hasten their decline.

In another British study[4] to which Meditel drew my attention, doctors performed post-mortem examinations on a group of HIV-positive haemophiliacs and compared the findings with post-mortems from a group of HIV-positive gay men. The study demonstrated that although some of the haemophiliacs were diagnosed as having died of Aids, the pattern of illness was very different from that in the other group. The main causes of death were intracranial haemorrhage (a major risk in haemophilia because of the blood clotting deficiency), and liver disease, also a major risk for all haemophiliacs because of their exposure to hepatitis viruses through blood transfusion. Unlike the other group, they had no Kaposi's sarcoma, and little evidence of the unusual opportunistic infections or of the central nervous system damage characteristic of Aids. This confirmed previous observations, the authors said, 'that a substantial burden of fatal disease occurs among haemophiliacs who are positive for HIV and not formally diagnosed as having Aids. If our cases of haemophilia are representative of others much of this fatal disease would seem to be accounted for by cerebrovascular and liver disease'. Other studies I came across had shown that although haemophiliac patients do run a higher than average risk of succumbing to illnesses such as pneumonia, their vulnerability can be related to underlying immune deficiencies associated with being a haemophiliac, as well as to Factor 8 treatment; there was no need to postulate that HIV was to blame.

Clearly, the case against HIV was nothing like as cut-and-dried among haemophiliacs as I had thought from reading the MRC report. I felt I should investigate further.

Over the next few weeks, I familiarised myself with the detail of Duesberg's case, and responses he had grudgingly received. This was when I found, to my surprise, that many of his criticisms of the HIV theory had gone unanswered, and that when they had appeared to be addressed, as with the haemophiliacs, closer examination of the arguments showed much room for uncertainty.

I also learned of important new developments highlighting uncertainties about HIV that until now had been mostly hidden from the public. Duesberg and Luc Montagnier, HIV's discoverer, were both to challenge the orthodox view of HIV as the exclusive cause of Aids at an 'alternative' Aids conference in Amsterdam. In a preview of his presentation, Montagnier told me in an interview at the Institut Pasteur that infection with HIV did not necessarily lead to Aids, and that Aids could develop in people who were not infected with HIV. He spoke of promising new lines of research based on seeing Aids as a process in which cells of the immune system that guard against infection become wrongly programmed and start killing themselves – they were not killed by the virus, as had been thought, though he felt there was 'a very strong case that HIV has something to do with Aids; without HIV, I don't think we would have Aids epidemics'.

Another important development was that nearly fifty scientists and other professionals had come together to form an international body, the Group for the Reappraisal of the HIV/Aids Hypothesis. Some were to take part in the Amsterdam conference, alongside Duesberg, although they did not all share his particular point of view. They were about to launch a newsletter, *Rethinking Aids,* to examine the scientific basis for claims made about Aids and HIV's role in the syndrome. The newsletter's editor was Harvey Bialy, the scientific editor of *Bio/Technology,* who agreed with Duesberg that up to now 'the virus theory has produced nothing'. Efforts based on the HIV approach, Bialy told me, had brought three results: 'A vaccine that doesn't exist; AZT, which is iatrogenic genocide; and condom use, which is common sense.'

All this made for a powerful news story, which was run across the top of the front page of the issue of 26 April 1992 under the heading 'Experts Mount Startling Challenge to Aids Orthodoxy'. Inside, two pages of text under the striking headline 'Aids: Can We Be Positive?' set out the detail of the challenge, the first time this had been done for a national newspaper audience anywhere in the world. An introduction spelled out what was at stake:

> Elizabeth Taylor launched the Freddie Mercury concert last Monday. It was watched by one billion people around the world and the proceeds went to Aids research. But suppose the researchers are looking in the wrong place.

> Suppose HIV doesn't necessarily equal Aids. Then we will have witnessed the biggest medical and scientific blunder this century.

The article explained the potential importance of the rethink for Aids patients, and for people who had tested positive for HIV. With some of the scientists, including Montagnier, suggesting the virus could be harmless on its own, but that it might play a part in throwing the immune system into disarray when other infections were present, it meant some HIV-positive people might never fall ill. That in itself was dramatically different from the view held for years by most Aids scientists, that the presence of HIV in the body was a time-bomb which sooner or later would explode, seeking out and destroying all the body's T-cells.

Other sceptics, such as Duesberg, went further, arguing that the virus was not new, that it was not normally sexually transmitted, and that it was almost certainly harmless. The reason it was usually present in people whose immune systems had failed was that those people had been exposed to special health risks that brought them into contact with many infectious agents. In the case of most gay men, it was the dangerous, drug-driven 'fast-track' lifestyle. Other victims, such as haemophiliacs, transfusion recipients and babies born to drug-abusing or otherwise sick mothers, had suffered illnesses that in the past would have been attributed to their physical condition or circumstances. Being exposed to other people's blood meant their chances of showing antibodies to a wide variety of infectious agents, including HIV, were much higher than average. So were their chances of falling ill – but not for reasons that need have anything to do with HIV.

The article described how the 'reappraisal' group had been trying to persuade a leading medical or scientific journal to publish a letter outlining its concerns. The letter stated:

> It is widely believed by the general public that a retrovirus called HIV causes the group of diseases called Aids. Many biomedical scientists now question this hypothesis. We propose that a thorough reappraisal of the existing evidence for and against this hypothesis be conducted by a suitable independent group. We further propose that critical epidemiological studies be devised and undertaken.

None of the journals approached had been willing to publish the letter, despite several distinguished signatories. 'It's frozen out,' said Dr Charles Thomas, the group's coordinator, a former professor of biological chemistry at Harvard who now headed the Helicon Foundation, a non-profit research organisation. Dr Kary Mullis, who was to receive the 1993 Nobel Prize for chemistry for inventing the polymerase chain reaction (PCR) technique, a breakthrough in genetic testing used world-wide in Aids research, said many experts were unwilling to question the HIV hypothesis because so many livelihoods and reputations depended on it. Yet he could not find a single virologist able to give him a set of references showing HIV to be the probable cause of Aids. 'On an issue as important as this,' he said, 'there should be a set of scientific documents somewhere, research papers written by people who are accessible, demonstrating this. But they are not available. If you ask a virologist for that information, you don't get an answer, you get fury.'

Asked why *Rethinking Aids* was needed, Bialy – who has a sharp way with words – said:

> The vast majority of instruments of public information, as well as the majority of scientists involved in biomedical research, have indiscriminately subscribed to a single hypothesis, that a virus called HIV is the cause of the disease syndrome called Aids.
>
> The hypothesis has become all things to all people. It violates everything we previously knew about virus disease, and allows any kind of therapy, any kind of research, to generate research bucks. What kind of science continues to place all its marbles, all its faith, all its research bucks, in such a theory?
>
> The answer I keep coming back to is that it has nothing to do with science; the reasons are all unscientific.
>
> We have taken sex and equated it with death, and into that mixture we have thrown money. What an ugly stew.

After summarising some of the arguments as to why 'HIV can no longer be considered a lone, infectious assassin', we recalled the razzmatazz that had surrounded the 1984 press conference 'launching' HIV, and how the scientific world had seemed hypnotised by Gallo's certainty that HIV alone explained the arrival of Aids – 'who needs co-factors when you've been hit by a truck'. Eight years on, however, Gallo's superstar status and scientific credibility had been undermined. The scientific community had now accepted that HIV was first isolated in 1983 by the group led by Montagnier, and had been sent to Gallo's laboratory for further testing. A National Institutes of Health inquiry panel had accused Gallo of 'intellectual misappropriation' of the virus. It said a 1984 article in *Science* contained 'misrepresentations or falsifications' of methodology and data, errors which Gallo had blamed on the rush to publish.

Meanwhile, Montagnier, the other 'founding father' of HIV, had been trying to signal to the world that HIV was not as dangerous as had been thought. 'We were naive,' he had said. 'We thought this one virus had been doing all the destruction. Now we have to understand the other factors in this.' He had first tried to make some of his views on these 'co-factors' known at the sixth international Aids conference in San Francisco nearly two years previously, seven years after his original discovery. He thought he had an important message, but it was not one the conference wanted to hear. Of 12,000 delegates present, only 200 went to hear his talk. By the time he had finished, almost half of those had walked out. His views were dismissed by leading American Aids scientists and public health officials. 'There was Montagnier, the Jesus of HIV, and they threw him out of the temple,' Duesberg had commented.

We explained how Duesberg had also been marginalised and 'defunded', and how although no one had been able to explain how HIV could be so devastating, most medical scientists believed the epidemiological evidence showed such a close link between HIV and Aids that the virus must be to blame.

But Duesberg had recently published an 8,000-word critique in the Paris-based journal *Biomedicine and Pharmacotherapy,* in which he maintained that not only the virology, but also the patterns of illness in the American and European Aids epidemics, failed to support the theory that HIV was responsible. In the seven years since HIV testing became available, the official estimate of the number of Americans carrying the virus had remained constant, and screening by the US Army among potential recruits had also shown a constant proportion of both men and women – 0.03 per cent – with antibodies to HIV. The explanation that best fitted those data was that they reflected a harmless background presence of the retrovirus in which it survived naturally, at a low level, by being passed from mother to children. It was unrelated to Aids, for which the vast majority of American victims were men.

The HIV-positive babies seen by health authorities were different: they came mainly from drug-abusing parents, and it was adverse emotional and physical circumstances, not HIV, that might prove lethal to them. When they came from good homes, or were adopted and well cared for, most stayed healthy. In fact, almost all Americans who developed Aids had been exposed to abnormal health risks. The virus acted as a risk 'marker'. The medical profession's mistake had been to jump to the conclusion that when that marker was present, the patient's illness was a consequence of it.

The article included a discussion of the special risks faced by haemophiliacs, and of the recent *Lancet* evidence that the ten Edinburgh patients who developed immune deficiencies differed from the others in that their immune systems were hyperactive *before* they became HIV-positive. The doctors had suggested that might be a genetic trait predisposing to 'HIV disease'. For Duesberg it supported the considerable body of evidence that haemophiliacs developed immune deficiencies because of their condition and its treatment.

If the real cause of haemophiliac Aids was haemophilia, how come their wives occasionally died of Aids after sexual transmission of HIV? The answer, according to Duesberg, was that they didn't. The US Centers for Disease Control had reported that a total of ninety-four wives of haemophiliacs had been diagnosed with 'Aids' diseases in the past seven years, on average about thirteen a year. Although HIV was difficult to transmit through vaginal intercourse, requiring on average about 1,000 sexual contacts, some of the wives did become HIV-positive. But about eighty deaths a year could be expected anyway in this group, on the basis of standard death rates*. And the wives did not get illnesses such as Kaposi's sarcoma, or dementia, or lymphoma, or wasting syndrome. 'What you see here are pneumonias, mostly, and a few other infections – typical diseases of older age. Normal morbidity and mortality may be the simplest explanation, but because they are the wives of haemophiliacs it is called Aids.'

* Duesberg assumed that out of the 15,000 HIV-positive haemophiliacs in the US since 1985, a third were married.

Developing his hypothesis that the explosion of 'recreational' drug use was the main cause of Aids, Duesberg said the ability of drugs to break down the immune system was well documented. But 'it's not one bath house party, or two, or even ten or twenty, but if you do it over and over and over again. One gay activist in New York says that when he was wild in the bath houses, he had 3,000 sexual contacts. You don't do that on testosterone [naturally occurring male hormone]. With testosterone you fall asleep after one or two contacts. But if they are flying on amphetamines and poppers they go in for two or three days, and with twenty or thirty contacts. Poppers sound so cute, but they contain a very reactive compound, which is mutagenic and carcinogenic.

'So they mutate and oxidise and damage their DNA and RNA, and they don't get any sleep, and in the long run if they go on harder drugs such as cocaine and so on they can't pay for their food any more and don't eat the vitamins and proteins they need to regenerate, and they come down in hospital with pneumonia... Then they give them AZT, which is inevitably toxic, and a year later you are definitely dead.'

The article concluded by saying that the drug theory left many questions unanswered, such as why homosexual victims who either never took drugs, or gave them up on learning of their antibody status, could still go into rapid decline. The scientists seeking a new look at Aids admitted their own ideas on its causes were speculative, the article said, but they were demanding that there should at least be more studies into the specific risks of drugs and other lifestyle factors.

In a separate column, readers were brought up to date with Montagnier's latest thinking on HIV and Aids. It was strikingly different from most people's picture of the disease. Montagnier insisted that HIV did not attack cells of the immune system directly, but that instead, when the virus infected the body in the presence of other microbes, it sparked a process in which some immune cells became wrongly 'programmed'. Faced with further attack, those cells failed to recognise the invaders as foreign. Rather than countering them, they regarded themselves as redundant and 'committed suicide'.

This ability to self-destruct, called apoptosis, was natural to many cells. It formed part of a system of checks and balances that enabled the body to maintain itself in good repair. But in people with Aids, the process had gone haywire. Immune cells were destroying themselves faster than they could be replaced. Laboratory tests had shown that about 10-20 per cent of the immune cells in HIV-positive people demonstrated a readiness to react in this abnormal way when challenged by other microbes, compared with almost none in healthy people. That still did not prove HIV was to blame; people infected with Aids had been infected with a lot of other 'foreign' agents as well. But it put it under strong suspicion of playing a part.

One important consequence of this way of thinking was that if activation by micro-organisms was important, HIV-infected individuals could reduce their risk of Aids by reducing their risks of being exposed to such microbes. Dietary advice and vitamin supplements were also likely to help. They could ease chemical stresses in the body, which had also been seen to provoke apoptosis. Another implication was that there should be great caution over the therapeutic use of any conventionally designed anti-HIV vaccine, as it might trigger the very process it should be preventing. This latter point was taken up the following week in an article about a British research team's efforts to develop a vaccine designed to de-sensitise the immune system, rather than trying to make it more reactive to HIV, as in the conventional approach.

I felt the *Sunday Times* had performed a useful service by setting out these doubts and uncertainties expressed by two world experts on retroviruses, and other scientists. That was not the way the medical or scientific communities saw it, however. A storm of protest followed the articles. Generally, the interview with Montagnier and the varying views of the reappraisal group scientists were ignored; the focus of hostile comment was on our temerity in having allowed a wider public to know of Duesberg's fundamental challenge to HIV.

Dr Kenneth Calman, Britain's Chief Medical Officer, wrote to say we had risked leaving readers with a misleading and potentially dangerous misconception. Duesberg's points had been 'refuted repeatedly by scientists worldwide'. There was an overwhelming scientific consensus that HIV caused Aids. The unifying factor which applied to all the disparate groups in which Aids was reported was the presence of HIV. In every population studied, infection with HIV preceded the appearance of Aids. Although scientists did not yet know exactly how HIV attacked the immune system or why the lag between infection and symptoms could vary so much, that did not mean HIV was not the cause. Follow-up of patients with HIV infection showed that after ten years, 50 per cent would have Aids and a further 25 per cent would have some symptoms of HIV infection. During the incubation period, infected people might show no symptoms and yet still be able to pass the infection on to others.

'I repeat these facts,' Calman said, 'which should by now be well known, because the greatest threats to public health are ignorance, complacency and denial. We also need an informed public because as yet our only defence against the disease is prevention. The media have a responsible part to play in this.'

At the time, I took this as an accusation that I had been irresponsible in writing as I had done, and, in the midst of all the other criticism, reacted defensively. Now that I am no longer in the thick of the controversy, I can see that Calman and his advisers were really quite restrained in their response, given the work that had gone into warning the British public about the perceived dangers of HIV. I also see now that I had been naive in hoping Calman would address the scientific issues raised. Instead – not surprisingly, in view of the subject's complexity – he cited overwhelming agreement among scientists as authority for the 'facts' stated. Nevertheless, I did feel strongly that the one point that came closest to a fact in his letter, in which he cited rates of death and disease totalling 75 per cent after ten years in HIV-positive people, was misleading. It was based on data from a cohort of gay men in San Francisco who, as Sonnabend and others had described, had brewed up a level of general infection and disease, as well as of chemically induced damage to the body, unprecedented in modern times and perhaps in human history.

Irresponsibility was the most common accusation. 'The overwhelming evidence is that Aids is caused by HIV. Promulgation of theories to the contrary is irresponsible and dangerous,' wrote a haemophilia doctor in Edinburgh. Dr Trevor Jones, Wellcome's research director, wrote of the importance of not discouraging HIV-positive individuals and those with Aids 'from using medicines which have been clearly and repeatedly demonstrated – under properly controlled, scientifically valid conditions – to provide benefit and extend life'.

'The spreading of a terrible myth,' said the headline on an article about the controversy by Steve Connor, science correspondent of the *Independent* newspaper, who some years previously had been responsible for dismissive coverage of Duesberg's case in the *New Scientist.* The rival *Observer* newspaper printed a story to the effect that a leading Aids charity had asked the Press Complaints Commission to investigate our 'irresponsible reporting' (we never heard from the Commission, which presumably gave the complaint short shrift). A spokesman for the Health Education Authority said all the evidence pointed to the fact that HIV was present in people who had Aids. 'To suggest otherwise against the weight of evidence is misleading and dangerous.' Robert Gallo wrote to say that he found the articles 'widely irresponsible both to myself and to HIV as the cause of Aids'. It was obvious that 'co-factors' might contribute to the rate of progression of Aids as they did to virtually every disease, 'but to deny HIV as the primary aetiologic agent was self-deluding in 1984. By 1992 it is an appeal to the dark ages'. A report by the *Guardian's* health page editor said the *Sunday Times's* recent reports on Aids 'have succeeded in uniting scientists and journalists' by resorting to 'appalling hype which alarms patients and confuses a complex issue'. There was also a furious attack on the *Sunday Times* in the *Lancet,* written by a *Guardian* leader writer, though I was grateful to the *Lancet* for publishing a long letter of reply.

After widespread press and television coverage of the 'alternative' Aids conference in Amsterdam, three Nobel prize-winners – Sir Aaron Klug, Cesar Milstein and Max Perutz, senior researchers at the Medical Research Council's Laboratory of Molecular Biology in Cambridge – wrote to the *Independent* applauding Connor's article, and declaring that there was no question in their minds that 'HIV is the cause' of Aids. The letter, which was also signed by Abraham Karpas, a leading Aids researcher at Cambridge University, said publicity for Duesberg's views 'can only serve to accelerate the spread of the virus'. Dai Rees, secretary of the MRC, issued a press statement headed 'Careless talk costs lives' which declared that 'there has been an epidemic of irresponsible and inaccurate media reports' publicising Duesberg's hypothesis. It was 'irresponsibility bordering on the criminal' to suggest, as Duesberg had done, that safe sex had not prevented a single case of Aids. Rees also poured scorn on Duesberg's suggestion that AZT was

'Aids by prescription'. The evidence for that was about as strong as saying that since many people with a toothache also take aspirin, aspirin causes toothaches. Careful clinical studies had shown AZT could benefit patients with Aids, he said.

In fact, because Duesberg's views on safe sex added nothing to the scientific argument, were controversial even among the scientists who agreed with him on HIV, and had a potential for causing harm, we did not mention them in our original coverage. Other media had aired those views as part of their coverage of the controversy, however, and Rees's outrage was therefore understandable, though again I felt surprised – foolishly, perhaps, even betrayed – at the lack of response to the wider issues raised.

Some of the delegates to the Amsterdam conference, including medical scientists Joe Sonnabend and Gordon Stewart, issued a statement dissociating themselves from Duesberg's disregard of the 'safe sex' drive. They emphasised that questioning HIV's role in Aids did not mean that practising safe sex was irrelevant to the spread of Aids.

Nevertheless, for those who were so ready to make accusations of 'criminal' irresponsibility, Sonnabend had some other food for thought. He told the conference that because scientists and health officials had single-mindedly promoted the idea that Aids was caused by one killer virus, they might be to blame for thousands of deaths. Nearly 300 of his own patients had died in twelve years of the epidemic, and eight years after HIV was identified, he still had nothing substantial to offer as treatment. The tragedy was the result of the total concentration of research funds on HIV and the 'criminal' suppression of other research possibilities.

Michael Callen spoke in similar vein about his researches among long-term survivors of Aids. He said they all mentioned lifestyle changes, including giving up drugs, alcohol and cigarettes, and switching to safer sex to avoid any further microbial infection. They also talked about 'emotional housecleaning' that had given them a commitment to life instead of a self-destructive lifestyle. And the overwhelming majority 'had somehow managed to resist the enormous pressure to take AZT'. Stewart, despite his distress over Duesberg's belittling of safe sex, welcomed the meeting as 'the first in Europe, or perhaps anywhere, which permitted the expression of facts and opinions contrary to those of the prevailing international consensus and censorship'.

Lauritsen and others spoke with considerable anger against the Aids 'establishment' at the conference. Was this simply a matter of denial, an attempt by Aids patients and those close to them to avoid unpleasant facts about HIV, as *Nature* suggested in a report from Amsterdam entitled 'Rage and Confusion Hide Role of HIV'? I posed the question myself in an article about the conference for the *Sunday Times*. Perhaps there was an element of that. Among those present, some were driven more by emotion than reason in their reaction to the presentations, which included measured argument from a group of Dutch researchers pointing to the very close links between HIV-positivity and Aids in concluding that 'HIV is the cause of Aids'.

But it had also become clear to me that emotions, and self-interest, were not confined to the anti-HIV camp. Data gathered by both sides were inadequate, and often coloured by preconceptions about what was going on. Again and again I saw false assertions from HIV's advocates which I only knew to be wrong because of having gone deeply into the scientific literature, and which previously I would have had to accept on trust. That was why it was so important, I wrote, 'to keep an open mind about Aids causes and research strategies until it becomes obvious that a particular approach is yielding benefit'. Montagnier made a similar point at the conference, beginning and ending his presentation with an appeal for tolerance and an end to dogma.

Faced with the immense welter of criticism, I took comfort from the occasional letter of support. David Lloyd, the senior editor at Channel 4 who had commissioned the Meditel programmes on Aids, wrote saying, 'We all – in our different ways – have got to keep this debate open rather than tight shut, as so many would wish. Do please keep it up!' Joe Bailey Cole wrote from Kensington, London:

> Hodgkinson's investigation into current medical treatments and research is the first time I have seen any major newspaper show an awareness of the crisis in current Aids affairs. Could we have more of this please? Because only the giants of the press, such as yourselves, have the clout to force governments, agencies, and even doctors themselves to seriously listen to the questions that many of us have been asking to otherwise deaf ears.
>
> I think this article will have upset a lot of people who under the guise of professionalism have forgotten what intellectual honesty is, and who

> will be forced now to bring their musty old prejudices out into the sunlight of public awareness.
>
> More! More! More!

At the end of June 1992, a fresh round of attacks greeted the *Sunday Times* after it punctured a huge scare story over alleged heterosexual transmission of HIV and Aids. A young, fast-living haemophiliac in Birmingham was said to have infected four female partners, one of whom had died of Aids. A week of headlines like 'Aids maniac on loose in city', 'My girl was killed by Aids lover', 'Aids connection sets off spiral of terror', and 'Aids nightmare spreads' sparked a national panic, prompting a renewal of warnings that everyone was at risk – and some finger-pointing at those who had questioned the validity of those warnings.

Robin McKie, the *Observer's* science correspondent, under the headline 'The comforters of a free-for-all lifestyle eat their cheery words', said the *Sunday Times* now faced a challenge of considerable proportions. How could the haemophiliac possibly have passed on the disease, except through being HIV-positive? And how did he come to be infectious in the first place, except by being infected with HIV-contaminated blood products given as treatment for his haemophilia? 'There are no effective answers to these questions,' McKie wrote, 'for one good reason: the cause of Aids is the HIV virus. Those who use their newspapers to say otherwise only promote ignorance and illness.' In another column, he wrote that 'the myth that Aids cannot be spread by heterosexual sex was painfully exposed once again' by the Birmingham case. 'For almost a decade, scientists have been aware that the virus responsible for acquired immune deficiency syndrome can be passed on like any other sexually transmitted disease. Yet their warnings have been consistently ignored.' Vaginal sex, he said, was the principal conduit. A single act of sexual intercourse could lead to a person becoming infected and developing Aids.

McKie's passionate advocacy of the conventional view reflected what he had consistently been told by the vast majority of Aids scientists, although I resented the distortion of our position – at no point had the newspaper stated that HIV was not the cause of Aids, and our coverage had brought lifestyle back into the picture rather than sanctioned a 'free-for-all'.

The same weekend, the *Sunday Times* came out with a story which, mercifully, brought that particular panic to an instant close. All week, the health authority at the heart of the scare, believing that it presented a useful opportunity to reinforce warnings about heterosexual spread, had declared that transmission of the virus resulted from 'straightforward heterosexual intercourse' and that other risk factors had been ruled out. By the weekend, however, reporters had discovered that one of the haemophiliac's former partners admitted having anal intercourse with him 'more often than not', while another was reported to have said it happened on one occasion (it was subsequently reported that a third girlfriend also said they had sex this way). Further, the young woman who died of 'Aids' – her actual cause of death was pneumonia – had been admitted to hospital in such a breathless state that she had to be sedated and put on a ventilator immediately. There was no chance to question her about her lifestyle before she died. Neither her parents nor her long-term boyfriend had been approached by health officials to learn more of the circumstances of her death. All she had told the doctors was that she had been out with a haemophiliac, on which basis she was tested for HIV antibodies and found to be positive – hence the Aids diagnosis.

We quoted Gordon Stewart as saying that the reports of anal intercourse – the commonest form of transmission of HIV among homosexuals – could be vital to understanding why so many women had apparently become infected from a single source. 'The public health people do not appear to have inquired into this, but it is terribly important,' he said. 'With normal vaginal intercourse, we know the transmission rate of HIV is low. Some studies show that less than 10 per cent of people who are HIV-positive are transmitting the virus to female partners through regular, unprotected sex. In the absence of other sexually transmitted diseases, it is difficult to get HIV and you certainly don't get Aids.' Anal intercourse involved physical trauma that was not present in vaginal intercourse: 'The rectum is fragile. The trauma can lead to rupture and bleeding and the disease-causing organism or organisms or sperm can get direct access to the bloodstream. In my view, that is what starts all the trouble.'

Stewart argued that the 'special treatment' given to HIV-infected and Aids patients was blocking effective understanding and counter-measures against the epidemic. 'The essence of controlling a communicable disease is obtaining as much information as possible about the source of infection and the way it spreads,' he said. 'The time, the person, and the circumstances – these are three cardinal approaches. And you must trace the chain of contacts... Are the women engaging in anal intercourse? When there is a lot of promiscuity and sexual adventurism, that sort of thing happens. Are the men involved completely heterosexual? Or is there a homosexual or bisexual aspect? These are very important points to clear.' He went on to make the crucial distinction – which all others seemed to have forgotten – between testing HIV-positive and developing Aids.

> Obviously, people can pick up HIV through sexual contact with an infected person. The big question is, do they get Aids without being in any other risk group? HIV is certainly heterosexually transmissible, though not very easily. You could expect some of a haemophiliac patient's partners to pick it up if practising unprotected sexual intercourse, though probably at a rate less than 10 per cent. But you then need to follow those infected partners very closely to see whether or not they get Aids.

Detective work of that kind did not exclude confidentiality, 'but the people entrusted with preserving public health must be able to talk directly to these people. It's not a job that can be done from an office'. He felt a change of direction was long overdue.

> Because of the sensitivity and 'politically correct' issues that surround it, HIV infection is being treated as a special case. It is exempted from all the normal security measures, but instead made the subject of national panic messages and misinformation. I think we are seeing these policies of untruths, which were developed with humane intentions, rebound in an adverse way. If there is a threat to health, people must know the precise nature of the threat. Anal intercourse, for example, unquestionably presents a far bigger threat than vaginal intercourse, but people have been mincing their words over this.
>
> The public health movement has lost so much of its momentum that the people in charge are not able or willing to square up to this kind of thing.

Even though our coverage on this issue left open the question of HIV's role in Aids, that did not stop John Maddox, the editor of *Nature,* from attacking us in his pages for 'putting consistency before correctness' by reporting that anal intercourse was present as a risk factor in the case. He also called the *Sunday Times* a convert to Duesberg's view that HIV was irrelevant to Aids 'and the comforting corollary that people have nothing to fear from heterosexual intercourse'. None of that was true, as I said in a letter of reply, asking 'Why is a journal dedicated to science so afraid of facts?' The letter added: 'We do however consider that Duesberg has raised some important questions. His claim that mainstream science has climbed on an HIV bandwagon which it defends in an unreasoning way is supported by your unwarranted attack on our coverage.'

Subsequently, *Nature* carried a letter from a Swedish researcher, Per-Erik Asard, emphasising that the relative risk of HIV transmission from men to women was increased by a factor of 5.1 in anal intercourse, compared to vaginal intercourse. Raw data from the European study concerned showed that an 'alarming' 46 per cent of women who had had anal intercourse with HIV-infected men became HIV-positive. But this important message, although well known within the Aids community, had not been clearly stated to the public. 'This information is especially important for women, because they are the main victims,' Asard concluded (actually, we learned later that his final line was, 'I think that the information the *Sunday Times* gave to the public in the Birmingham affair was of utmost importance,' but that was edited out). Four years previously, a very similar letter, published in the *Lancet,*[5] stated: 'It is unfortunate that anal sex has not been considered separately from other practices as the main mode of HIV transmission, regardless of the gender of the partners. Calls for abstinence and warnings that all forms of heterosexual activity are equally dangerous are invalid. Warnings that anal intercourse is dangerous are valid, can be understood by most lay people, and could save many lives.'

Up to now, the *Sunday Times* had experienced a truly enormous volume of criticism for doing little more than raise questions. As the headline on one of our reports from the Eighth International Aids Conference – the 'official' Aids conference in Amsterdam, in July 1992 – put it: 'The truth is, we don't know what causes this disease.' But the climate of opinion was such that our questioning was considered an intolerable intrusion on the authority of science. Since it was difficult for our critics to say that, they persisted in attacking us for positions we had not taken up. I found this behaviour very suspicious.

When an individual is suppressing from awareness some embarrassing or threatening fact, he reacts with excessive emotion to any challenge in the area of sensitivity. I began to wonder if the community of scientists, including those who identified with that community in the media, was behaving in the same pathological way. Could Duesberg be right, and the entire medical and scientific world have got it wrong? I still felt instinctively that his alternative theory, the drug-Aids hypothesis, was inadequate, though common sense dictated that the explosion of drug use which he and Lauritsen had highlighted had a lot to do with Aids. However, from a starting point in which I had simply believed that the challenge to HIV had not been properly answered and deserved a wider audience, I now began to feel I might have stumbled upon one of the most extraordinary stories in the history of science – that there really was some fundamental flaw in the HIV hypothesis. But would anyone ever believe that? We had achieved the object of setting the 'dissident' arguments before our readers, but there had been precious little support – virtually none from doctors or scientists in the UK. Where were we to go from here?

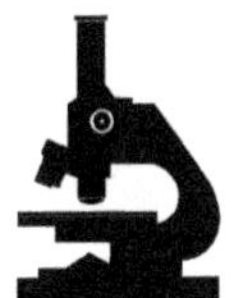

8: THE CASE AGAINST HIV GROWS STRONGER

The second half of 1992 passed slowly. I had been widely criticised for writing about the challenge to HIV, but I felt that the reactions to our coverage – as with earlier responses to the HIV critique – were short on reasoned argument. There was more to the story, I was sure, and I wanted to continue with it. But how? Within the office, several colleagues were uncomfortable. It was one thing to set out the challenge and report on the growing demand for a reappraisal, but if we kept returning to such a controversial story, it would look as though we had joined the 'dissident' cause. At this point neither the editor nor myself were ready to believe for sure that so monumental a mistake had been made. Questions needed to be asked, but no one knew where the truth lay. Had I taken the newspaper down a blind alley? Repeated assertions by our critics that millions of heterosexual Africans were in the pipeline of death because of HIV, demonstrating the virus's potential to wreak indiscriminate havoc elsewhere in the world, were unanswerable in the absence of first-hand data or authoritative information. The editor had taken a big risk in publishing the 'dissident' case. No matter how much we might justify doing so on grounds of openness, if the HIV theory, and the apocalyptic predictions based on it, turned out to be true, we would still look pretty stupid, to say the least.

Despite having tried for some years to improve my ability to work according to conscience, and not to be put off by adverse opinion, my self-confidence had been shaken by the vehemence – and near-universality – of the attacks. Had I blundered? Was Duesberg a maverick, already thoroughly discredited?

That was how *New Scientist* described him in a report of a June 1992 meeting in London of the All-Party Parliamentary Group on Aids, a group of concerned MPs, held to 'clarify' the HIV issue. 'Researchers and journalists in the US and Europe are bemused by what seems to be a peculiarly British preoccupation with the maverick scientist,' Phyllida Brown began her report on the meeting at the House of Commons. To the general reader – and indeed to the MPs – the arguments levelled against Duesberg (who was not invited to attend the meeting) may have seemed persuasive.

I now knew, however, that as with previous 'rebuttals' of Duesberg's case, there were reasoned replies to the points raised, certainly deserving respect rather than ridicule. Although it is tedious to detail arguments only to have to explain why, in my view, they are ill-conceived, I shall do that with this short *New Scientist* report, as it typifies how mainstream science held the HIV theory in place for much longer than it deserved.

Jonathan Weber, professor of communicable diseases at St Mary's Hospital Medical School in London, was invited to speak to the MPs, and his comments, which were in line with mainstream thinking, formed the bulk of the *New Scientist's* report. He found the media's fascination with Duesberg 'bizarre'. 'There is no unifying theory being put forward by him,' he said. In the US, where 1 million people had HIV and more than 200,000 had developed Aids, few people paid attention to him. 'Such is the size of the problem that these arguments are purely academic.' I knew, however, that the essence of Duesberg's case was that the imposition of a unifying theory – HIV – on a syndrome that in reality had a variety of causes was the very reason why the problem continued to grow.

Duesberg's claim that drugs were a direct cause of Aids was discounted, Phyllida Brown wrote. 'Weber repeated the results of a study published in *Nature* two years ago showing that drug users infected with HIV died earlier than those who were not infected. If drugs caused Aids, there should be no difference.' I knew about this 'study'. It was actually data presented in a short letter to *Nature* by Weber and others, published on 27 September 1990. It stated that out of 194 HIV-positive homosexual men followed since 1984, Aids had developed in sixty-eight, and there were forty-eight deaths from all causes; but none of a group of 120 HIV-negative men had developed Aids, and none had died. According to the letter, information about sexual behaviour and recreational drug use had been obtained at recruitment and follow-up visits, 'and the two groups were closely matched'. Among a group of patients with severe haemophilia, followed since 1979, the HIV-positive ones showed similar rates for Aids and deaths, whereas none of the HIV-negative group had developed Aids or died.

On 7 March 1991, Duesberg had pointed out in a letter of reply in *Nature* that the data was unpublished (in the sense that it had not been submitted as a scientific document to a peer-reviewed journal). Before he could accept the conclusion, he wrote, he would need to know for what drug use the two groups were matched, since cohort studies were biased by those who recruited and by those who volunteered to be recruited. He would also want to know what Aids-linked diseases they developed. It was surprising that among 120 HIV-negative 'sexually active homosexual men' and fifteen HIV-negative subjects with severe haemophilia, not even one developed any of the twenty-five indicator diseases of Aids in six years. 'Could it be that these diseases were not listed because in the absence of HIV they are called by their own names?' he asked. Indeed, recent studies had shown that HIV-free haemophiliacs had the same immunodeficiencies as HIV-positive controls, and HIV-free male homosexuals had the same Kaposi's sarcomas and some of the same T-cell deficiencies as HIV-positive controls. This, in Duesberg's view, was why it was necessary to conduct randomised, controlled studies, instead of studying selected cohorts, to determine whether health risk factors could cause Aids without HIV, and whether HIV could cause Aids without such factors.

I checked one[1] of the haemophilia studies (from Michigan State University, East Lansing) referred to by Duesberg. It stated that no correlations were found between HIV infection and immune abnormalities, and even patients who had not received any Factor 8 treatment showed an underlying immune deficiency, although the abnormalities grew more profound in those who received treatment. It was a small study, with only fifteen patients, but a careful one involving measurement of a range of immune system parameters. Perhaps it was misleading, but I knew also from the Edinburgh haemophiliac study that the story was not as simple as the MPs were being led to suppose.

Third, the *New Scientist* stated that 'in response to Duesberg's claim that Aids is an old disease, Weber said that in 1979 there was widespread sexually transmitted disease among gay men but no deaths. By 1989, the number of cases of conventional STDs had fallen, but deaths from Aids had risen into the thousands'. In fact, there *were* deaths among promiscuous gay men in the 1970s, from Aids-type diseases such as pneumocystic pneumonia and Kaposi's sarcoma, although they were not classified as Aids at that time. But in any case, it was nonsense to say Duesberg claimed that 'Aids is an old disease'. He accepted that the epidemic of immune deficiency was new, but linked it to the cumulative effects of an epidemic of long-term drug abuse rather than to HIV.

Fourth, it was stated that 'Duesberg rightly points out that no one has proved, in direct molecular terms, that the virus causes Aids. But a purified cloned version of the simian immunodeficiency virus, HIV's closest relative, causes immune deficiency in laboratory monkeys'. Duesberg, however, had also pointed out that SIV was totally harmless in monkeys in the wild: 50 per cent of African green monkeys carry it, and illness has never been seen to be caused by it. In the artificial circumstances of laboratory injections with the cloned version, the animals did not have a chance to produce an immune response, and rapidly became ill.

Fifth, Weber said scientists accepted that other infections, such as certain herpes viruses, might enhance HIV's effects, but that did not make HIV 'innocent' and in any case was not unique to HIV. But this argument was irrelevant to Duesberg's case, since he believed drugs were the prime cause of the epidemic. It was not even doing justice to Montagnier's position on 'co-factors', because the French scientist was not simply saying that other infections made HIV disease worse, but that HIV might be harmless in the absence of these other factors.

Weber's next point was that although the virus might infect only small numbers of T-cells, 'there is evidence that HIV triggers other destructive effects on the whole of the immune system... for example, the virus may increase the normal tendency for some T-cells to "commit suicide" – a process known as apoptosis'. But in my interview with Montagnier, he had been quite clear on this: although apoptosis was seen more frequently in HIV-positive people, that correlation was as far as the evidence went. It was only a theory that HIV, rather than the many other risks to which HIV-positive people had usually been exposed, was causing the apoptosis.

Finally, Duesberg had said HIV could not be isolated from everyone with antibodies to the virus. According to Weber, 'this was true once but it is no longer the case because of better techniques for detection. The amount of HIV in the blood also increases as Aids progresses, strongly implicating it as the cause'. In fact, Duesberg had explained that the 'better technique' was the polymerase chain reaction (Kary Mullis's invention) which did not isolate or even detect active virus, but simply showed the presence within cells of genetic material thought to be related to HIV. And as Sonnabend and others had long argued, the easier detection of this material as Aids progressed could be a consequence of the immune deficiency rather than a cause.

None of this meant Duesberg was right and the HIV hypothesis wrong. What was striking was that *New Scientist* should regard this as another example of how 'scientists have argued convincingly against' Duesberg and that the case against HIV could therefore continue to be dismissed, and Duesberg's requests for better evidence disregarded. To me, it demonstrated yet again how doctors and scientists – and science journalists – had become so emotionally bound by the dynamics of the Aids emergency that they were unable to see or think clearly. The evidence was confusing and sometimes contradictory, but no one seemed willing to admit that.

Haemophilia Findings

In November the same year (1992), after several frustrating months in which the *Sunday Times* made no further reference to the controversy, I came across a development that renewed my sense of something being very wrong with the HIV paradigm. Directors of Britain's haemophilia centres were rebelling against attempts by National Health Service administrators to prevent them prescribing an expensive but potentially lifesaving new treatment. They wanted to switch their patients, particularly all those who were HIV-positive, to a new, very high-purity version of Factor 8, the blood-clotting agent, following studies showing it could slow or halt what was thought to be a key component of the immune system decline that led to Aids.

In the latest research,[2] to be presented the following month at a meeting of the American Society of Haematology, twenty patients in the US who had been transferred to the new treatment three years previously had experienced, as a group, no decline in their immune status as measured by T4 ('helper') cells. But a similar group given an 'intermediate' purity product had the classic signs of progression towards Aids. Over three years, their mean T-cell count fell from 400 to 200, while the high-purity group stayed at around 400. I found that almost identical results had been published in the journal *Blood* the previous year by a group of Italian researchers.[3]

Despite similar results from other studies, regional health officials in several parts of Britain were blocking a switch to the new treatment, saying they could not justify the extra expenditure. On average, it cost the health service about £30,000 a year to treat patients with severe haemophilia, and that could rise to more than £50,000 with the new product. As a result, well over half of Britain's 1,000 surviving HIV-positive haemophiliacs remained on the 'intermediate' purity product. A Health Department ruling that cash earmarked for Aids could not be used to pay for the new product had even led to some patients being taken off it and put back on the 'old' Factor 8. Subsequent advice urged health authorities not to withdraw funds abruptly if that would harm patients, but the department was insisting that 'like any other new treatment, it should be funded from mainstream NHS allocations' and that it was up to the regional authorities to decide how fast to introduce medical advances.

The haemophilia doctors were upset by this decision, particularly so because they saw some health authorities awash with cash earmarked for Aids because of over-estimates of Aids cases. Six months previously, a scientific committee they had set up to review the Factor 8 evidence urged in a report that all their HIV-positive patients should receive the new product. Other haemophiliacs should receive it too, the committee said, though in their case the need was less urgent. John Marshall, an MP who helped win compensation for HIV-positive haemophiliacs, had written to the Prime Minister urging him to intervene. 'The state, through the NHS, was responsible for infecting these patients; it owes a duty of care, kindness and courtesy to ensure they get the best possible treatment known to science,' he said. 'There is no doubt that if they were given this treatment it would extend their lives by at least three years, and perhaps avoid the onset of Aids altogether.'

In the light of all the trouble already suffered by haemophiliacs, I was surprised to learn of this red tape surrounding the introduction of a treatment that could certainly be expected to delay the onset of Aids. After all, it was the decline in T4 cells seen in HIV-positive haemophiliacs that was originally held to confirm HIV's deadly potential. What was particularly strange was the reluctance of health administrators to use Aids cash to delay or prevent Aids by paying for the improved clotting factor treatment. It was as if they were afraid that by doing so, they might be admitting to a weakness in the idea that HIV was doing all the damage. I wrote a story about the row, and although it was not published, the newspaper's interest may have helped to bring about a rethink, because almost immediately afterwards a more liberal policy was implemented.

For me, however, the particular interest in the findings was the scientific light the studies cast on HIV's role in Aids. Many of the patients – nine out of ten in one study – showed an upsurge in T4 cell counts during their first year on the high-purity treatment. They tended to fall back in the second year, and then to stabilise around the level they had started with during the third year. I rang one of the study coordinators to check what had happened to them since: she said it was now known that although there were big individual fluctuations, the mean for the group remained stable for up to four years.

This had dramatic implications. If T4 counts were a reliable predictive factor for Aids, as a number of studies had suggested, HIV-positive haemophiliacs might not after all be under sentence of death. Furthermore, the findings provided strong confirmation of Duesberg's longstanding claim that haemophiliacs had been dying as a result of side-effects of their treatment, not as a result of HIV infection. The more I found out about the treatments, the more likely this seemed. The differences in quality between old and new were enormous, although the haemophilia doctors, struggling with cash restraints, were usually less than frank about this with their patients. The so-called 'intermediate' purity product contained only about five units of Factor 8 per milligram of blood extract, the rest being unwanted blood proteins; whereas the new, manufactured by a technique that isolated the pure Factor 8 and set it in a neutral base, provided up to 4,000 units per milligram. The old product was made from concentrated extracts from the blood of thousands of people; a typical patient receiving forty to sixty treatments a year could be exposed to blood from up to 2 million donors annually.[4] Not surprisingly, and contrary to the claims of Duesberg's detractors, several studies had suggested immune deficiencies in haemophiliacs before the HIV era, with reports of increased deaths both from pneumonia and cancer.

Although haemophilia itself is linked with certain immune system abnormalities, the rate at which patients progress towards Aids is linked to the rate at which the T4 cell count falls.[5] If the decline can be stopped and even reversed, there are good grounds for hoping that the principal 'Aids' risk which these patients used to face has been removed. I have spoken about these findings with haemophilia doctors, and never been given any good reason why the patients and their relatives are not being informed of this dramatic improvement in their prospects, only comments about the position being more complicated than I realise and the need to avoid raising false hopes. It seems that the need to remove false predictions of impending disease and death carries less sway.

A 1994 paper in the *British Medical Journal*[6] attracted news headlines with the prediction that up to a quarter of HIV-positive haemophiliacs may remain free of Aids for twenty years or more after first becoming positive. In fact, the proportion may be higher, because the basis on which this 'extension' of lifespan was calculated neither acknowledged nor took into account the role played by improvements in the quality of Factor 8. In a comment on the paper, the *BMJ's* editor stated: 'For years we have assumed that everybody infected with HIV would eventually die of Aids if they didn't die of something else first. In retrospect it seems strange that we should have made such an assumption – perhaps we were reacting to the hysteria that surrounded the world coming to recognise the disease.' That rare piece of frankness, though welcome, still did not go far enough in lifting the HIV 'hex' inflicted upon haemophiliac patients.

In good faith, because of believing what they had been told about HIV's deadly potential, haemophilia doctors gave their HIV-positive patients to understand that sooner or later, almost all were likely to die of Aids – 'the most sinister, terrible disease to afflict mankind since the plague', as Dr Max Perutz, of the Medical Research Council's Laboratory of Molecular Biology at Cambridge, put it in a 1990 letter to the *Guardian*. Equally in good faith, because of believing what they had been told about AZT's benefits and HIV's perils, the doctors prescribed this toxic drug to many haemophiliac patients whose only problem, as Duesberg said, may have been their haemophilia and its treatment. It is questionable, however, whether it can really be called 'in good faith' that they have continued to let these patients believe they are infected with a deadly virus, and continued to prescribe them what is, for healthy people, an unquestionably useless and probably dangerous drug, after such clear evidence became available that it was the challenge to the immune system from repeated administration of blood proteins – from up to 2 million donors a year – that was previously contributing most to their T-cell decline, and not HIV.

A change of *Sunday Times* newsroom executives at the beginning of 1993 brought an opportunity to resubmit a story about these developments. It appeared in the issue of 21 February under the headline 'Factor 8 hope in HIV battle'. In it, we stated that about 1,200 of Britain's 5,000 haemophiliacs had become infected with HIV from contaminated transfusions in the early 1980s, and 200 had since died, with HIV-Aids usually given as the cause of death. But others thought to be under sentence of death because of HIV 'have had their decline towards Aids halted by a dramatically improved treatment for their blood disorder'. Gordon Stewart did not pull his punches on the implications of the findings, which he regarded as 'immensely important'. He commented:

> If this work is confirmed, it means the patients may not get Aids at all. It also gives us an immense clue to the mechanism of Aids. We now know that if the haemophiliacs are infused with impure concentrates, they get changes that resemble Aids; and if they get the high-purity product, they don't get those changes. So the probability is that the haemophiliacs' response is to the foreign protein in their treatment, and not to HIV. The allegation that haemophiliac patients get Aids because of being infected by HIV has to be questioned*.

* A 1995 study confirming higher death rates in HIV-positive haemophiliacs did nothing to counter these hopes, since it included deaths only to 1992, and so as the authors stated, 'does not permit examination of data following widespread use in the UK of high purity factor concentrate'.

As far as I know, Stewart was the only British doctor to speak out publicly about the importance of these findings in relation to the HIV/Aids hypothesis. But he was surely right to do so. The data had implications that went beyond the hope that HIV-positive haemophiliacs might now be spared the threat of Aids. They raised the question of whether any haemophiliacs could properly be said to have died of Aids, or to be at risk of Aids, since from its earliest days the definition of the syndrome required an immune deficiency that was unexplained by any 'history of either immunosuppressive underlying illness or immunosuppressive therapy' (Centers for Disease Control, 1982). In 1985, after HIV (LAV/ HTLV-3) had been accepted as the cause of Aids, the CDC redefined the syndrome as requiring one or more opportunistic diseases, in the 'absence of all known underlying causes of cellular immunodeficiency (other than LAV/ HTLV-3) and absence of all other causes of reduced resistance reported to be associated with at least one of those opportunistic diseases'.

Now, as described, doctors had some evidence of an underlying tendency to immunosuppression caused by haemophilia itself, and very clear evidence that therapy for the condition had been – and still was – immunosuppressive for those receiving the 'intermediate purity' treatment. In fact, this had been known for many years. In 1986, *Aids Research* (while still under Joe Sonnabend's editorship) published an article by a group of Greek doctors showing immune abnormalities in both HIV-positive and HIV-negative haemophiliac patients, and noting that the HIV-positive patients had consumed more Factor 8 than those who were seronegative. In the same year, CDC researchers concluded that 'haemophiliacs with immune abnormalities may not necessarily be infected with HTLV-3/LAV, since factor concentrate itself may be immunosuppressive even when produced from a population of donors not at risk for Aids'.[7]

Transfusion and Other Victims

Although the 21 February story was not prominently displayed, it was the first of a run of articles published in the *Sunday Times* during 1993 that was to help bring about a crisis of confidence within the scientific world over the validity of the HIV hypothesis.

On 14 March, under the challenging headline 'Aids truth falls victim to virus of ignorance', a review article that I wrote about a book by Robert Root-Bernstein, associate professor of physiology at Michigan State University, was carried on the news feature pages. The news 'peg' was an enormous fuss that had blown up about HIV-positive doctors. To try to calm the row, health officials rightly insisted that there was not a single documented case anywhere of a doctor, nurse or midwife passing the virus on to a patient. Yet across the country, as the article pointed out, health authorities were spending millions of pounds disseminating the idea that Aids was caused by a new microbe which, once in a person's blood, would gradually but inexorably destroy their immune system until they became prey to a multitude of other diseases. Not surprisingly, patients became fearful when they learned they might have been treated by a doctor carrying this deadly disease.

Did Aids put everyone at risk, or didn't it? The problem, as Root-Bernstein spelled it out in *Rethinking Aids – The Tragic Cost of Premature Consensus,*[8] was that the medical and scientific community simply did not understand what was going on. There was no definitive evidence that HIV could cause Aids by itself – a point Montagnier had tried to drive home for years. There was definitive evidence, however, that everyone who developed Aids had multiple challenges to their immune system other than HIV – and in some cases they didn't even have HIV. Healthy people living normal lives did not get Aids, he argued. It took a multiplicity of factors, which together threw the immune system into such a state of confusion that it began attacking itself. One possibility was that antibodies to one's own immune system cells, rather than to HIV, might be the true cause of Aids.

All who indulged in anal intercourse were at risk, because semen and blood were themselves immunosuppressant, as were the bacteria, viruses, fungi, yeast and parasites to which that form of sexual activity exposed both partners. Having unprotected sex with a person with full-blown Aids could be particularly disastrous, not necessarily because of the risk of transmission of HIV, but because of the cocktail of infections that might be transmitted. Root-Bernstein presented much evidence that such co-infection had a synergistic effect on the immune system and could be particularly hard to treat.

Aids in the homosexual community had accompanied the unprecedented levels of promiscuity and drug use that accompanied the 'gay lib' revolution of the 1970s. Habitual drug users were exposed to numerous infections from needle use. The drugs themselves and the lifestyles to which addicts might become drawn also damaged the immune system.

Blood transfusions depleted immunity and carried a variety of risks apart from HIV, in people whose health was already compromised by the illness or injury that necessitated their transfusion. About 2 per cent of Aids cases were associated with transfusions, but the typical patient who developed Aids had received an average of twenty-one units of blood or plasma during their hospital stay – four to five times the general average. Among those who received blood that was subsequently thought to have been contaminated with HIV, the disease rate was thirty times higher in patients transfused with more than ten units compared with those who received less than that. Because of the association between HIV and other infections, HIV-contaminated blood was much more likely to be contaminated with other immunosuppressive viruses transmissible in blood, such as cytomegalovirus, Epstein-Barr virus and hepatitis viruses.

In *Rethinking Aids,* Root-Bernstein presented data demonstrating an astonishingly low survival rate among transfusion patients generally, regardless of HIV or Aids. A CDC-associated study[9] found that of 694 recipients of HIV-contaminated blood, 331 (48 per cent) died within a year of transfusion – which in the absence of comparative data would have seemed like dramatic confirmation of HIV's deadly role. But, uniquely in all studies of transfusion-associated Aids, these researchers also provided data for an HIV-negative group – and their death rate was just the same. Out of 146 recipients of blood components from a random selection of donors, seventy-three died in the year after transfusion. Several other American studies pointed in the same direction. 'Statements ... to the effect that transfusion patients prove the necessity and sufficiency of HIV as the cause of Aids are wishful thinking,' Root-Bernstein commented.

What about the babies and young children who had died of Aids? What risk behaviours could foetuses indulge in, as Anthony Fauci, one of the NIH Aids 'barons', had asked? The answer was that 80 per cent of infant Aids cases were born to drug abusers, 10 per cent had required blood transfusions, and 6 per cent were haemophiliac. In fact, less than a third of babies born seropositive went on to develop Aids. But among those that did, the immune-suppressing factors in evidence were the same as those that had long afflicted the children of addict mothers: foetal malnutrition, prematurity, low birthweight, small head size, distress at birth, jaundice, underdeveloped thymus, anaemia, and neurological, behavioural and developmental deficits. Problems like these caused death rates among such infants to be three times the national average during the 1970s. Many of the deaths were from pneumonia.

There was even a syndrome, first described in 1971, that was almost indistinguishable from Aids in infants. It was widely seen in the children of poverty-stricken and drug-abusing mothers, who often turned to prostitution and who sometimes passed on multiple infections to their babies as a result. It was known as TORCHES, which stood for congenital infections caused by TOxoplasmosis, Rubella, Cytomegalovirus (CMV), HErpes simplex virus and Syphilis. The symptoms were all found in Aids infants, who differed only in that they were also known to have tested HIV-positive. The data implicating CMV in infant Aids was particularly strong: most women with Aids were carrying active CMV infection, which they typically passed on to their babies via breast milk, and babies with CMV and HIV were much more likely to develop full-blown Aids and die by the age of twenty-four months than those without CMV.

'History suggests that such children have existed for as long as drug abuse and poverty have existed,' Root-Bernstein said. 'Treating them and their mothers only for HIV infection will hardly decrease their health risks. At best, eradicating HIV will only allow them to die of virtually identical problems, categorised under other names. That is the true tragedy of Aids infants.'

He kept open the possibility that HIV was a contributory factor in Aids. Although the probability of passing most sexually transmitted diseases from person to person was 'hundreds or thousands of times higher' than it was for HIV, when those other infections were present they made it more likely that HIV would be transmitted and that it would become active. They also expanded the range of cells that could become infected by HIV, thereby allowing it 'to create much more havoc than it could otherwise do'. It became a marker of people who might have multiple infections – including HIV itself – which put them at risk of Aids. Almost all had been infected repeatedly or chronically with several disease agents before developing the syndrome. Urging Aids researchers to widen the scope of their inquiries, he wrote: 'At best we have half the story; at worst, we missed the boat.'

Benefits of Behaviour Change

The enormous importance of this wider look at Aids was brought home by studies showing that regardless of HIV-positivity, the risk of developing Aids could be drastically lowered by health-promoting changes in behaviour. Such changes in the lives of HIV-positive gay men and former drug users had so strengthened the immune system that Aids was either prevented or its onset considerably postponed compared with those who kept exposing their bodies to the same risks.

One of the clearest examples of this phenomenon was that of Dr Maurizio Luca Moretti, of the Florida-based Inter-American Medical and Health Association, who has been collaborating with colleagues in Italy on a study of 508 former intravenous drug abusers. The men, all HIV-positive, were voluntarily confined to a rehabilitation centre where their lives were under the daily management of staff. Most were found to be severely malnourished on arrival, 397 of them chronically so. Their nutritional status was returned to normal, their drug use ended, and their sex lives curtailed – the centre is a monastery in which the patients sleep in small groups under supervision. Among 139 individuals who had been using heroin daily for an average of more than five years, all were still free of Aids symptoms after an average of more than four years since they first tested positive. This is a phenomenal success rate compared with the US, where 32 per cent of HIV-positive addicts develop Aids within two years and more than 50 per cent within four years. Similarly, a Swiss study found that the risk of developing Aids was three times higher among HIV-positive addicts who continued to inject drugs than among those who stopped.

Root-Bernstein's analysis had important implications for every aspect of the public health approach to Aids. It did not mean we would have no reason to be concerned about doctors with HIV or Aids, because in either case there could be a risk of passing on multiple infections. But checking for

HIV-positivity in anyone, doctors or others, without attending to the co-factors that led to Aids, might be worse than useless. It would not identify which patients were likely to go on to get Aids, nor would it identify treatable causes. But it would terrify those told they were positive for the virus, and their contacts, even though many HIV-positive people had immune systems that were in just as good shape as those who were HIV-negative.

Summarising his arguments in an article for the *Wall Street Journal* of 17 March, Root-Bernstein wrote that perhaps the most striking data concerned female prostitutes in western nations. Early in the epidemic, it was assumed that these prostitutes would become the vectors by which HIV and Aids would spread to the heterosexual community. A single, HIV-infected female prostitute might, it was thought, infect dozens of heterosexual men, and equal numbers of women through those men. In fact, although up to 10 per cent of female prostitutes tested HIV-positive in major US cities such as Los Angeles and New York, almost all were intravenous drug abusers. Cases of sexually acquired HIV were almost unknown among prostitutes who did not take drugs. Furthermore, there was literally only a handful of cases in which female prostitutes were thought to have transmitted HIV to a client, and drug abuse by both the prostitute and client had been documented in almost all of those cases.

As a result, every major review of female prostitution by the medical authorities of western nations had concluded that drug-free female prostitutes were not susceptible to HIV and would not be the means of infecting the general population. This data, along with findings that haemophiliacs had also not become vectors for heterosexual spread on any scale, argued that immunologically healthy people seemed immune. 'This is hardly the behaviour expected of a typical sexually transmitted disease,' he concluded.

In the UK, Root-Bernstein's scholarly, 500-page work was ignored by almost all of the lay and scientific press. The *Sunday Times* even came under attack in the *Observer* the following weekend for having reviewed it. Robin McKie, the science correspondent, accused me of indulging in a propaganda campaign, 'unsupported by credible scientific evidence', that argued 'without qualification' against Aids being caused by HIV. He interpreted my article as having claimed it was a person's lifestyle that did the damage — 'and serve them right for overdoing things'. The diatribe continued:

So, for the benefit of Mr Hodgkinson, and other pundits similarly affected by an acquired intelligence deficiency, let us state, slowly and clearly, that the prime cause of Aids is HIV.

Yes, Mr Hodgkinson, there are other factors involved in the disease's spread and no, not all are known. But there is one unequivocal connection. When, and where, you have HIV infections, you have Aids.

Take the example of Africa (conveniently ignored by Hodgkinson). Ten years ago, the disease was unknown there. Today the continent has several million cases of Aids. Are we seriously expected to believe that these are all victims of an epidemic triggered because they suddenly became unhealthy? In other words, Africans must either have suffered from crippled disease immunity centuries ago – in which case we would have identified Aids long ago – or their immune systems have suddenly crashed. Only HIV explains the latter event.

Doubts Cast on African Epidemic

I did not recognise our coverage as having sought to exculpate HIV, but, rather, to draw attention to information that pointed strongly to the need for a rethink. From my perspective, we were simply reporting facts that hardly anyone else seemed able to see. But from the reactions our reports sparked, it was becoming increasingly clear that *anything* said or written that questioned HIV was liable to be interpreted as putting you in some kind of enemy camp – right-wing, homophobic, fundamentalist Christian, or whatever.

If writing about Root-Bernstein's measured critique had been enough to trigger rage, our next article, the following Sunday, must have provoked apoplexy. For the first time, we dared to question the claims about Aids in Africa. It was bad luck for McKie, whose 1986 book *Panic: The Story of Aids* concluded with a quotation from a British professor that 'If you wanted to design a bug for a horror science fiction film, you couldn't really top the Aids virus', that the same weekend as the *Observer* published his attack accusing us of ignoring this issue, the *Sunday Times* ran a prominent article, filling most of page two, headlined 'Epidemic of Aids in Africa "a tragic myth"'.

In it, we described an authoritative challenge, mounted in a new Meditel documentary to be screened by Channel 4 that week, to the idea that the continent was in the grip of an Aids epidemic. The film would outrage much western medical opinion, we said, because of the belief that 'heterosexual Aids' in Africa was a warning of what could happen elsewhere. But a growing body of expert opinion believed that false claims of devastation by HIV were leading to a tragic diversion of resources from areas of genuine medical need such as malaria, tuberculosis and malnutrition. Some of the 'heretics' were even saying there was no evidence of a new sexually transmitted disease in Africa, but that instead, death rates had increased in some countries because of civil war, and because of poverty and malnutrition linked to economic decline. Predictions by the World Health Organization (WHO) and other agencies that millions would die because of HIV were based not on scientific evidence, but on unfounded assumptions about the extent of HIV infection in Africa and its links with Aids.

The documentary, produced and directed for 'Dispatches' by Joan Shenton, was based on a two-month investigation in Uganda and the Ivory Coast, thought to be epicentres of what agencies were calling a 'pandemic' of Aids. According to the WHO, 7.5 million people were infected with HIV in sub-Saharan Africa, and Aids would be killing 500,000 people a year there by the end of the century. But Dr Harvey Bialy, of *Bio/Technology,* who worked as a tropical disease expert in Africa for many years and who accompanied the television crew, had concluded that there was 'absolutely no believable, persuasive evidence that Africa is in the midst of a new epidemic of infectious immuno-deficiency'.

'Dispatches' argued that because international funds were available for Aids and HIV work, politicians and health workers had an incentive to classify people as Aids sufferers who previously would have been diagnosed as having other illnesses. The Ugandan government could afford less than US$1 a head on health care from its funds, but the previous year it received $6 million for Aids research and prevention from foreign agencies. Of that, $750,000 came from WHO, against $57,000 for the prevention and treatment of malaria, which killed an estimated 1 million people in sub-Saharan Africa every year.

Part of the problem was that HIV testing was frequently misleading in Africa, as the tests reacted to antibodies to other diseases, producing high rates of false positives. Furthermore, most Aids diagnoses in Africa did not involve an HIV test, but were based on a WHO definition that relied on clinical signs including weight loss, chronic diarrhoea and prolonged fever. The scope for misclassification was enormous. A recent *Lancet* report from Japanese doctors working in Ghana showed that out of a group of 227 diagnosed 'Aids' patients who had all three of those signs, as well as other 'Aids-related conditions', 59 per cent showed no trace of HIV in their blood.

Bialy, whom I interviewed for the article, told me that people were frightened of going to see a doctor, because they believed they would be diagnosed as having Aids – and feel condemned to death. 'It has become a joke in Uganda that you are not allowed to die of anything but Aids,' he said. 'A favourite story is that a friend has just been run over by a car; doctors put it down as Aids-related suicide.'

The only 'utterly new' phenomenon he had seen was in the drugabusing prostitutes in Abidjan in the Ivory Coast. The girls came from Ghana, from families of prostitutes who were brought in by the busload. 'They have been doing this for generations, and never became sick until now. What is new is that these girls are addicted to viciously adulterated, smokeable heroin and cocaine. It completely destroys them. They look exactly like the inner-city crack-addicted prostitutes of the United States.

'Otherwise, I have seen malaria, tuberculosis, diarrhoeal diseases, which arguably have got more severe; but by all the laws of scientific reasoning this is caused by the general economic decline in these countries, the decline of health care and development of drug-resistant strains. All these things can explain exactly what is going on much more efficiently and persuasively, and to much greater good for the public health than saying the diseases are being made worse by HIV.'

Our story also quoted a British expert puzzled by a disparity between apocalyptic warnings about the spread of Aids in Africa and her own observations. Professor Beverly Griffin, director of virology at the Royal Postgraduate Medical School in London, had been receiving blood samples of hundreds of children in Malawi for the past seven years. The proportion that were HIV-positive had remained unchanged, at between 1 and 2 per cent.

That cast doubt, she felt, on claims elsewhere that Malawi was in the grip of an HIV epidemic, with about a fifth of its population infected. The claims might be right for a small group of people in an urban setting, 'but my figures suggest you should not extrapolate from that to what exists in the country as a whole'. Although, at her request, 1 did not state it in the article, Griffin had long had reservations about the HIV theory of Aids and had been an early member of the group of scientists seeking a reappraisal of the hypothesis.

The article produced a long letter of response, dated 23 March, from Dr Geoff Garnett and Professor Roy Anderson, of the department of biology at Imperial College, London University. They reiterated the close association between HIV-positivity and Aids, and claimed that 'two carefully controlled studies' published that month had shown drug use to be no more frequent in gay men who developed Aids than in those who did not. I knew Duesberg was attempting to challenge these findings, but this was certainly an issue that deserved exploration.

However, when it came to Africa, their argument was less specific. The body of evidence which charted the emergence and rapid growth of the Aids epidemic in Africa – and other regions of the developing world – over the past twelve years was 'detailed in many hundreds of scientific publications,' they wrote, asserting that the current generation of HIV tests were 'highly reliable (100 per cent specific)'. As for 'a Dr H. Bialy' whom I had cited, a search for papers published by him in 1992 revealed one on transgenic wheat and another on pathway analysis in plant cells. 'If the *Sunday Times*' views about Aids are to be seen as anything more than sensationalist then it should choose its "experts" more carefully.' In fact, those articles were both commentaries in *Bio/Technology*, for whom Bialy, a microbiologist, worked as research editor. My dealings with him to date told me he did not deserve these belittling remarks. On the contrary, I felt, his long experience of Africa, allied to his scientific credentials, gave him considerably more authority than the large numbers of western scientists and other workers whose first exposure to the continent was brought about by Aids. There was certainly a big question mark over what was going on in Africa.

'The Cure That Failed'

Two weeks after that challenging report, another piece of the jigsaw fell into place. First results from the four-year Concorde trial of AZT showed no clinical benefit in symptom-free HIV-positive individuals, either in terms of living longer or in delaying progression towards disease. In a full-page article, 'The Cure That Failed', the *Sunday Times* set this failure in the context of the enormous dominance of a single focus – HIV – for research, prevention and therapeutic efforts, to the exclusion of other approaches.

We talked to Jody Wells, a fifty-two-year-old gay man living in London, HIV-positive since 1984 and diagnosed as having Aids in 1986, who had seen scores of HIV-positive friends die while taking AZT. He had become convinced, like Duesberg, that the drug was a poison that harmed more than it helped, and could even kill, producing symptoms which doctors misinterpreted as Aids. He felt so strongly that he was working up to eighteen hours a day establishing a charity, Continuum, 'an organisation for long-term survivors of HIV and Aids and people who want to be'.

The group emphasised nutritional and lifestyle approaches to combating Aids, arguing that those factors had been grossly neglected in the ten years since HIV was declared to be the cause.

To most within the Aids community, we said, the announcement had come as an unpleasant shock. It meant that a decade of the most intensive research ever mounted by the medical and scientific community against a single virus had left doctors empty-handed in therapeutic terms.

AZT, some doctors had declared, was the 'gold standard' of Aids treatment.* They believed in it so strongly that many patients had come under heavy pressure to take it, and to join trials liberally funded by the Wellcome Foundation, its manufacturer. At the last count, more than fifty

* This was despite a December 1988 study in The Lancet, from the Claude Bernard Hospital in Paris, which found that AZT was too toxic for most patients to tolerate, and left patients with fewer T4 cells than they started with. Although they noticed a clinical improvement at first, they concluded that 'by six months, these values had returned to their pre-treatment levels and several opportunistic infections, malignancies and deaths occurred'.

hospitals across Britain were involved in such studies. It was even being given to HIV-positive children: one advertisement, with the slogan 'Helping keep HIV disease at bay in children', said it had been shown to be generally well tolerated in children, that it improved their cognitive function, gave survival rates similar to those in adults, and improved their growth and well-being. That was very strange, in the light of the Concorde findings (which actually showed it to be worse than useless, with more deaths and side-effects in the treated group compared with controls). AZT had become big business. It earned Wellcome more than £200 million in 1992, and £131 million in the six months to February 1993.

As the *Sunday Times* had first reported as far back as 1989, with a meticulous investigation by reporter Brian Deer, some scientists had argued against the huge concentration of resources on AZT, and in particular had questioned the wisdom of putting symptom-free patients on to a drug for the rest of their lives that was originally developed as chemotherapy for cancer. 'It is an Alice in Wonderland world,' Wells said.

> There are so many uncertainties, and yet this extremely toxic drug has been given to thousands of people, many of whom are completely well apart from having antibodies in their blood to HIV. It is outrageous that they should have been put at risk in this way.

How had it happened? We recalled how in the mid-1980s, researchers at America's National Institutes of Health (NIH) were under huge pressure from a panic-stricken homosexual community to fast-track anti-Aids drugs on to the market. Gallo's colleague Sam Broder, at that time associate director of the National Cancer Institute's clinical oncology programme, had steered the drug through regulatory procedures from test-tube to patients in a record nineteen months, feeling every move scrutinised and criticised by Aids lobbyists. 'I've had to recognise that we cannot approach this problem in the usual scholarly way,' he had said.

We described how AZT was granted its licence by the FDA, with licensing authorities around the world soon following suit, on the basis of a single, multi-centre study that was beset with problems of protocol violations and bad data. It involved 281 Aids patients who were supposed to be tested for twenty-four weeks, but was called off prematurely, when only fifteen had run the full course, because only one of those receiving the active drug had died compared with nineteen in the placebo group, a phenomenally high death rate never seen again in any comparable group (there was also a swift acceleration in deaths in the treated group after the trial was stopped, and it emerged later that many had been kept alive by repeated transfusions). We told of how a flood of reports then started appearing claiming various benefits for AZT, but mostly based on individual clinicians' observations rather than arising from scientifically sound trials. As millions poured into Wellcome's coffers from AZT, the company sponsored an ever-growing number of research projects, as well as Aids 'educational' materials and public relations campaigns. Mercifully, however, after another major NIH-sponsored trial that appeared to halve the rate at which a group of HIV-positive patients became ill had also been stopped prematurely, the Concorde trial organisers had resisted pressure to do the same. Now, we said, armed with the exposure of the weakness of previous claims provided by the clear-cut Concorde results, the licensing authorities must surely review whether AZT was fit to be prescribed to patients with Aids as well.

To date, no such review has taken place. The reason appears to be that AZT is so closely linked with the beleaguered HIV paradigm, and so important to the pride of those who have adopted that paradigm, that the clear evidence of an understandable but enormous mistake having been made just cannot be acknowledged. 'The apparently well-founded discovery that AZT is not a useful drug for the treatment of people infected with HIV does not mean that it is useless in the treatment of those with Aids,' said the heading to a *Nature* commentary on the Concorde announcement, in which John Maddox said there was no case for abandoning that treatment. This seemed to me to be a really extraordinary statement from a scientist, since from my own reading of the evidence there was no scientific case at all favouring such a toxic drug. Concorde, and a few other well-conducted studies, had demonstrated that the claims made for AZT's use in HIV-positive people had been wishful thinking. The presumption should be that a similar process had been at work in *all* the many studies that claimed to show an excess of benefit over risk, especially in the light of what was now known of the original trial in Aids patients. Maddox, however, detected 'a note of hysteria' in British press reports on the findings, especially in the *Sunday Times*. For him, a more important development for the future pattern of Aids research had been provided by two recent articles in *Nature* claiming that the body's lymph nodes 'sequester replicating HIV particles' during the long latency period in Aids. His commentary concluded: 'All that, of course, would be based on what the sceptics insist on calling the "HIV hypothesis": there is no other, and thus no choice.'

Once again, Gordon Stewart was the only leading British doctor or scientist we knew of who recognised the wider implications of the Concorde findings. That week, the *Lancet* published a letter from him pointing out that previous Aids projections for 1992 had been up to ten times higher than the actual figure, largely because of false assumptions about heterosexual spread. 'I have been trying to put this across for nearly four years,' he said. 'I have tried numerous journals. The response has either been rejection, or silence.' His efforts, he said, had included letters to several government bodies arguing that the medical establishment had 'jumped the gun' in using AZT so widely. 'I received no comment whatever in response,' he said. 'They were all persuaded HIV was the sole cause of Aids, that an anti-viral drug would destroy viral replication, and thereby delay the onset of Aids. They wouldn't consider any alternative reasoning.'

Since AZT did not help, what were HIV-positive people to do? In a follow-up article to try to help fill the gap, we pointed to the work of a newly established Office of Alternative Medicine, set up within the National Institutes of Health complex in the US. Dr Larry Dossey, co-chairman of its panel on mind-body interventions, said preliminary assessments pointed to behaviour and lifestyle as crucial determinants of who stayed well. 'There are a lot of people with Aids and HIV who refuse to take AZT, and some of them do quite well or never get sick,' he said. 'This should alert us to the fact that there are other possibilities for treatment that are non-pharmaceutical.' There might not be one specific intervention, but rather, 'they clean up their lives,' according to Dossey. 'They stop using illicit drugs; they exercise and sleep; they take care with their diet; and they engage in visualisation exercises to build a positive outlook. Many also devote themselves to helping others.'

Those observations, we reported, were in line with results from a preliminary trial of 'alternative' and lifestyle approaches conducted in Seattle two years previously. Sixteen people who were already unwell with Aids-related conditions received a pot-pourri of health advice covering such factors as diet, nutritional supplements and behaviour. After one year, none had died or progressed to full-blown Aids. The study needed scientific confirmation, but such striking results 'would have had everybody excited if it had been a drug trial,' said Earl Baldwin of Bewdley, joint chairman of the Parliamentary Group for Alternative and Complementary Medicine, which had heard a presentation on the study at one of its meetings. Two comparable AZT studies, he said, showed much worse results, with 28 per cent and 36 per cent progressing to Aids.

Lack of Heterosexual Spread

The following Sunday, 18 April, a scoop: we discovered that British government advisers were finalising a report showing that fears of a hidden spread of HIV into the heterosexual population were proving unfounded (although that was not the interpretation they put on it). Far from running into millions, as had been feared back in the mid-1980s, there were still only 20,000-30,000 HIV-positive people in Britain (the best estimate was 23,000) – fewer than in official estimates six years previously, when the figure was put at between 50,000 and 100,000. The new figure was based on an 'excellent' HIV surveillance system put in place by Medical Research Council workers, after much thought, several years previously. We reported that Aids cases in homosexual men, the group hardest hit, were approaching a plateau of about 1,000 cases a year, and that numbers in heterosexuals outside the known risk groups were still tiny – only 63 to date, out of a cumulative total of 6,929 Aids cases since the epidemic began ten years previously. There had been no cases of Aids reported in London prostitutes who were not also drug abusers, even though some had several hundred partners a year.

The report gave projections for the course of the epidemic over the next four years to help health officials and ministers plan their responses to Aids. It confirmed that projections made in 1989 for the subsequent four years, tentatively revised downwards from earlier predictions of an exponential spread, had proved accurate. The 1989 projections included a wide range of other possibilities, but with four more years' experience the experts were growing increasingly confident that Aids was not going to break out of the established risk groups. That feeling, however, had not yet been reflected in the picture given to the public by health educators or ministers – or in any reduction in Aids spending, currently £200 million a year, a phenomenal sum for a disease taking just 800 lives annually.

The official view of the new figures was related by the *Independent*'s Steve Connor, who in articles on 21 May headlined 'Heterosexual HIV epidemic predicted' and 'The truth about growing menace of heterosexual Aids' reported that several thousand HIV-positive heterosexuals had been identified as having 'caught' the virus through sexual intercourse with the opposite sex. In fact, this was an assumption, and a very shaky one at that. The confidential screening survey that gave rise to these figures did not allow for detailed follow-up to establish precise mode of transmission; hence, 'as many as eight out of ten of these infected heterosexuals are unaware they carry the virus'. According to Duesberg's thinking, with such a stable background incidence of HIV-positivity, cases in which no clearly evident risk factors were identified were far more likely to have resulted from the virus being passed harmlessly from mother to child at birth, rather than from sex.

Nevertheless, Connor was able to quote Cambridge statistician Professor Nick Day, who chaired the scientific committee that produced the report, as saying that as the pool of HIV-positive heterosexuals got bigger, the chances of the virus spreading 'even faster' increased. 'The more there is, the more difficult it will be to control.' Connor did not mention that the figure for total numbers of HIV-positive people was now a half to a quarter of earlier (admittedly approximate) estimates. Oxford University's Professor Richard Peto was quoted as saying that observations of HIV's spread in other countries were the clearest warning yet that Britain faced a 'monstrous' heterosexual epidemic. 'It shows we are dealing with a virus that can spread in the heterosexual population,' he said. 'It is going to be magic if this virus doesn't spill out into heterosexuals and what works against magic?' This coverage earned Connor the 1993 Association of British Science Writers Award for best entry on the theme 'Improving Human Health in the 1990s'. The awards are for writers and broadcasters 'who have done most to enhance the quality of science journalism'. They are sponsored by Glaxo, developers of the anti-

HIV drug 3TC, and now, since their 1995 takeover, the owners of Wellcome.

Science is supposed to work against magic. Health educators had been understandably alarmist while they had in front of them the seemingly frightening US example of about 1 million HIV-positive people, in a population of 270 million; and the predictions that most HIV-positive people would develop Aids. But now, the picture was changing. After ten years, latest estimates of HIV-positivity in America were down, not up, and it had become clear that many HIV-positive people were staying well. Aids experts in the US, and advocates for people with Aids, had been shocked by a recent National Research Council report which concluded the disease was having little impact on most people's lives. An eleven-member panel of the council, in a 300-page study prepared for the National Academy of Sciences, found that many geographical areas and population groups were virtually untouched by Aids, and probably never would be. Instead, they said, it had remained largely confined to the 'socially disadvantaged' such as homosexuals, drug users, the poor and the under-educated. The report concluded that 'instead of spreading out to the broad American population, as once feared, HIV is concentrating in pools of persons who are also caught in the "synergism of plagues": poverty, poor health and lack of health care, inadequate education, joblessness, hopelessness and social disintegration converged to ravage personal and social life'. These findings, we said, from one of the nations worst afflicted by Aids, strongly supported the argument that the disease might be as much a product of lifestyle as of a new virus.

References to 'lifestyle' in the context of Aids tend to elicit an emotional reaction among HIV protagonists, not only because of the challenge to HIV, but because of the belief, embedded in the debate on Aids causation from the very beginning, that to discuss non-viral possibilities is equivalent to saying 'serve them right for overdoing things', as Robin McKie put it in the *Observer*. But I have never encountered that 'serve them right' attitude among the 'dissident' Aids scientists. Their efforts to draw attention to the facts as they see them are motivated at least partly by a genuine concern that the present use of resources is tragically misplaced. The billions of dollars poured into HIV research, and into broad-based propaganda campaigns, could, if redirected, extend a life-saving helping hand to many of those caught in the 'synergism of plagues' identified by the NRC. It isn't homophobic to try to change research and prevention strategies based on faulty premises.

There was also, it seemed to me, a simple concern for truth, and for the future good name of the medical profession as its leaders continued to keep their heads in the sand. In a letter of encouragement dated 23 April, Gordon Stewart wrote:

> Congratulations on your piece last Sunday. Deep suspicion about the duplicity of the health authorities over Aids is very widespread. Young as well as older people are asking me why doctors are so scared of telling the truth about Aids. In this regard, have you read the *British Medical Journal* of 10 April? On page 949, they use the science correspondent of the *Independent* to analyse a highly technical article, and conclude that HIV can cause Aids, all by itself. On the same page, a staff writer acknowledges 'doubts' about the prophylactic efficacy of AZT. On page 947, two laboratory scientists derive 'cautious optimism' from a mass of negative experimentation in chimpanzees with vaccines prepared from an 'unrepresentative' strain of HIV, and then proceed to justify 'large-scale trials' overseas after 'small-scale trials' of efficacy of three doubtful vaccines in 'pregnant mothers and young children' – the very groups in which all speculative trials are explicitly banned! Another example of the exemption of Aids from all the safeguards of ethical medicine and public health.
>
> I could, of course, write to the *BMJ* instead of to you about this but my past experience is that they would hold it for weeks or months before rejecting it and that, even if published months later, there would be no response... The behaviour of the medical and scientific press is overdue for exposure.

In a column in the *Guardian* about the differing interpretations of the same UK statistics, Colin Spencer, who at the time was writing a history of homosexuality, argued that 'moral zealots' had seized on the new report as evidence that Aids was a threat limited to gays. 'If Aids did not exist the homophobic instinct would have had to invent it,' he wrote, adding that Aids was 'the perfect affliction to be called up by the concept of the wrath of God... Disease and sin for many centuries have been fused together in the minds of the self-righteous.' Heterosexuals were at increasing risk, and official campaigns must still target them.

The other side of the debate was expressed in the *Daily Telegraph*[10] by columnist Geoffrey Wheatcroft, who said the coming of Aids coincided with the arrival of homosexuality as a politically correct cause and a politically organised lobby.

> It cannot be doubted that the medical profession was, for the most part, desperately concerned not to offend this lobby. There was an undisguised concern not to be censorious or, as we now say, judgmental, or to say or do anything that might encourage the ostracism of minorities. To which I would say only that a dislike of bigotry and persecution is a very good motive in general, but a poor starting point for a public health campaign.

The *Telegraph's* medical expert, Dr James Le Fanu, a London GP, had been one of the first commentators to point to the lack of heterosexual Aids, the risk of which he likened to being struck by lightning.

The following month, four years after it had first become clear to Gordon Stewart that a heterosexual epidemic was unlikely, Virginia Bottomley, the Health Secretary, announced a shift in the government's attitude and priorities over Aids. The Health Department said it would no longer aim costly 'safe sex' campaigns at the population at large. Instead, it would target its prevention efforts at those known to face special risks such as promiscuous homosexuals and drug users. It also withdrew the 'special priority' status previously accorded to Aids, which had earned it £886 million in state cash over the past seven years, an enormous sum for a disease whose UK cases numbered just 1,000 a year, on average, over the same period.

A *Sunday Times* article on 9 May about these developments, 'New Realism Puts the Brake on HIV Bandwagon', welcomed Bottomley's statement not only as marking the beginnings of a return to sanity in Aids funding, but also as a signal to the public that the scare was now being officially downplayed. Even so, we said, some powerful voices had yet to comprehend the reality of the situation. In a live television debate that Thursday with *Sunday Times* editor Andrew Neil on the popular *Frost Programme*, Jerry Hayes, vice-chairman of the All-Party Parliamentary Group on Aids, accused Neil of 'condemning thousands of young heterosexual men to death' by questioning the view that everyone was at risk. 'For the first time we are now seeing that heterosexuals are seriously at risk,' Hayes said.

The tiny numbers of Aids and HIV cases – ten-year cumulative totals of sixty-three and 214 respectively attributed to sex between men and women, without known risk factors, bore witness to how out of touch this view had become. It was also wrong to declare, as both Hayes and Imperial College's Roy Anderson had done on the programme, that HIV-positive people were going to die. Thousands of HIV-positive haemophiliacs had lived for more than ten years with HIV, we said, despite regular immune-suppressing injections, and there were good grounds for hoping that with the new, purified treatment, some might achieve a normal lifespan. Africa had millions who tested HIV-positive but the figures for deaths from Aids in that continent – thought by some to be grossly overestimated – had totalled about 200,000 in ten years.

Today, it is clearer than ever that 'straight' sex carries a minimal risk of Aids – even less than the chances of being struck by lightning, as the chairman of the US Society of Actuaries Aids task force puts it. Another British newspaper, the *Sunday Telegraph,* has been at the forefront in reporting recent developments confirming the myth of heterosexual Aids, as first documented by Michael Fumento. Ambrose Evans-Pritchard reported from a meeting of research scientists in Washington in December 1993 the results of the first large random screening survey for HIV-positivity in the US. Of nearly 8,000 people tested, twenty-nine tested positive, including just one white woman. 'These figures are stunning,' Evans-Pritchard commented. They gave the lie to claims that Americans were riddled with HIV, 'complacently incubating the disease that will eventually wreak havoc in the suburbs'. HIV was confined to specific pockets of the population. Infection rates were much higher than average among blacks and Hispanics, chiefly because of drug use among the poorer strata and untreated diseases such as syphilis – sixty-one times more prevalent among blacks than among whites.

These figures came from Dr Geraldine McQuillan, of the National Center of Health Statistics. Yet 'the dogma of heterosexual Aids has possessed the American establishment from top to bottom... So, instead of targeting funding on those at risk, the money is scattered around the country indiscriminately. Programmes for sexually transmitted diseases in the inner cities, an effective way of controlling the spread of HIV, have been gutted to help pay for Aids awareness campaigns for Mormons in Utah and Baptists in the Bible Belt... The heterosexual Aids scare is one of the great scandals of modern journalism and modern science.'

The *Sunday Telegraph* returned to the theme in June 1995 with an interview in which Luc Montagnier declared that Aids had stabilised and was even declining in parts of northern Europe. It was time the public was told the truth, he said: there was no 'explosion' of Aids in northern Europe. It was wrong to frighten people into thinking that there was a high risk of catching the disease, because that only caused a backlash when it did not appear.

In New York City, where intense surveillance provides data difficult to obtain elsewhere, a recent increase of Aids in women (arising mainly from the expanded list of Aids-qualifying conditions introduced in 1993) has still left the disease almost exclusively confined to the risk groups identified by the NRC, as the tireless Gordon Stewart pointed out in a 1995 letter published by the *Lancet*.[11] Sixty per cent of all female cases were identified as drug users. A further 28 per cent were thought to have acquired Aids through heterosexual transmission; closer monitoring showed that all these women reported sex either with men with Aids (30 per cent), or with drug users (61 per cent) or bisexuals (8 per cent). Eighty-six per cent of the women were black or Hispanic, and in this group all other sexually transmitted diseases were very common.

Of about 5,800 Aids cases in children in the US since 1982, 1,391 (24 per cent) were in New York City, and all but twenty of those – which were still under investigation – were born to mothers in risk groups: 54 per cent to mothers 'at high risk of injecting drugs during pregnancy', 11 per cent to mothers with Aids, and 27 per cent to mothers who were the partner of a man at high risk. Stewart took other *Lancet* correspondents to task for 'generalising' that Aids was increasing faster in women than in men. 'To imply that this is so in all women denies to those few at uniquely high risk the special attention that they need, while ringing alarm bells everywhere for enormous numbers of women who are not and need never be at risk.'

The continuing almost exclusive association between Aids and special risk groups, after fifteen years of the epidemic in one of the hardest-hit cities in the world, gives powerful confirmation to the hypothesis that Aids is not an infectious disease in a conventional sense, but that it may be a *transmissible* syndrome caused by a package of immune-suppressing risks, including multiple infections and drug toxicity, which tend to be shared by people in certain sub-groups of American society. This distinction was not grasped by the *Lancet* editors who, without consulting Stewart, changed the heading on his letter from 'Transmission of Aids in women' to 'Transmission of HIV in women'.

'Aids by Prescription'

During 1993, instead of respecting my role as a science correspondent reporting newsworthy developments, many of the doctors, scientists and other journalists involved in the field increasingly came to regard *me* as the problem, along with Andrew Neil as the editor who was allowing me to write such dangerous nonsense. Letters such as the following, from the executive director of the Christian Aids charity ACET (Aids Care Education and Training), one of our most persistent critics, had a wearing effect, all the more so because I knew it came with a lot of feeling:

> Once again Neville Hodgkinson is allowed to put his side of the HIV story without challenge.
>
> Yes there is evidence to show that the HIV rate is levelling off in the UK; that the epidemic is restricted to certain behaviour and sometimes to groups; that AZT is not a 'miracle cure'; that due to the unique and relatively new appearance of the virus there have been miscalculations with the result of over (and under) financing. However, the suggestion that the African Aids catastrophe is an invention or that AZT causes Aids flies in the face of all the scientific and medical evidence.
>
> This kind of reporting is a gross dis-service to the thousands ill or dying or indeed at risk that agencies like my own are involved with world-wide.

For the moment, the African story was an unknown. The claims about AZT, however, unlikely as they seemed, were supported not only by intelligent and well-informed observers like Michael Callen and Jody Wells, but by harrowing case histories that came our way from time to time. These served to reinforce our will to continue to press for an open debate about Aids and its treatment.

The 'New Realism' article began and ended with a sad story that brought home the enormity of what might be happening. Sue Threakall, former deputy head of a primary school, was convinced that her husband Bob, a haemophiliac who had died two years previously, had been killed not by HIV, as his doctors thought, but by AZT. She was now suing Wellcome for damages, alleging that the company promoted the drug without adequate evidence of safety or effectiveness. She had written to Duesberg in May 1992 to ask for advice, and with her permission he had recently passed the correspondence on to me. Her case subsequently attracted further publicity when it was announced that she had been awarded help with legal costs from public funds. It is notoriously difficult to obtain damages for drug disasters through the British courts, but whatever the final outcome, her courage in speaking out will have helped to hasten the process of disillusionment with AZT for many doctors and patients. Although 'anecdotal' – based on her own observations – her account of what happened to her husband and a friend probably came closer to the truth than the numerous 'scientific' studies, subsequently negated by the Concorde trial, which had purported to show that AZT was beneficial in HIV-positive patients.

'Dear Professor Duesberg,' Sue Threakall began:

Having already seen you on television and been most interested in your views on HIV and Aids, I have finally decided to write to you following an article last week in the *Sunday Times* newspaper, which outlined at great length your ideas and those of some of your colleagues.

I am thirty-nine years old, heterosexual and as far as I know not carrying HIV. My husband, who died last February, was a severe haemophiliac, and in 1985 we were told that he was HIV-positive, and it was presumed that he had contracted the virus in 1983. The only advice given to us at that time was to use a condom when making love, and for me not to get pregnant for at least two years! Since that time I have relentlessly pursued anyone and anything that can add to my understanding of the subject, to the extent that recently I have been finding things out that were new even to some of the doctors treating our haemophiliacs.

> My husband was in reasonably good health, apart from grossly enlarged lymph glands, and remained so for some time. His only other health problems were bouts of sinusitis and cold sores, also tonsillitis – complaints which he had always suffered from but which appeared to come more frequently.
>
> He underwent regular blood tests to assess the state of his immune system and was eventually put on AZT – twelve a day, which I now believe to be the maximum recommended dose.
>
> Steadily his health deteriorated until in November 1990 he finally stopped work owing to severe weight loss, thrush, stomach upsets, poor sleep patterns, sore mouth, continued sinus infections, weakness, breathlessness, loss of appetite etc. At the time we all put this down to the effects of HIV, though my husband himself apparently told a friend at this time – 'never take AZT, it will kill you'.
>
> He was admitted to hospital in February 1991 and died three days later – confused, delirious, wasted, constant diarrhoea, unable to swallow, and with hardly any normal lung tissue left.

Threakall has many close friends in the haemophilia community, and she wrote that she was particularly concerned for one of these, a man of only thirty-nine, who was also HIV-positive and thought he was going to die.

> Apart from some thrush in his mouth, however, he remains well, though the doctors were concerned at his low T-cell count and advised AZT, which he agreed to try for a short time – and, Professor Duesberg, it nearly killed him. In only a few weeks he suffered severe chest pains, constant indigestion, loss of appetite, weight loss, joint pains, muscle pains and wastage, headaches and vomiting. He was a changed man – until he decided to stop taking the tablets, from which point he slowly reverted back to the man we knew, left only with occasional indigestion.
>
> Between us we discovered that AZT should not be taken with analgesics, especially paracetamol – and my friend, like many other haemophiliacs, was on high doses of this for joint pains. It seems that the side-effects of AZT had been magnified, and also the painkilling qualities of the paracetamol reduced.

My friend and I, along with several friends in the haemophiliac community, have severe misgivings about current HIV and Aids theories and on reading the article about you found so much to relate to – at last here were some people thinking along the same lines. Our main points of concern are as follows:

- Does HIV on its own cause Aids? We believe that most, if not all deaths from haemophilia/HIV among our friends have occurred in people who have already been exposed to other viruses, in particular hepatitis B.

- Transmission. Some of the haemophiliacs' wives have tested positive, but so far I believe they are all fairly well. All my blood tests were negative until six months after my husband died, despite having regular unprotected sex at the beginning of his infection. I now refuse to have another test, because at the moment I fail to see what it will achieve.

- Lifestyle – we believe that a healthy life, with good food and, most of all, lack of stress is crucial.

- AZT – we share your views entirely! Professor Duesberg, please would you help us? Please know that there is a small but growing group of people here in the UK who would be sympathetic to your views and would I am sure be willing to help you if we could. What hope would you offer to us? I am very sorry for the length of this letter, and hope I have made myself understood. Good luck with your work, the future of people like me, my friend and my eight-year-old son may depend on you.

Duesberg replied:

I was very touched by your letter. It is a masterpiece of descriptive scientific analysis and, unfortunately, human tragedy. I enclose a package of material on Aids and HIV. Please read it, then contact me any time for further questions.

> Clearly, you are on the right track in rejecting AZT. No AZT! – and your friend will live a normal life for a haemophiliac, which is over fifty-five years now. I enclose for your information a paragraph on haemophilia Aids and on AZT toxicity from a paper I am preparing on Aids.

A few days later, I received a letter from Steve and Cheryl Nagel, of Minneapolis, to the effect that they also hoped to sue Wellcome, and wanted to establish contact with Threakall. Their adopted daughter, Lindsey, born in Petrosani, Romania in October 1990, was brought back to America that year and found within weeks to test HIV-positive. Although she had no symptoms of illness, she was put on Retrovir syrup – AZT, as marketed for children's use – for twenty-two months until 'by the grace of God, we determined that the drug was making her very ill,' Steve Nagel said.

For her first eighteen months, Lindsey's general health declined. She became hyperactive, as though 'she did not feel comfortable in her body'. She did not eat properly, avoided milk, and suffered nausea and diarrhoea. Then for three months in 1992, the two-year-old 'would wake up in the middle of the night grabbing her knees and screeching; she was in severe pain'.

'We had read a couple of articles about Peter Duesberg, and sent him a letter asking him for his advice,' Nagel wrote. 'He responded promptly, saying that we should get our daughter off AZT immediately, or that she would die a "death by prescription", just as Kimberley Bergalis had.' The Nagels sent me an article about their case by Tom Bethell in the *National Review,* in which he recalled that Bergalis was believed to have been infected with HIV by her dentist, although there was much contradictory evidence on whether that had really been the case. She also had a yeast infection, common among women, but one of the CDC's ever-expanding list of 'indicator diseases' for Aids. 'With a yeast infection plus HIV, Miss Bergalis became an Aids patient by definition, and was duly prescribed AZT. Within a year she was in a wheelchair,' Bethell wrote. She died in 1991. The same plight befell Rudolf Nureyev towards the end of his life, and he, too, took AZT; as also did Arthur Ashe. After Ashe's death, *New York Daily News* columnist Earl Caldwell reported that Ashe had wanted to break away from his treatment, but was worried about giving offence. 'What will I tell my doctors?' he said to a friend.

It isn't nice to put stories like these before the public. Aids physicians have told me subsequently of the confusion, distress and distrust they cause. I'm sorry if there were times when I could have reported the facts with more sensitivity. But about 100,000 people were taking AZT in America at the time, and world-wide sales had exceeded £200 million. When doctors and scientists appear to have taken leave of their senses, and intelligent individuals like Threakall and the Nagels have apparently come to theirs, if the press won't publish, what hope remains?

We did not even tell the full extent of the nightmare the Nagels experienced. Lindsey had to be taken every six weeks for tests at the University of Minnesota, and after the screaming bouts started, her parents informed the doctor. 'She just grunted, and left us with the impression, "What do you expect, this kid is dying of Aids." She didn't really acknowledge it,' Steve Nagel told me. 'We didn't see this as being an immune deficiency problem. We saw it as one of the side-effects of AZT.' After receiving a packet of literature from Duesberg, and reading about what he said AZT was doing to people, the couple recognised the symptoms as 'exactly what was happening to Lindsey'. They took her off the drug immediately. Two days later the cramps stopped, and 'she has not looked back since'. Nagel added: 'I am convinced at least 45 per cent of her life was gone. She had lost all her muscle tone – she would look like an Aids person right now, without a doubt. That was the direction she was headed in. As it is, she is perfect. Her health is 100 per cent.'

The couple had Lindsey's records transferred to another doctor who had a reputation for taking a holistic approach to disease, putting a big emphasis on nutrition. But the university doctor was angry. 'She threatened to have Lindsey removed from our home. She wrote saying we were responsible for the health of that child and that taking her off AZT would hasten her decline and death. She also called the holistic doctor, and told her she had no right seeing this child, and that there are foster homes out there for children whose parents don't go along with the medical community.' The couple took it very seriously, and made efforts to find a lawyer who could protect them, but in fact did not hear from the university hospital again. Steve Nagel added: 'One thing that is really peculiar to me is that the homosexuals and HIV-positive public don't want to think AZT could do anything to harm them. It's a terrible thing that is going on here.'

The late Derek Jarman, a British film-maker diagnosed HIV-positive in 1986, took AZT for two years between 1990 and 1992. He told Simon Garfield of the *Independent on Sunday*: 'My feeling about AZT is that I'm glad I took it, even though I can't prove to you that it did anything. You can say that if it helps someone psychologically then it must be doing some good. I think the doctors generally feel that it does some good. But how do you know?' Garfield, in an even-handed review of AZT's extraordinary history,[12] published on 2 May 1993, told of how Nureyev, who died the previous January, had demanded to go on AZT against his doctor's advice; and of how Earvin 'Magic' Johnson, the basketball star who tested HIV-positive in October 1991, accepted medical advice to take AZT immediately, 'as a preventative'.

He described the anger felt by several young homosexual men, founders of a London group called Gays Against Genocide (GAG), who had suffered severe side-effects on AZT. They felt betrayed by Wellcome and their doctors when they 'woke up to the news that the drug didn't work on HIV at all', and that their suffering had been avoidable.

Wellcome, meanwhile, were reiterating why AZT might still be beneficial, pointing to studies that had reached different conclusions from Concorde's. 'The number of people who have shown aggression against us concerns us no end,' Dr Trevor Jones, the company's director of research, told Garfield. 'About three years ago we started to open our labs to people with HIV and their carers, contrary to the advice of my security and other colleagues. You then realise the uncertainty and the frustrations involved in that act of taking a tablet for the very first time. When people with HIV came through the door of the lab I could almost touch their anger. But I realised that the anger was not really about Wellcome or me, but about their mortality. They were frustrated, and saying, "Please, please what can I do?" These were genuine *cris de coeur*.' Jones, a member between 1985 and 1989 of the government's Medicines Commission, which advises ministers on drug licensing, added:

> People say we're purely acting out of commercial interests, but it is not in our commercial interests to do anything else but get this drug right. We wanted to show people that we are working night and day, weekdays and weekends trying to develop better medicines. Otherwise we look like ogres and robber barons all the time. That's the whole history of our business; if

> you've got a problem with a product, you must, you *must* tell people. The criticism hurts a lot; our integrity as a scientific body is important to us... You have to believe that the integrity of science is good.

But the integrity of science was *not* good. The fear that Jones remarked upon had been put into HIV-positive patients by science itself, which was refusing to admit its mistakes and correct its errors. AZT's benefits were being exaggerated and its side-effects underplayed by doctors such as Lindsey's, who did not want to lose their control over their patients, or their tenuous hold on Aids – and the accompanying HIV theory of its origins – by recognising that the drug was worse than useless. Professional ego was at stake. It was small wonder that some patients were angry.

Money was a factor too, as the *Sunday Times* clearly demonstrated in an article on 30 May headed 'How giant drug firm funds the Aids lobby'. The Wellcome Foundation, we said, was facing growing criticism over the pervasiveness of its influence on Aids education, treatment and research. The company stood accused of using a unique position of power in the British medical establishment, via its close links with the Wellcome Trust, the world's richest medical research charity, to establish AZT as the 'gold standard' of Aids treatment, despite strong question marks over its safety and effectiveness. Until recently the Trust owned 100 per cent of shares in the company. In 1985, after AZT's arrival, its holding was reduced to 75 per cent and in 1992, in a further massive sales of shares, to 40 per cent, but these changes had left it with more than £200 million a year for distribution. Although forbidden to support the company's activities, some of the Trust's work had a direct bearing on HIV and Aids, and according to critics its enormous power of patronage had helped foster a climate in which the anti-viral approach to Aids had squeezed out almost all other lines of inquiry.

The issue was being taken up in Parliament by George Galloway, Labour MP for Glasgow, Hillhead, who commented: 'The British health service rolled over on its back for Wellcome, spending millions of taxpayers' money on this drug. The hegemony Wellcome have built up, which has also been based on the natural desire of people to clutch at straws in the face of the horrendous problem of Aids, may turn out to be one of the greatest medical scandals of the century.'

Some of the Wellcome Trust's work had a direct bearing on HIV and Aids. It had recently set up the Wellcome Centre for Medical Science, which had just run a conference for teachers and school governors called Aids Education in Schools – the Way Forward. The main scientific speakers were Professor Anthony Pinching, who conducted early AZT trials, and Roy Anderson of Imperial College, a Wellcome grant recipient and a governor of the Trust.

In addition, as sales of AZT had grown, the company itself had extended its funding and support operations to a huge range of Aids organisations. Those included the All-Party Parliamentary Group on Aids, which over the past five years had received £65,000 from the Wellcome Foundation, plus extra help for specific projects, such as a London conference on HIV and Aids for European parliamentarians. The group had provided MPs with large amounts of information through its newsletter, the Parliamentary Aids Digest. But not everyone agreed it had achieved its stated aim, of promoting 'balanced and effective policies on HIV/Aids'. At a 1991 meeting of the group to discuss Aids research, organised jointly with the Medical Research Council, four of the six speakers were linked to Wellcome, including Dr Jones. In its 1990 report, the group made clear that its idea of balance did not include serious attention to the arguments raised by the 'dissident' Aids scientists. It said the year had been 'characterised by a degree of scepticism, particularly in the media. For example, there was a series of articles in the press arguing that heterosexual Aids was a "myth" and on Channel 4 a programme called "Dispatches" disputed whether HIV really caused Aids and argued that in any case it was not infectious. In both these cases the group coordinated a response to try and repair the damage done by misinformation of this kind.'

Another opinion-forming recipient of Wellcome Foundation cash was the British Medical Association Foundation for Aids. It received a grant of £144,000 in 1988. The company also helped the Terrence Higgins Trust to set up a fund-raising division, and backed production of four 'health education' booklets. The first of those, *Understanding Aids,* described AZT as 'the first drug shown to be effective against HIV'. The fourth, *HIV Infection and Its Treatment,* contained nine pages about AZT and its purported benefits.

Not content with earning a fortune from a drug with known high toxicity and whose risk-benefit ratio had never been properly established in scientific trials, Wellcome had sought to get still more AZT into Aids patients by telling its salesmen how to overcome medical reservations on dosage levels. Guidance issued to sales representatives in 1987 addressed the question: 'There seems to be conflicting evidence when it comes to choosing the optimum dose of Retrovir [AZT] for long-term use – 500 mg per day seems quite adequate and perhaps too much in some patients.' The strategy to be pursued if this question was raised went as follows:

1. Establish actual situation and find common ground

    - What in particular are his concerns that some of his patients may be receiving 'too much' Retrovir?
    - What problems, if any, has he seen in any of his patients that he could attribute to Retrovir dosage?
    - What 'conflicting evidence' is he referring to?

2. Reassure and gain agreement

    - It is true to say that there is no standard dose of Retrovir that can be used in all patients in all circumstances. However, in no way does this amount to 'conflicting evidence'.
    - In most clinical studies, optimum benefit has been achieved with a dose of 500 mg per day or above. In the recently initiated MRC Combination Studies, a dose of 600 mg per day is being recommended. Is it therefore reasonable to use a lower dose in mono-therapy?
    - Many clinicians now accept that the dose of Retrovir may need to be increased to 800 or 1000 mg per day as the disease progresses. This is to ensure that sufficient Retrovir crosses the blood brain barrier to protect against neurological damage. 500 mg per day is widely felt to be inadequate to achieve this.

3. THE CHALLENGE

To convince the doctor that:

- 500 mg per day of Retrovir is not 'too much' and should be regarded as the minimum dose in most situations. Many clinicians now regard 600 mg per day as a more suitable dose.
- He should seriously consider increasing the dose to 800 or 1000 mg per day as the disease progresses to protect against possible neurological damage.
- Identify with the doctor any patient who is currently on a dose of less than 500 mg per day with a view to increasing it as appropriate.

Even after Concorde, the world's biggest study of AZT, had shown that it brought no benefit to HIV-positive people, Wellcome persisted in attempting to promote sales by citing company-sponsored studies that reached a different conclusion. One of these, led by Professor David Cooper of the University of New South Wales in Australia, was claimed to have shown that AZT could halve the rate at which Aids-related diseases developed.

How could such a different result from Concorde's be reached? The answer probably lies in the fate of a US study, also supported by Wellcome but conducted in thirty-two units of the National Institute of Allergy and Infectious Diseases, that reached similar positive conclusions, widely publicised both by NIAID and Wellcome but later withdrawn. The trial was halted prematurely in 1989 on the grounds that it had already shown such benefit that it would be unethical to continue. It appeared to show that the rate of progression to Aids-type diseases, in participants with fewer than 500 T4 cells, was roughly halved by AZT. Tony Fauci, NIAID's director, said in a press release that August: 'This study has clearly demonstrated that early treatment with [AZT] can slow disease progression *without significant side-effects* [my italics] in HIV-infected persons with fewer than 500 T4 cells who do not yet have symptoms.'

Four and a half years later, however, a new analysis of the trial data[13] reached a similar conclusion to Concorde: that AZT was essentially useless. This very different picture came after investigators paid more attention to the drug's side-effects, which can include anaemia, liver damage, fatigue, nausea, headaches and sometimes a collapse in white blood cells, making patients more prone to disease. The researchers looked at the average time patients experienced neither a progression of disease nor an adverse effect. Those treated with low doses of AZT were found to suffer a reduction in quality of life 'due to severe side-effects of therapy' that approximately equalled any benefit from slowing down the disease; people on higher doses suffered even greater ill-effects, outweighing the supposed benefit.

As Duesberg commented, it was clear that the original claims of benefit 'without significant side-effects' were completely ill-founded. 'The opposite interpretations of the same data lead me to conclude that those responsible are not acting as scientists; they are acting as politicians. When the time is ripe to say that AZT is detrimental, that it actually hurts, the interpretation will change again.'

The Concorde results failed to halt a trial of AZT in HIV-positive babies, even though a preliminary study had shown that out of thirty-five given the drug, fifteen developed blood disorders because of a toxic effect on their bone marrow. (In seven, the effect was serious enough to require blood transfusions.) The trial, known as the Paediatrics European Network for Treatment in Aids (Penta), was set up by Britain's Medical Research Council and its French equivalent, Inserm. In an information sheet for families, paediatricians associated with the trial said: 'We hope this study will help doctors to decide when is the *best* time for children to begin treatment with AZT.' But as Dr Richard Nicholson, editor of the *Bulletin of Medical Ethics,* told the *Sunday Times:*[14] 'What on earth is the point of continuing with a trial to find the correct time to start AZT in HIV-positive children when you haven't conclusive evidence that AZT does the children good at *any* stage?' Two HIV-positive mothers whose children had also tested positive told the newspaper that they had been put under pressure from the trial organisers to cooperate. One said she had received ten letters from Great Ormond Street Children's Hospital in London encouraging her to give her four-year-old daughter the drug.

Post-Concorde hopes for AZT were also kept alive by 'combination' trials, in which it was felt that if AZT alone was not enough to bring benefit, adding it to another powerful drug or drugs might do the trick. 'The company is probably right... to say that several drugs in combination are likely to be involved in more effective drug therapy,' wrote John Maddox in a kind of *apologia* for AZT in *Nature.* But Concorde trial doctors, who were upset at the way Wellcome tried to negate their findings, were alarmed by moves to give Aids patients an AZT drug cocktail as if it were already an established therapy. 'There's a suspicion of more toxicity if you combine it with other treatment,' said Professor Ian Weller, the principal British investigator in the Concorde trial. 'We are a long way from showing an important clinical benefit, or that it is safer than AZT on its own. There are physicians who are jumping the gun.'

At the time of writing, the latest, desperate moves to salvage some value from AZT seem, from the perspective of this author, to demonstrate the ultimate HIV folly: the drug is being promoted for use by HIV-positive pregnant women and their newborn babies, in the belief that it will help protect the infants against HIV and Aids. In late 1995, magazines and newspapers in the United States began running advertisements, part of a campaign by the Paediatric Aids Foundation, showing a baby lying on a quilt, superimposed with the words, 'The only thing worse than losing a child to Aids is finding out you didn't have to'. The US Public Health Service has suggested that all pregnant women voluntarily receive HIV testing, on the basis that 'there is now an effective means of preventing HIV from being transmitted to their infants', as a report in *Science* put it.

The basis for this campaign was a 1994 'interim analysis' of an NIAID study which found that 8.3 per cent of babies exposed to AZT were born 'infected with HIV', compared with 25.5 per cent of a group treated with placebo. (Other studies, not using anti-viral drugs, have shown that between 15 per cent and 40 per cent of babies born to HIV-positive women are born HIV-positive themselves, though many later revert to HIV-negative.) To achieve the apparent reduction, the mothers took AZT five times a day for an average of eleven weeks prior to giving birth, and received AZT intravenously when they went into labour. In addition, the newborns were given the drug in syrup form four times a day for six weeks.

This 'Aids research victory', as *Science* called it, leaves many questions unanswered, and is based on some unproven assumptions. What are the short- and long-term side-effects of the treatment? There is evidence that AZT can cause bone marrow changes that are not readily reversed when the drug is withdrawn.[15] Will the AZT-treated HIV-negative babies do any better than those born HIV-positive? In the light of the history of HIV-positive babies reverting to negative, how do the scientists know that the babies are genuinely HIV-infected? If they are, how do we know that AZT has genuinely prevented transmission of the virus, rather than simply suppressed its expression? (A

1990 study[16] in mice showed that HIV infection was suppressed during AZT treatment, but was detected in all the animals after the treatment was stopped.) In view of the fact that in the US most HIV-positive babies are born to drug-abusing mothers, where are the studies showing that HIV, rather than the ill-effects of drugs in pregnancy, is responsible for putting babies at risk of Aids?

Despite the lack of answers to these questions, several trials of AZT in pregnancy are now being organised by US, French and World Health Organization researchers. The WHO's Global Programme on Aids intends to administer the drug with 3TC, another experimental anti-HIV drug, to 1,900 women in Tanzania, South Africa and Uganda – notwithstanding the fact that even if it were successful, it could never be afforded by countries like Uganda, where per capita spending on health care is about $2 a year, roughly the retail price of two AZT capsules in the US. The trial drugs are being donated by Glaxo Wellcome, a conglomerate formed after the 1995 takeover of Wellcome by Glaxo, another giant British pharmaceutical company.

By June 1993, the persistent airing of the dissident case had begun to have an impact on the Aids establishment, and its confidence in the HIV hypothesis. In the week of the Ninth International Aids Conference in Berlin, *Nature* displayed nervousness. In a commentary, Dr John Moore of the Aaron Diamond Aids Research Center in New York argued that the event 'has shot its bolt as a worthwhile forum for scientific debate; it is far too large, unfocused and glitzy for many scientists' tastes. But it does attract the media, on the look-out for stories'. Supporting Moore's argument that the conferences should be stopped, an editorial stated: 'For those who wish to catch public attention, say for an untested candidate vaccine, the announcement of a research collaboration or the denunciation of the "Aids hypothesis", Berlin will be a splendid venue.' The editorial admitted, however, that with seven years having passed since the first conference, 'the Aids virus has turned out to be a more obdurate agent than originally expected'. It would be in the public interest if the disappointment were more openly acknowledged. 'Then the research community would be less easily pilloried than at present, which would then make for more seemly open conferences.' In the event, while Wellcome had a massive public relations operation under way at the conference to try to sidestep the Concorde trial results (described by one

Harvard researcher as 'an intellectual earthquake'), a small band of people who set up a stall with literature challenging the AZT/HIV paradigm were thrown out by the organisers. In any case, there was no interest as far as most of the mainstream media were concerned. As yet, the challenge to HIV was a complication they would rather do without.

Moore rewarded the *Sunday Times's* efforts with abuse. 'It is a common perception that inappropriate press coverage of Aids issues is the fault of journalists,' he wrote. 'Except for some tabloids like the London *Sunday Times,* this is usually not the case. Journalists working for specialist science magazines and most quality newspapers are generally responsible professionals who report the field fairly and accurately.'

But the consequences of dissent and controversy were now apparent, at least in the UK, 'where hostile press comment may have contributed to the recent change in government Aids policies'. This would be to the detriment of those infected with HIV and those yet to be infected, as well as everyone involved in Aids research and education. 'The "Murdoch" press has run a highly slanted campaign parroting Peter Duesberg's line that HIV is not the cause of Aids and that the risk to the heterosexual population is minimal. The subliminal message of these newspapers is that "normal" people *(Sunday Times* readers?) don't get Aids. There is dirty politics at work.'

Nature need not have worried (yet). My own story from the conference, under the innocuous headline 'Vaccine helps HIV sufferers', concerned a treatment developed by the late Dr Jonas Salk, discoverer of the polio vaccine, which had been shown to boost the immune systems of some HIV-positive people, though no one knew yet whether that would translate into protection against Aids. The underlying theory behind this 'therapeutic' vaccine was in line with Gene Shearer's findings*: that many more people, perhaps millions more, encounter HIV than just those who become HIV-positive, but that healthy people have a natural reaction against it which either destroys the virus or keeps it dormant inside infected body cells.

I also included a paragraph about a presentation by Luc Montagnier, in which he showed slides of the T-cell counts of HIV-positive haemophiliacs whose immune systems had almost declined to the point of Aids, but returned

* See Chapter 3

to normal after they were switched to high-purity Factor 8. Montagnier put these up at the end of a rather general talk, without much explanation, and I am not sure how many of those present understood their significance. It seemed to me this was another example of a dilemma Montagnier has faced for several years, of trying to have his cake and eat it: signalling to the world that the HIV story is not what it once seemed, and even that HIV may be harmless, and yet not wanting to let go altogether of a role in Aids for the virus that brought him so much fame and fortune.

The genie was out of the bottle, however, and as far as most of the world was concerned, HIV was still a huge threat to everyone, even if a little more distant than had been believed. As *Guardian* readers were told in the introduction to a major feature on 19 June, 'Aids is a virus. It is not homophobic. It has nothing against heroin addicts. It doesn't care how many people its host has slept with. It kills indiscriminately.' Wherever the exact truth lay, Procrustes was still definitely playing havoc with it.

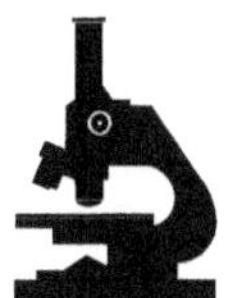

9: SCIENCE FAILS THE 'AIDS TEST'

When *Bio/Technology's* Dr Harvey Bialy told me of his conclusion that there was 'absolutely no believable, persuasive evidence that Africa is in the midst of a new epidemic of infectious immuno-deficiency', my confidence in his view was boosted by an astonishing statement he had made about the HIV test. *Bio/Technology* had a paper in press, he said, which did more than highlight a problem with false positives: it challenged the very basis of the test as indicating the presence of a specific virus, HIV, arguing that it had never been validated against the accepted 'gold standard' for a diagnostic test, isolation of the virus itself.

The implications were so enormous that I was once again nervous of the hostility such a revelation could arouse, and I did not pursue the story immediately. Indeed I found this conclusion hard to digest, simply by virtue of what it meant for the entire edifice of understanding that had been erected around HIV and Aids over the past ten years. But during subsequent weeks, I studied the paper concerned and corresponded with the main author, Eleni Papadopulos-Eleopulos, a biophysicist at the Royal Perth Hospital. To my growing amazement I found that there was indeed a mass of evidence, pulled together in Eleopulos's enormous review article, that what had come to be called 'the Aids test' was scientifically invalid. The proteins used in the test kits were not specific to a unique retrovirus. Positive results were produced in people whose immune systems had been activated by a wide variety of conditions, including tuberculosis, multiple sclerosis, malaria, malnutrition, and even a course of flu jabs. Patients with Aids, and promiscuous gay men leading lives likely to expose their immune systems to multiple challenges, were certainly much more likely to test positive than healthy Americans, but for reasons that need not have anything to do with a deadly new virus.

The possible relevance of this paper for an understanding of Aids in Africa was particularly clear. African countries were those where the tests might be at their most meaningless, because of the widespread ill-health caused by malnutrition and associated chronic diseases. Had an entire continent been panicked by western scientists into believing it was in the grip of a deadly epidemic, on the basis of a test that had never been shown to be valid for the retrovirus whose presence it was claimed to detect? The paper's claims were of course also vitally important to people who had tested HIV-positive anywhere, for whatever reason.

The review article, which was the first of its kind and carried hundreds of references, was co-authored by Val Turner, emergency physician at the Royal Perth, and John Papadimitriou, professor of pathology at the University of Western Australia. It was headed, 'Is a Positive Western Blot Proof of HIV Infection?' To understand the significance of the challenge that was being mounted, one first needs to distinguish between the two main types of HIV test in use, called western blot and Elisa. Both purport to show whether or not a person has been infected by HIV on the basis of detecting the presence in their blood of antibodies to various components of the virus.

The western blot test employs a selection of proteins thought to belong to the virus, separated and immobilised by the test's manufacturer, usually on a strip of nitrocellulose paper. The strip is then incubated with a dilution of the blood or blood components to be tested. If antibodies to those particular virus proteins are present in the blood, they bind at the appropriate points on the surface of the nitrocellulose strip. Unbound materials are washed away, and a colouring agent stains the strip where antibody is present, producing characteristic bands indicating the presence of the viral proteins. Because this test is thought to identify individual proteins that are specific to the virus – that is, which only HIV produces – it is widely believed to be so accurate as to mean that a positive result is synonymous with HIV infection.

The other main type of antibody test used, called Elisa (enzyme-linked immunosorbent assay), again uses a variety of proteins thought to be representative of HIV, and bound to a solid support, but as a group rather than separated from one another as in the western blot. The original tests of this kind were made from 'whole virus lysate' – that is, from materials obtained from cell cultures thought to be infected with and growing HIV. It is now accepted (although I knew nothing of this before reading the article) that these materials often contained normal cell proteins as well, which confounded the test results, producing large numbers of positive results even when the person was not actually infected with HIV (false positives).

Later generations of Elisa tests, made with proteins manufactured synthetically or by genetic engineering techniques, have been claimed to be more reliable. Nevertheless, the Elisa test is still generally considered more prone to produce false positives than the western blot. In the US, for example, the Centers for Disease Control designate the Elisa a 'screening' test, to detect suspicious blood samples, rather than as a 'confirmatory' test, the role usually given to western blot. The CDC state in guidance issued in 1993 that Elisa results 'should never be used alone to report a final positive result'. Instead, if two or more blood tests are 'reactive' on Elisa, 'then the results are "confirmed" using a second more specific antibody test such as the western blot'. This more specific second test can tell the difference, the CDC says, between HIV antibodies and other, non-HIV antibodies that react to the Elisa. 'Results from this two-part testing are greater than 99 per cent accurate.' Today in the US, people are only told they are positive if they are repeatedly reactive by Elisa, and are confirmed by western blot (there are other test systems, but these two are the ones in widespread use).

The significance of the *Bio/Technology* review article, which was published in June 1993, was that it not only presented evidence confirming the Elisa test's unreliability, but demonstrated that the western blot was also incapable of determining whether people were really infected with HIV. Yet as the authors said, 'A positive HIV status has such profound implications that no one should be required to bear this burden without solid guarantees of the verity of the test and its interpretation.'

To show that an antibody test for HIV is scientifically valid and reliable, the paper said, requires four steps. The first of these is to identify a source of HIV-specific antigens – the protein components of the virus to which antibodies bind. Here, one of the first surprises is that because HIV is extremely difficult – and perhaps impossible – to isolate in a clear-cut way, there is no guarantee that the method used really does obtain the virus or its components. I shall be discussing these problems of isolation in a later chapter, but for the moment suffice it to say that the manufacturers of the tests do not have an unequivocal collection of HIV viruses, visible through electron microscopy, which can then be broken down into their various components. Instead, a multi-step procedure has to be followed involving a variety of assumptions, each of which is questionable. The final assumption is that some material which bands at a particular density (1.16 grams per millilitre) when spun in a centrifuge represents 'pure' HIV proteins and RNA from which to make the antibody test, or which can serve as a template from which to manufacture the proteins.

These proteins are then exposed to blood from patients with Aids, or at risk of Aids, and those to which antibodies attach become the basis of the HIV test. If other patients show similar reactions, they are considered to be HIV-positive. The proteins (p) are numbered according to their molecular weight. On this basis, those considered to be most important in triggering production of antibodies to HIV have been identified as p120, p41/45, p55, p31/32, p24/25 and p17/18.

In the *Bio/Technology* paper, Eleopulos went through each of these in turn and showed that in most instances there were alternative explanations for the presence of the proteins, which did not require HIV. The p41 protein, for example, one of those detected by both Gallo's and Montagnier's groups in the first 'HIV' isolates, could be accounted for by actin, a protein found in all cells as well as bacteria and several viruses. Montagnier and his colleagues, in fact, had seen that serum from Aids patients reacted with a p41 protein both in HIV-infected and in non-infected cells, concluding that the p41 band 'may be due to contamination of the virus by cellular actin which was present in immunoprecipitates of all the cell extracts'. Actin is known to play a key role in activity at the surface of a stimulated cell, and for that reason the binding of actin antibody to such cells has been proposed 'as a sensitive marker for activated lymphocytes'. There is also evidence that two other bands, p120 and p160, are simply oligomers (multiples) of p41.

The p31/32 protein has been shown to be identical to one coded by the major histocompatibility complex (MHC) set of genes. It is described as an MHC class 2 protein, which plays a part in controlling the reactions of T4 (helper) lymphocytes, so again there is a logic as to why it should be found in people whose immune systems are under pressure much more than in those who are healthy.

The p24 protein has been considered to be extremely specific for HIV infection, so much so that it is considered to correlate with the progression of 'HIV disease' and is used to quantify virus levels. Until 1987, according to CDC criteria, the presence of a p24 band alone in the western blot test was considered sufficient to confirm HIV infection. However, it then became apparent that healthy blood donors at no risk for HIV infection were often showing up positive on this band – fourteen out of 100 donors (who were negative on the Elisa test) had antibody to p24 in one 1989 study. Among the recipients of blood from such donors, 36 per cent showed a similar reaction on the western blot test six months after their transfusion – but so did 42 per cent of individuals who received western blot-negative blood. Both donors and recipients remained healthy. The authors of this study[1] concluded that such patterns are 'exceedingly common' in randomly selected donors and recipients and do not correlate with the presence or transmission of HIV.

The p24 thought to represent HIV may in fact be a protein of the same weight that is present in the outer lining of platelets, particles that circulate in the blood and whose main job is to clump together to stop bleeding. Antibody to it may be especially high in regular blood donors, arising as a harmless consequence of their blood loss. Most homosexual men with Aids and pre-Aids have been shown to carry an antibody that reacts with this protein. The reason is unknown, but may relate to platelet activation. In any case, the reaction seems to be very variable, contrary to what one would expect if the cause were HIV infection. In one study quoted by Eleopulos, the authors found that 'In half of the cases in which a subject had a positive p24 test, the subject later had a negative test without taking any medications that would be expected to affect p24 antigen levels ... the test is clinically erratic and should be interpreted very cautiously'.

Finally, there is evidence that p18, which along with p24 is most often detected by western blot in healthy blood donors, is also associated with immune system activation. Blood from Aids patients reacts with a p18 protein in HIV-infected T-cells that have been stimulated into dividing, but not with uninfected, unstimulated T-cells. However, when the uninfected T-cells are stimulated, the same reaction appears, so it would appear that the antibodies are binding to a protein associated with cell division and activation rather than with HIV.

In view of these observations, Eleopulos wrote, 'It is difficult to defend the view that the bands p41 (and thus p160 and p120), p32, p24 or p18 represent specific HIV proteins.'

Even if it could be shown that they really did belong to HIV, it could not simply be assumed that someone with antibodies reacting with them was infected with HIV. From the first antigen-antibody reactions performed by Montagnier and Gallo, it was found that not all the 'HIV' proteins reacted with all sera from Aids patients, or even sera from the same patients obtained at different times. Other factors were evidently involved, so a second criterion of test validity had to be met, that of standardisation. There needed to be some criteria as to what constituted a positive western blot, so that a given test result had the same meaning in all patients, in all laboratories, in all countries.

That was not the case, however. An FDA-licensed western blot kit, used by a minority of laboratories, required a positive result on three different bands, p24, p31, and either p41, p120 or p160. When these stringent criteria were used, less than 50 per cent of Aids patients tested HIV-positive. The Consortium for Retrovirus Serology Standardisation, however, defined a positive western blot as the presence of antibodies to at least p24 or p31/32, and p41 or p120/160. Using these criteria, the proportion of Aids patients testing positive increased to 79 per cent. Other laboratories and organisations used still different standards. Moreover, even with the most stringent criteria, 10 per cent of control samples, which included specimens from blood donation centres, showed positive on western blot.

In the scientific literature, no strips had been published of a standard positive western blot. Interpretation, even with a single kit, left much to the subjective experience of a particular clinician or laboratory. For instance, one early instruction manual which reproduced examples of strong, weak and non-reactive patient sera, went on to warn: 'This example shows typical reactive patterns only, and is not to be used as a reference for comparison with results from unknown serum samples... Patient samples may show varying degrees of reactivity with different proteins, thus showing different band development patterns... Each laboratory performing western blot testing should develop its own criteria for band interpretation. Alternatively, band interpretation may be left to the clinician.'

The difficulties went still further. Other workers had shown that the patterns obtained depended on many factors including temperature, and the concentrations of a chemical used in the preparation of the 'viral' material for the test.

The third criterion for a valid test was that it should be reproducible, but, perhaps partly because of the above, there was evidence that even first-class laboratories could produce widely differing conclusions concerning the same samples. In addition, according to a 1989 CDC report, many laboratories were still using unlicensed western blot kits because of cost and the 'stringent criteria required for interpreting the licensed test'.

Once an antibody test was thought to have met the criteria described above, Eleopulos said, its specificity for HIV infection had to be determined. For that, an alternative, independent method of establishing the presence of the infection for which the test is employed was needed. 'This method, often referred to as the gold standard, is a crucial *sine qua non,* and represents the tenet upon which rests the scientific proof of validity.' The only possible gold standard for the HIV antibody test was HIV itself. In other words, to be sure that the test was valid, you would need to show that HIV was present in people who tested positive, and that it was not present in people who tested negative.

This has never been done! Instead, some studies purport to validate one test by seeing how well it performs against another, but since the tests are usually based on similar principles, if the principles are wrong it means all such tests are wrong too. Other studies have used the clinical syndrome of Aids as a 'gold standard', so that a test is considered valid if it can distinguish between serum from Aids patients and serum from healthy people. Thus, back in 1987, the CDC's Aids definition accepted a positive Elisa, without confirmation by western blot, 'because a repeatedly reactive screening test result, in combination with an indicator disease, is highly indicative of true HIV disease'. However, since most Aids patients have many physiological abnormalities, especially affecting their immune system, it is not surprising that many test positive for proteins which, as described above, are associated with immune system activation. Assuming that these proteins represented HIV was an unwarranted step.

All 'HIV-Positive' Tests May be False Positives

Since no one could say with any certainty whether the antibodies detected by the 'HIV' test related to HIV or to these other proteins, *all* HIV-positive test results might be false positives, Eleopulos argued:

> Since individuals from the main Aids risk groups, that is, gay men, drug users and haemophiliacs, are exposed to many foreign substances such as semen, drugs, Factor 8, blood and blood components; and individuals belonging to the above groups commonly develop infections unrelated to HIV; one would expect these individuals to have high levels of antibodies directed against antigens other than HIV. In fact individuals with Aids, Aids-related complex, and those at risk have circulating immune complexes, rheumatoid factor, anticardiolipin, anti-nuclear factor, anti-cellular, anti-platelet, anti-red cell, anti-actin, anti-DNA, anti-tubulin, anti-thyroglobulin, anti-albumin, anti-myosin, anti-trinitrophenyl and anti-thymosin antibodies. Anti-lymphocyte auto-antibodies have been found in 87 per cent of HIV-positive patients, and their levels correlate with clinical status.

There was evidence that apart from specific cross-reactions with the 'HIV' proteins used in the test, the general burden of immune system reactivity, with consequent heavy load of circulating antibody-antigen complexes, increased the chances of testing HIV-positive. A 1985 study[2] found that in healthy Africans, the probability of a positive test result increased significantly with increasing immune-complex levels. The authors concluded that 'reactivity in both Elisa and western blot analysis may be non-specific in Africans... the cause of the non-specificity needs to be clarified'. A similar possibility was raised in relation to intravenous drug use, when researchers tested stored serum samples from 1,129 users, and eighty-nine controls, dating back to 1971-2. They found that seventeen of the samples from the drug users, but none of the controls, tested positive. The study authors commented:[3] 'On the basis of our positive western blot data, it appears that parenteral drug users may have been exposed to HTLV-3 [HIV] or a related virus as early as 1971. An alternative but equally viable explanation is that the HTLV-3 seropositivity detected in these specimens represents false positive or non-specific reactions.' A 1988 study[4] demonstrated that in drug addicts there was a strong association between high serum globulin, which includes immunoglobulins (the antibodies responsible for the immune response), and a positive HIV antibody test. This was 'the only variable which remained significant' in statistical analysis.

In Eleopulos's view, the link was a cause-and-effect one: the immune system activation in such cases was causing the 'HIV' test to show up positive. The reaction was similar to one that can confound testing for syphilis. Known as a 'biological false positive' (BFP), it has been described by syphilis researchers as often being 'a marker for an unidentified disorder of the immune system that predisposes to auto-immune diseases'.

Several other pieces of evidence were cited in the paper in support of the idea that a positive HIV antibody test may be the result of a challenge to the immune system other than HIV.

- HIV was thought to be transmitted by infected needles, yet a higher percentage of prostitutes who use oral drugs (84 per cent) than intravenous drugs (46 per cent) tested positive, according to a 1988 study published in the *Lancet*.[5]

- Mice exposed to T-cells from another mouse strain were shown to make antibodies against two 'HIV' proteins.[6]

- Recipients of HIV-negative blood have been shown to become HIV-positive and develop Aids, while the donors stayed healthy and seronegative.[7]

- In healthy individuals, partners of HIV-positive individuals and organ transplant recipients, a positive HIV-test may revert to negative when exposure to semen or immunosuppressive therapy ends or clinical improvement occurs. (Several similar cases have since been reported in haemophiliacs.)[8]

- Hospital patients in the US (twenty-six hospitals studied), who were not at risk of developing Aids and who did not have any infectious diseases, tested HIV-positive at a high rate on western blot (1.3 per cent to 7.8 per cent). That might either mean HIV was spreading to the general population, or that the HIV antibody tests were nonspecific. The latter seemed more likely, in view of the fact that by 1992 in New York only eleven men were reported to have acquired Aids through heterosexual infection.

- Amazonian Indians with no contact outside their tribes, and with no Aids, were found to test HIV-positive with western blot at rates varying from 3.3 per cent to 13.3 per cent depending on the tribe. In another study by the same researchers, 25-41 per cent of malaria patients in Venezuela had a positive western blot, but no Aids.

All such problems could be avoided by use of the only suitable gold standard, HIV isolation, the paper argued. So why had the HIV tests not been validated in that way? The answer, set out in four more pages of closely argued and extensively documented text, was even more astonishing. It was that Aids scientists, including Montagnier and Gallo, had been unable to isolate HIV in an unequivocal way.

Various indirect molecular, biochemical and genetic findings had been interpreted as meaning virus isolation, but none of these had offered conclusive evidence. In other words, the entire HIV story, with all the problems it had brought in its wake, might be a monumental error – a monstrous self-deception. It was not just that HIV was harmless, as Duesberg insisted. If Eleopulos was right, the HIV emperor did not just have no clothes, he had no body, no identity. He was not even a little man making a big noise, as in *The Wizard of Oz*; according to this evidence, HIV had never been shown to exist!

When I first read the paper, I did not have enough knowledge of molecular biology to comprehend fully the argument on virus isolation. It is only after another two years of familiarising myself with the field, including a period spent in Perth with the paper's authors, that I have gradually appreciated the significance of what they are saying. There are also limits to the human being's ability to grasp ideas and arguments – no matter how logically presented – when those arguments flatly contradict not just what one has previously believed oneself, but what the rest of the world believes too.

I was even reluctant to write a news story about the challenge to the HIV test until I could find some further support for it, although after several readings I felt the review article had certainly made a very powerful case. I faxed the article to four experts in case some glaring error invalidating its reasoning had been missed by *Bio/Technology*, although the article had been peer-reviewed before publication.

One did not send any response to the article. He told me when I first called him that if false positives had been a common finding, 'I think we would have spotted them. One would have been erroneously diagnosing HIV; patients will sue, and make a few millions'. Another preferred not to comment, but referred me to a third, Dr Philip Mortimer, of the Virus Reference Division at Britain's Central Public Health Laboratory. Mortimer wrote a courteous reply acknowledging that the article 'does make some fair points about the weakness of the western blot test when it is used incautiously and without follow-up'. He added, however, that 'the situation it describes is not typical of this country where initial positive serological (antibody) screening tests are confirmed by (i) further investigations, usually a combination of different Elisa assays but sometimes including western blot and (ii) a test of a follow-up specimen. Only if the positive reactions on both specimens are confirmed, usually in a reference laboratory, is a positive report issued'. Perhaps this more stringent procedure helped to explain why Britain had only some 23,000 seropositive people, compared with an estimated 1 million in the United States and multi-millions in Africa.

But Eleopulos *et al.* had not just criticised the western blot test. They had cited evidence indicating huge numbers of false positives with the Elisa test. In Russia in 1990, for example, out of 20.2 million such tests performed, there were 20,000 false positives and only 112 'confirmed' positive results. A similar study in 1991 confirmed only sixty-six out of approximately 30,000 positive test results. Reporting these findings in the *Lancet* on 20 June 1992, Alexander Voevodin, of the Institute of Pulmonology in Moscow, said the severe consequences could largely be avoided 'if the HIV status of screening-test positives is clarified rapidly, but this does not happen in Russia. The time scale for completing confirmation tests ranges from weeks to months and field epidemiologists often embark on contact tracing without waiting for the confirmation. Also, personal information on results of HIV tests is often leaked, resulting in discrimination and stigmatisation both of HIV-infected individuals and the large number of false positives.'

Clearly, by using multiple tests giving very different results, false positives would be greatly reduced. But this still did not answer Eleopulos's charge that there was nothing in the literature to indicate why *any* of the tests should be considered reliable as indicating the presence of a specific retrovirus. Even if the damage done by false positives was being reduced in the UK and elsewhere by repeated testing, that was no comfort to those still left with a false diagnosis. Nor was it any help with regard to the situation in Africa, where because of cost considerations, most HIV diagnoses were being made on the basis of a single test. As Eleopulos told me, 'The paper really shows that we have to question all types of the antibody test, especially in Aids patients, who have all types of infectious agents in them. How do we know that a positive test in Aids risk group patients is due to antibodies directed against HIV, and not against the many infectious agents to which Aids patients have been exposed? If the test is no good, you can repeat it a thousand times and it still won't be any good. When the principle of the test, the basis of it, has not been established, it doesn't matter how many times you repeat it, you still won't prove anything.

'The only way to show an antibody test is good, that it is telling us something specific, is to have a gold standard. For that, they have to have HIV; and it doesn't matter what they say, nobody has done that. So instead, when any other test is introduced, they have had to use the western blot as the gold standard. If the western blot is no good, no other test is any good either.'

Mortimer also commented that diagnostic capability had recently been advanced by the introduction of a commercial polymerase chain reaction (PCR) assay for detecting minute quantities of HIV genetic material. 'Comparison of results using this procedure with those obtained by antibody tests show a very close correlation confirming the reliability of HIV antibody tests,' he wrote. However, as the *Bio/Technology* paper pointed out, this correlation might be the result of some quite different cause common to both the PCR test and the antibody test. PCR signalled the presence of only a small stretch of genetic material; perhaps it was picking up the presence of a sequence made detectable by the same stimulus as that which caused a person to test antibody-positive, a stimulus which need not have anything to do with 'HIV'. The *Bio/Technology* paper cited evidence in support of this idea. For example, a positive PCR reverted to negative when exposure to risk factors was discontinued; and cells from HIV-positive patients in which no HIV DNA could be detected, even by PCR, became positive for HIV RNA after immune activation by co-cultivation with activated T-cells.

The fourth expert was Professor Robin Weiss, head of the Chester Beatty Laboratories at the Institute of Cancer Research, London, who with Dr Richard Tedder, a virologist at the Middlesex Hospital in London, developed and patented Britain's first HIV test in conjunction with the drug company Wellcome. Weiss had invited me to visit his 'blinkeredly orthodox' HIV research laboratory – 'if you dare to expose yourself to possible contamination by orthodox views' – after the original 'Aids: Can We Be Positive?' article. He had spent two hours trying to explain why he thought Duesberg was wrong. Although my experience of the meeting was mainly of being berated for having had the temerity to write as we did (I remember him showing me a front page headline from the *Daily Mirror* that week, 'Your Surgeon Has Aids – Hospital Sends Shock Letter to 200 Patients', and telling me it was a more responsible story than our own) his exasperation had been laced with humour and besides, he had been involved with Aids research from the start.

Weiss told me on the phone that 'I have always bemoaned the fact that western blots became the gold standard, I have never liked them'. He then took the trouble to write a two-page letter concerning the *Bio/Technology* paper. His tone was set in the first paragraph: 'It is the sort of paper I would have stopped reading by paragraph 5 if you hadn't requested an opinion.' Later, he commented: 'Sorry, if the authors were my students, I'd mark this essay B-minus. Of the 1,000 or so papers on HIV/Aids that must have been published in the last six months, I'd put this in the bottom 10 per cent for being worth reporting ... I wonder if you will report it all the same. That would confirm my opinion that the *Sunday Times* is not interested in genuine controversies about Aids, which are, of course, in plenty.' He quarrelled with some of the technical points raised, although he acknowledged that the paper might have had some merit if it had been published around 1986/7, as 'there were serious difficulties and much variation in assessing western blot data, and some of the Elisa tests were still giving false positives'. But since then, he argued, the tests had been greatly improved because almost all the commercial companies had switched to using HIV antigens produced in bacteria by recombinant DNA technology, rather than isolated from sera taken from Aids patients.

It seemed to me that he had not answered the central complaint, that no one had ever established that the proteins held to indicate the active presence of HIV really are related to the virus in people who test positive, as opposed to other possibilities raised by the *Bio/Technology* authors. I wrote back along those lines, adding: 'This is extremely important, surely. If they are right, it provides a perfect explanation of why "HIV-positive" haemophiliacs who are switched to purified Factor 8 cease declining towards immune system failure. I have not heard any other explanation for this phenomenon.'

On 1 August 1993, the editor ran our most challenging story to date across the top of the front page. The headline read: 'New Doubts Over Aids Infections As HIV Test Declared Invalid'. The story began:

> The 'Aids test' is scientifically invalid and incapable of determining whether people are really infected with HIV, according to a new report by a team of Australian scientists who have conducted the first extensive review of research surrounding the test. Doctors should think again about its use, say the authors. 'A positive HIV status has such profound implications that nobody should be required to bear this burden without solid guarantees of the verity of the test and its interpretation,' they conclude. The findings, likely to cause intense debate in the medical fraternity and anguish for many HIV-positive people, are contained in an article published by the respected science journal, *Bio/Technology.*
>
> Many people who appear to be infected by HIV, say the researchers, can be suffering from other conditions such as malaria or malnutrition that produce a positive result in the test. Even flu jabs can produce the same effect. As a result, predictions by the World Health Organization that millions are set to die because of being HIV-positive may be wildly inaccurate.
>
> The paper also lends powerful support to the theory, held by growing numbers of scientists, that HIV is not the true cause of Aids. One of its authors, Eleni Eleopulos, a biophysicist at the Royal Perth Hospital, said

> this weekend: 'There is no proof that people labelled as "HIV-positive" are infected with such a retrovirus. We should really question the role of 'HIV' in the causation of Aids.'

After setting out key aspects of the case against the test, the article noted that the World Health Organization – which was seeking an extra £2 billion a year for its Aids prevention programme – estimated that about 14 million people had been infected with HIV world-wide. The WHO claimed the total would reach 30-40 million by the year 2000, and that most would eventually contract Aids. Developing countries were said to face the biggest threat, with Africa alone already having an estimated 8 million HIV-infected people.

However, according to the *Bio/Technology* report, those were the countries where the tests might be at their most unreliable because of widespread ill-health caused by other diseases. Severe malnutrition and multiple infections were especially likely to produce a misleading result in the test. Claims that current Aids tests were virtually 100 per cent accurate were based on studies using *healthy* subjects as controls.

We also quoted Peter Duesberg as welcoming the report, on the grounds that it helped to explain how 'a false correlation' had been found between 'HIV' antibodies and Aids. 'The whole virus hypothesis of Aids is based on this correlation,' he said. 'Its proponents have nothing else: no mechanism whereby HIV could do the damage attributed to it, no animal tests, no cure, no vaccine, no virus activity. They have nothing conventional in terms of virus-disease argument, except this correlation with antibodies. If this study is correct, and I have no reason to doubt it, it means that even that is now falling apart.'

The article added that the findings had led to a call by the *New York Native* for legal action against the American government by relatives of people who had killed themselves, or suffered toxic effects from taking AZT, as a result of positive HIV tests.

Circular Reasoning Means Test Remains Unvalidated

Having already had to cope with so much protest over previous articles reporting on the calls for a reappraisal of HIV's role in Aids, I expected this fresh challenge to provoke a new wave of criticism and comment. After all, the claims were completely at odds with conventional thinking on this enormously important subject. But this time, there was hardly a word of protest, let alone any arguments of rebuttal. No scientific papers to validate the tests. And no comment elsewhere in the media. I felt sure we were being privately criticised by the Aids experts to whom specialist writers turn for advice on such issues, but perhaps they now felt it better that there should be no public debate.

Robin Weiss wrote again on 2 August, as follows:

> Yes I did answer their central complaint – you chose to ignore it:
>
> - Since ~ 1988, most tests including western blots, slot blots and other variants of antibody blotting have used HIV antigens recombinant DNA methods and the bands are therefore nothing other than HIV.
> - Ref (3) by Pinter et al., the major complaint was misunderstood. The gp120 was genuine gp120 and the gp160 a mixture of gp160 and gp41 tetramer – in both cases, real HIV antigens.
> - Western blots are only *ever* used as part of a panoply of confirmatory tests, not as screening tests.
>
> It is difficult to believe you are as slow a learner as you make out. I cannot respect the integrity of yesterday's article, including again a gratuitous, petty and wrong smear on the Wellcome Trust (which does not fund my lab's Aids research).

Weiss was wrong in his challenge to Eleopulos's claim that p120 and p160 had been found to be multiples of the p41 protein, and therefore did not qualify as separate indications for HIV infection in the western blot test. In a letter to the *New England Journal of Medicine* (11 May 1989) Dr Abraham Pinter and co-authors stated that they had 'unexpectedly' found that these two viral antigens 'are primarily multimers of the HIV transmembrane glycoprotein gp41 that react with antibodies to gp41. Confusion over the identification of these bands has resulted in incorrect conclusions in experimental studies. Similarly, some clinical specimens may have been identified erroneously as seropositive, on the assumption that these bands reflected specific reactivity against two distinct viral components'. Tests indicated that some true gp120 was also present, but *no* gp160.

Weiss's last sentence was referring to an AZT story written by another reporter the same weekend, and apart from allowing Weiss to let off some steam, had nothing to do with the question of the HIV test's validity. I replied:

> I am getting used to your style and now rather like it. However, please have patience with this slow learner and explain how the bands which you say are 'nothing other than HIV' are the equivalent of virus isolation as a gold standard for testing the specificity of the diagnostic kits? The purity of the bands overcomes one of the complaints in the *Bio/Technology* paper, that the proteins previously came in a mixed soup; but there was a lot of evidence in the paper that pure or not, the proteins are not specific to HIV and that therefore the test should be proved effective by comparing positive results with virus isolation.

Weiss responded: 'As I wrote, that might have been a valid argument six years ago, but not today as the proteins have been specific for some years.'

We were getting nowhere, except that I now felt more confident than ever that Weiss had no effective response to the Perth team's criticisms of the test. Like so much in HIV/Aids thinking, his argument was circular. Philip Mortimer, despite being more generous towards the *Bio/Technology* paper, seemed to have fallen into the same trap. In a 1991 *Lancet* paper[9] he had favoured new Elisa tests 'based on recombinant and peptide antigens', which, as Weiss said, overcame the problem of not knowing precisely what antigens were present in the test kits. But even if those antigens were HIV-related, one still needed to distinguish between reactions caused by HIV antibodies and cross-reactions caused by antibodies from other sources. It was not much use knowing what had gone into the tests if you still did not know whether or not those antigens specified the presence of HIV.

This, surely, was exactly what had happened. As Mortimer said, the western blot was used as a 'gold standard' for the other HIV antibody tests. Yet his paper, entitled 'The Fallibility of HIV Western Blot', concluded that 'western blot detection of HIV antibodies began as, and should have remained, a research tool'. Earlier, in a 1989 article,[10] he had written:

> Diagnosis of HIV infection is based almost entirely on detection of antibodies to HIV, but there can be misleading cross-reactions between HIV-1 antigens and antibodies formed against other antigens, and these may lead to false-positive reactions. Thus it may be impossible to relate an antibody response specifically to HIV-1 infection. In the presence of clinical and/or epidemiological features of HIV-1 infection there is often little doubt, but anti-HIV-1 may still be due to infection with related retroviruses (e.g. HIV-2) which though associated with Aids, are different viruses.

Mortimer revealed here another important indication of why HIV-positivity has appeared to be so closely correlated with Aids risk groups, apart from the fact that for several years a positive HIV test has formed part of the definition of Aids: clinical and epidemiological features are sometimes, perhaps commonly, invoked as part of the diagnosis. Thus, a gay man with a given test result may be judged positive, while a heterosexual with the same test result may not be burdened with an HIV 'diagnosis', unless some risk factor can be identified. This policy, reflecting the difficulties Aids scientists have encountered as the non-specificity of the test became more evident, was spelled out by the Consortium for Retrovirus Serology Standardisation in 1988: 'For symptomatic individuals clinical evidence of infection with a positive western blot test provides criteria for diagnosis. However, for asymptomatic individuals, other criteria including history, high-risk behaviours or results of other virological or serological studies may be necessary for the diagnosis of HIV infection.'[11] The consortium added that 'the western blot test result is highly dependent on the technical skill and subjective interpretation of the experienced laboratorian... The establishment of even the most rigorous criteria will not completely eliminate the subjectivity and variability inherent in western blot testing'.

In another big critique of the HIV test,[12] Eleopulos and her co-authors have pointed to evidence which could also help to explain why in Africa as well as elsewhere, HIV-positivity in healthy people tends to concentrate in certain age groups. The scientific literature 'abounds' with data, they say, demonstrating cases of mistaken identity when researchers thought they had found retrovirus causes for diseases such as cancer, only to discover that the antigens they had detected did not belong to retroviruses at all, but were of a naturally occurring 'heterophil' (general) type. This type of antibody, which may be related to growth spurts as well as generalised stress, peaks at about three years of age and at about thirty-five years. Levels are also influenced by tumour growth and chemotherapy, and have been seen to be raised in older people suffering from several types of cancer. One group of authors said that their findings 'emphasise the need for extensive controls in determining the specificity of human antibody recognition of viral protein determinants'. The need was especially great when radioimmunoprecipitation (RIP), a third, ultrasensitive type of antibody test was used.

The idea that the HIV antibody tests are non-specific – that is, that positive results can be triggered by a wide variety of conditions – may answer a number of puzzles in Aids research, Eleopulos says. For example, researchers have found that TB responds just as well to treatment in African patients who are HIV-positive as in those who are not. The reason may be that the HIV-positivity is a false positive reaction. TB itself can produce symptoms that mimic Aids, including a decrease in T4 cells and prolonged, depressed immunity.

Scientists in Nairobi have been surprised to find that many prostitutes stay HIV-negative despite continuing to have unprotected sex with HIV-positive men. The idea that they have some kind of special resistance to the virus has been discussed, attracting world headlines. The real reason may be that the HIV-positivity in their clients is a non-specific reaction that therefore does not put the prostitutes at risk of becoming infected with a deadly virus.

Those prostitutes who themselves test HIV-positive may similarly not be infected with any such virus. This would explain the puzzlement of researchers who reported on 'Aids Virus Infection in Nairobi Prostitutes' in

1986 in the *New England Journal of Medicine.* They found that two-thirds of female prostitutes from an economically depressed neighbourhood tested positive, just under one third of prostitutes from a better-off area, 8 per cent of a group of men treated at a clinic for sexually transmitted diseases and 2 per cent of medical personnel. But they added: 'The high prevalence of [HIV] antibody among the prostitutes was a surprising finding in view of the paucity of cases of overt Aids diagnosed in Kenya... The prostitutes whom we interviewed did not describe any deaths within the prostitute community during the past five years that were suggestive of Aids.'

In 1985, Robert Gallo and colleagues reported how they tested sera dating back to 1972/3 from seventy-five healthy children from the West Nile district of Uganda. Both Elisa and western blot tests were performed. Two-thirds of the samples were positive. Since the children, whose mean age was 6.4 years, were presumed infected by their mothers, the authors expected at least an equal percentage of adults to be infected, raising the question of 'why the incidence of Aids in the Ugandan population (and neighbouring Zaire) has gone unnoticed for so long ... it is possible that Aids existed in African populations without being recognised as a separate disease entity'. That point of view, Eleopulos said, was inconsistent with the conventional idea of HIV as being an extremely infectious agent with an incubation period for Aids of about four years in African victims. 'The Ugandan population should by now ... be drastically reduced – perhaps decimated. This is not the case and it would seem prudent to accept that the majority, if not all of the positive tests, were false positives induced by other diseases endemic in the area of study.' Tragically, however, after whole nations had been panicked by these false test results into believing they were about to be decimated by HIV, many of the traditional causes of death became redesignated 'Aids' in Africa.

Also in 1985, US and French researchers reported that the wife of a haemophiliac Aids patient who was found to have low T4 cells and to be HIV-positive reverted to normal after exposure to her husband's semen (vaginal, oral and anal) was stopped. According to the researchers, 'her discontinuation of sexual exposure [to HIV], or her lack of antigenic stimulation or both, may have played a role in her conversion to seronegativity and increase in the number of T-helper lymphocytes'. According to Eleopulos, since semen is known to be capable of provoking antibody production as well as causing immune suppression, especially in anal intercourse, it may have been the original cause both of the decrease in T4 cells and of the HIV-positivity, 'irrespective of HIV infection'.

All of this evidence, she and her co-authors conclude, makes it likely that in healthy people as well as Aids patients a positive test does not indicate HIV infection but represents a non-specific marker for a variety of unrelated conditions. 'Consequently, the general belief that almost all individuals, healthy or otherwise, who are HIV antibody positive are infected with a lethal retrovirus, has not been scientifically substantiated.'

Just as when Joe Sonnabend received the cold shoulder – and worse – for his multifactorial theory of Aids; and just as Peter Duesberg had met months of total silence, and ultimately utter rejection by the Aids establishment, for demonstrating his belief that HIV was harmless; so Eleopulos *et al.* have been unable to engage the scientific mainstream in any open debate on the dramatic possibilities they have raised – though I suspect that behind the scenes, discomfort over what to do about the HIV test is growing acute.

Was it possible that, as Robin Weiss tried to persuade me, 'the authors could have written a similar paper about any virus save, perhaps, measles, and found similar discrepancies; polio, herpes simplex, CMV, influenza'? 'There is nothing special here about HIV,' Weiss wrote. 'Their whole concept of a gold standard is bizarre, as technology moves forward and tests are better now than five years ago.'

That was not how Harvey Bialy saw it. *Bio/Technology* is a journal whose specialities include the validation of diagnostic tests, which was the issue at the heart of the Eleopulos paper. According to him, Eleopulos was absolutely right in her analysis of the circular reasoning surrounding the attempts to validate the HIV test by reference to other, similar tests.

Besides, I knew that during the second half of the 1980s, as the world was being driven into a panic by virologists over HIV's allegedly rapid heterosexual spread in Africa, there had been no public acknowledgement of inadequacies in the HIV test. Weiss had been among those responsible for this panic: in a February 1985 *Lancet* paper that he handed to me when we first met in 1992 – without any reservations about the quality of the data – he and his co-authors stated: 'In Africa HTLV-3 [HIV] appears to be transmitted through heterosexual contact or exposure to blood through insect bites or scarification.' The paper included the devastating information that a fifth of 'control' samples taken in Uganda from healthy people as well as hospital patients tested HIV-positive, and declared that 'the serological tests are highly specific'.

WHO Meeting Hears of Test Unreliability

Although it had never been made plain to the public, experts knew from an early point that there were exceptional problems with the HIV test. Some of these doubts and uncertainties came up at a meeting at the WHO's headquarters in Geneva on 14-16 April 1986, called to discuss the safety of blood supplies and issues related to antibody screening. There were more than 100 participants, from thirty-four countries. The proceedings were published by the WHO as a book, *Aids: The Safety of Blood and Blood Products,*[13] the following year, priced at £39.95. It was an academic publication and I never heard about it at the time, but came across a copy several years later.

Dr James Allen, assistant director for medical science in the CDC's Aids programme, told the meeting that the importance of eliminating technical errors was emphasised 'by the high proportion (66.7 per cent) of initially reactive specimens in blood donors that give negative results when the tests are repeated'. Another source of error derived from the inability of some manufacturers to provide uniformly reliable test kits and reagents. The result was variations in the rates at which screened specimens were repeatedly reactive by Elisa. Additional reasons for false positive test results included non-specific reactions, particularly antibody in specimens that cross-reacted with non-HIV antigens in the test system. 'This latter problem has proved to be both real and annoying for blood collection agencies which find that less than 20 per cent of donors who are repeatedly reactive by EIA [Elisa] also have a positive western blot.' Studies suggested that some people were reacting to components of the cell line used to grow HIV for many of the test kits licensed in the US. Other cross-reactivity was occurring because of antibodies to naturally occurring cell surface proteins, the so-called HLA antigens.

Allen gave a warning that the problems could be magnified in areas of the world that did not have the sophisticated facilities of the United States. Blood centre laboratories that were not routinely processing large numbers of specimens might find the tests uneconomical and technically difficult. 'In addition, laboratories that are not equipped to handle the dilutions, critical incubation times and temperatures, and washing procedures required, or that do not have a constant and dependable electrical supply for automated readers, may have trouble obtaining accurate and reproducible results. Blood centres that do not have refrigerated storage facilities for donated blood may find the delay of several hours required to perform the test unacceptably long.' Other problems that needed to be assessed included the impact of variable shipping and storage conditions on the test kits and reagents, and potential problems of non-specific cross-reactivity of sera collected from donors in different areas.

Allen added that although the tests licensed for screening blood supplies were sensitive enough to detect most infected donors, a highly specific confirmatory test was needed to distinguish which people with a repeatedly reactive result had genuinely been infected with HIV, and which had a non-specific reaction. 'To date, no entirely satisfactory confirmatory test has been developed, standardised and licensed to help resolve this dilemma, although it is probable that such tests will be available in the future.' Later, challenged about the CDC's criteria for determining test results, he said: 'A major part of the problem in reading western blots is that methods are not standardised and interpretation is subjective. It varies from one laboratory to another, depending on how the gels and the blots are set up, on the source and amount of antigen that is used, and on multiple other technical factors.'

The CDC had spent many hours of discussion with groups and different laboratories trying to establish the definition of a positive western blot. It had ended up deciding that most infected people had antibody against the p41 and p24 proteins, and that therefore the presence of one or both of those bands could be interpreted as a positive result, although 'if the only band present is p24 we are reluctant to call the blot positive, and we try to get an additional specimen to repeat the blot'. That led Professor F. Deinhardt, director of a microbiology institute in Munich, Germany, to say that in his unit, non-infected cells had been shown to produce a false-positive band in the p41 region, so even that could not be trusted on its own. 'We ourselves would never report a sample as confirmed positive if we do not have at least two virus-specific bands which we can be sure of. We would also further investigate before we let the axe fall on the poor individual and tell him he is anti LAV/HTLV-3 [HIV] positive.' He felt it would be 'highly dangerous' to license a western blot test so that any laboratory could start running it, because of the technical difficulties and the pitfalls in interpretation.

Dr Thomas F. Zuck, from the FDA's office of biologics research and review, commented: 'Dr Deinhardt's concerns are the same concerns we have; interpretation is as much a part of the test as are the physical reagents one uses for it. So we have difficulties at this point deciding what is going to be required to validate a claim a manufacturer may make that a test is confirmatory.' Later he added: 'One of the difficulties we have in looking at "claims" for confirmatory tests or designing systems to validate what in fact is going to be "confirmatory", is determining how you define and validate it... What will be confirmatory? What claims are we permitted to make? It's going to take some time for us to sort through this and to do the appropriate clinical trials.'

In his own presentation, Zuck emphasised that an initial positive reaction using the Elisa test meant very little, 'unless the test is highly reactive or the subject is known to be at high risk' for HIV infection. Only 3.8 per cent of initially reactive sera from more than 2.5 million blood donors screened by American Red Cross centres could be confirmed by western blot. Surveys conducted jointly by the College of American Pathologists and the American Association of Blood Banks, covering more than 5.5 million donations, produced a similar result, with a confirmation rate of 4 per cent. He went on: 'Because knowledge of the degree of risk [for HIV infection] of the person being tested is of such importance when interpreting test results, an additional more specific test, such as western blotting, is needed to interpret the meaning of repeatedly reactive sera from people of unknown risk.' If tests were interpreted that way, few diagnostic errors would be made. 'Further, because a positive test has such enormous social, medical, and psychological implications, persons with sera reactive by additional more specific tests need medical evaluation and counselling.'

Similar difficulties with false positive reactions were raised by Dr John Barbara, head of microbiology at the North London Blood Transfusion Centre in England. Because the virus replicated by budding through the wall of an infected cell, it carried cell antigens with it. 'In addition to this, viral purification for preparation of reagent antigen can never be perfect.' As a result, non-specific but repeatable 'cross-reactions' were a considerable problem. There was a big need for a definitive confirmatory test. 'It is important to remember that the western blot (commonly used as a confirmatory method) is itself an antiglobulin assay. It is liable, therefore, to the same kind of false-positive reactions as the screening test it might be confirming.' Barbara also pointed out that when (as with HIV in blood donors) the prevalence of an antibody is very low, even a test that sounds highly specific may still produce a high rate of false positive results. For example, if the true prevalence were one in 1,000, a test with 99.8 per cent specificity would find one true-positive and two false-positives in every 1,000 samples – 'a 67 per cent false positive rate!'

Commenting on the difficulties of separating the virus from normal cell components, Dr M. V. O'Shaughnessy, head of viral surveillance at the Laboratory Centre for Disease Control at Ottawa, Canada, said that when the proteins from an HIV preparation were electrophoretically separated and stained using ultra-sensitive techniques, 'more than thirty individual proteins can be recognised'. Several large Canadian studies had shown extensive non-specific cross-reactivity, especially in haemophiliacs and in North American native populations. He also reported problems with cross-contamination. The western blot procedure was so sensitive that some positive sera could be diluted up to a million times and still be clearly positive. Accidental transmission of one microlitre (one millionth of a litre) of diluted sample from one well to another in the incubation tray could result in a false-positive being reported. O'Shaughnessy added that new tests based on genetically engineered or synthetic antigens were now being evaluated, which had the theoretical advantage of not being contaminated with proteins from the host cells or from the cell line in which HIV was grown. 'However, these second-generation procedures will almost assuredly result in a second generation of problems for the diagnostic laboratory.'

Today, with the advantage of hindsight, distanced from the madness that surrounded discussion of Aids in the mid-1980s, one can feel sympathy for the experts who struggled to the best of their ability with the tangled web of issues surrounding blood testing. The more I read of their difficulties, however, the more it seemed that Eleopulos might be right, and that the root of their problems could be that the deadly new virus they had assumed they were dealing with was itself a 'false positive' – a mistaken concept. Questioning that root assumption was not a part of their agenda at that time.

Nevertheless, sympathy comes still more readily for all those people who have been falsely given to understand that they are infected with HIV. Because of its ability to detect a generalised immune system activation, the Elisa test helped clean up blood supplies, but it was never suitable for more than that. Regardless of whether or not the virus is a real entity, it is clear that in the early years at least, the uncertainties surrounding the HIV test were so great as to render it unfit for diagnostic use.

The FDA's Thomas Zuck admitted as much at the WHO meeting. Indications for the use of the Elisa kits in the US had expanded beyond those for which they were designed and initially licensed, he said. 'Consistent with the data obtained in support of test licensure, use of the test was intended to be limited by phrases in the package inserts stating, "the primary use of the HTLV-3 antibody test is to screen blood and plasma donations ... it is inappropriate to use this test as a screen for Aids or as a screen for members of groups at increased risk for Aids in the general population".' However, 'enforcing the intent of this language would be analogous to enforcing the Volstead Act which prohibited alcoholic beverage sales in the United States in the 1920s – simply not practical'.

Broad application of the test was evident, he said. The non-specificity of the test would cause difficulties when indications for its use were expanded, particularly when diagnostic and policy decisions might be based on the results. But he took some comfort from the fact that Elisa testing 'to slow the spread of...infection may serve the public health well', backed up by additional more specific testing, such as western blot, of all repeatably reactive sera. 'Public policies about confidentiality of test results, economic and social decisions based on the results of these tests, and uses dictated by public health needs must be determined by judicial bodies rather than control authorities.'

In fact, as Gordon Stewart has constantly emphasised, the public health has been ill-served by an infectious disease paradigm, with a non-specific diagnostic test at its heart, that told the world it was in the grip of a deadly new disease putting everyone at risk. As well as inflicting great psychological and physical damage on 'HIV-positive' people, the test led to the misappropriation of billions in public funds. Science disgraced itself by adopting the test on the basis of inadequate evidence, allowing its indiscriminate use, and by failing to make the non-specificity of the test absolutely clear to policy-makers, physicians and individuals as soon as this flaw became apparent, as it clearly had done to the experts who gathered in Geneva as far back as April 1986.

Are Today's Tests More Reliable?

According to the *Bio/Technology* analysis, the lack of validation of HIV antibody tests was an intrinsic defect. No matter what permutations manufacturers developed with the proteins used in the tests, they would still be in difficulties as long as they did not check how well the tests performed against the gold standard of virus isolation – which they were unable to do, because they could not isolate the virus. Robin Weiss, on the other hand, had told me that 'the proteins have been specific for some years'. Who was right?

Evidence that the HIV test is still beset with major difficulties is contained in the latest comprehensive guide to the subject, the 1994 edition of *Aids Testing,*[14] a 400-page textbook edited by two CDC experts, Dr Gerald Schochetman and Dr J. Richard George. There are bland assertions that the tests are 'highly sensitive and specific', just as used to be said of the earlier tests. But the science tells a different story.

In a chapter on FDA regulation of the tests, Dr Jay Epstein, of the agency's centre for biologics evaluation and research, comments on 'a continuing controversy' surrounding the inconsistency of some screening test kits 'because of the familiar problem of false-positive reactions' with non-specifically 'sticky' antibodies. 'Such a problem has been observed for several blood donor screening Elisa tests following immunisation for influenza,' he says. Another concern with screening tests is the accuracy of rapid tests introduced in recent years, which require subjective interpretation by the operator. 'Poorly trained operators can easily misinterpret test results.'

The western blot remains by far the most widely used procedure for 'confirmatory' testing, Epstein says. With this, 'the greatest concern has been the high prevalence of nonspecific banding patterns, resulting in indeterminate test results. Unfortunately, this phenomenon is intrinsic to the technology due to a variety of causes that include antibodies in the patient sample that bind to non-viral proteins in the viral antigen preparation and antibodies of unknown specificity that cross-react with viral proteins.'

Furthermore, the FDA has actually relaxed its criteria for a positive western blot, to get over the embarrassing fact – spotted by Eleopulos – that with the first kit licensed for confirmatory testing, which required a positive result on three different bands, fewer than half of Aids patients tested HIV-positive. 'Currently used criteria are less stringent and have resulted in tests that are more sensitive but have a higher false-positive rate,' Epstein admits. His justification for this move sounds legalistic rather than scientific. 'The FDA has accepted product amendments for revised western blot interpretative criteria that are consistent with the prevailing scientific view and the recommendations of the Public Health Service.'

It has also 'attempted to reduce the occurrence of falsely reactive bands by close attention to quality control issues in manufacturing and through lot release criteria'. This seems an inadequate recompense for reducing the stringency of a test which, as Eleopulos has demonstrated and as the UK's Philip Mortimer and other experts have agreed, was already severely flawed.

Epstein adds that the FDA has become 'increasingly concerned' about the sale of unlicensed confirmatory test kits. Initially, it did not act against them because of a lack of availability of licensed kits, and because of 'the pressing public health need for a means to validate HIV screening test results'. Now that licensed tests were widely available, action would be taken against unlicensed products. Again, with hindsight, it seems extraordinary that such action, to reduce the margin of error in a procedure with such devastating potential impact on a person's life, should have been delayed for so long.

In a review of the various testing methods used, George and Schochetman reiterate the need not to tell people they are HIV-positive, or take medical decisions about them, based on Elisa testing alone. This is because of the continuing risk of false-positive results. 'Testing by the sensitive EIA

[Elisa] is done to identify those persons who need additional, more specific supplemental testing. Counselling and medical decisions are made based on the results of the supplemental assay, not on those of the screening test alone.' Apart from Elisa, they say, probably the most widely used screening test is one called SERODIA-HIV, made in Japan. It is not licensed by the FDA but is widely available in most other countries, particularly those in Asia, Australia, Latin America and Africa. It works on a principle known as agglutination. Particles such as gelatin or latex, coated with viral proteins, settle into distinctive patterns depending on the presence or absence of antibodies attributed to HIV in the patient's sera. False positive reactions are slightly more of a problem than with Elisa, the authors say, though the factors that trigger them seem to be different.

A variety of rapid screening tests are also on offer, many performing comparably to the Elisa, but some of which 'have been developed and offered for sale at low prices in developing countries without being validated through clinical trials or reviewed by any recognised institution'.

Problems also clearly remain with the western blot. Production of the strips for this test is not a precise process, George and Schochetman say. 'Differences in protein concentrations, identities, and positions are observed between manufacturers and even between lots from the same manufacturer.' Since the first recommendation, in 1988, by the US Public Health Service that Elisa-positive specimens should be further tested by western blot, 'there has been extensive debate over the appropriate interpretive criteria for this assay'. As Eleopulos pointed out, even within the US the criteria recommended by various organisations still differ considerably. Outside the US, the expense of confirmatory tests – they can cost US$60-100 in some African and Latin American countries – means that they are often not used at all.

A chapter on quality control makes plain that there are concerns in that area, too. 'Each year the number of tests performed and the number of laboratories performing tests increase in the United States. Yet programmes for quality control of laboratory testing have not kept pace.' Standard panels of serum for quality control and evaluation of Elisa and western blot tests are not generally available, the authors say. Quality control is more difficult for western blot than for Elisa, the major reason for the difficulty being the need to compromise 'between what is scientifically necessary and what is commercially feasible'. Measures to guard against deterioration of the kit, proficiency testing and performance evaluation, and daily monitoring and routine maintenance of the refrigerators, freezers, waterbaths, incubators, microplate readers and washers and pipettes are all needed to prevent inaccurate results being given to doctors and patients.

The polymerase chain reaction (PCR), which can amplify DNA a million times or more, is increasingly used for direct detection of genetic sequences attributed to HIV. However, because of its exquisite sensitivity, and the huge amplification it employs – it can multiply even a single molecule up to detectable levels – it is also very vulnerable to error, both in terms of procedure and interpretation. In a chapter concerning such techniques, Schochetman and Dr John Sninsky, of Roche Molecular Systems, say that PCR 'does not have an intrinsic analytic or diagnostic sensitivity and specificity. The diagnostic sensitivity and specificity are inextricably linked to the laboratories performing the procedure. As a result, the confidence in the reported results is directly proportional to the experience and critical interpretive criteria used by the laboratories performing the assay'. Factors that make a dramatic difference to results include the genetic sequence 'primers' chosen to start the reaction off, the probes used to analyse the results, the concentration of the various reagents used, and the temperature and time over which the reaction is run. False positives result from cross-contamination of samples and reagents, and 'carryover' of PCR products from previous reactions. The latter is the usual reason for false positives, because of the number of copies of a particular genetic sequence that it generates – anywhere between a million and a million million, for example.

Manoeuvres such as PCR, which are replete with opportunities for confusion, have had to be invoked in HIV research because, as *Aids Testing* says, the virus cannot be detected directly by conventional molecular biology techniques. The reason usually given for those difficulties in detection is that the virus is very inactive. The book cites estimates that generally only 1 in 10,000 to 1 in 100,000 lymphocytes in the peripheral blood of infected people are actively replicating virus. That in itself puts HIV – should it exist – in a very different category from most other viruses for which diagnostic testing has been developed.

'HIV-positive' is also a very different diagnosis from most in that HIV and Aids have been invested with so much fear and prejudice. 'No other disease, except perhaps leprosy from the beginning of the millennium to the 1800s, has brought so much societal pressure on its victims and caused such cataclysmic social consequences over such a long period,' says Dr Ann James, another of the contributors to *Aids Testing.*

It is a rare individual who has the strength and good fortune – and good humour – enabling them to fly over the cuckoo's nest of an HIV diagnosis. One such is Christine Maggiore, from Los Angeles, who told her story in the March/April 1994 issue of *Rethinking Aids*, the newsletter of the group seeking a reappraisal of the HIV/Aids hypothesis. She wrote:

> I am writing to thank you for your commitment to reason, science and truth amidst all the compromised interest and hysteria that surround Aids, and to let you know of my own adventures in the wacky world of HIV.
>
> I was diagnosed as positive in March of 1992 after having been annoyed into an antibody test by a gynaecologist who relentlessly recommended testing to all her new patients. I finally consented even though I had been in a mostly monogamous relationship for over seven years, did not fit into any of the groups described as high risk and had even tested negative in 1990 to qualify for life insurance. The news that I was suddenly positive devastated me. I knew nothing about HIV except that everyone that had it was supposed to die and end up on a quilt.
>
> I immediately saw an Aids specialist who had me retake the test since only two of the seven bands on the western blot were reactive. A week later, for reasons he never explored or explained, the test was completely reactive. At that point I was considered positive beyond a doubt and began to live as if I were going to die within the five to eight years officially allotted me. Fortunately I had (and have) a high T-cell count, so none of the many doctors I went through pushed me to start AZT or any of the other alleged antivirals.
>
> Since all the experts I met with told me there was nothing I or anyone could do to halt the inevitable and unattractive demise of my immune system, I started looking for solutions on my own. This led me out of

mainstream medicine and away from the typical Aids-think supported by those depressingly helpful groups and foundations.

Somehow I stumbled upon Dr Duesberg's telephone number (I had no idea who he was or that the entire world was mad at him) and the conversation we had made a tremendous and irrevocable impact on my life. Mostly because he told me I could expect to have one [a life] if I stayed away from AZT and other such drugs. He generously sent me copies of all his writings and news articles which I reviewed with the same sceptical interest I now applied to everything about this subject. What I understood shocked and amazed me: HIV was a runaway hypothesis that grant money had turned into a belief system and that science had never bothered to substantiate! No wonder all those doctors made no sense to me – there was no sense to be made of any of this!

Christine read books and contacted alternative organisations that were challenging HIV and Aids, and started to think differently about what Duesberg referred to as a 'boring' retrovirus 'that seemed to be doing nothing but make finding dates and insurance coverage difficult'.

I began to wonder what, if anything, was going on in my body one year into 'HIV disease'... I took all my tests all over again and found I still had the same T-cell count but was now considered 'undetermined' for HIV: certain bands previously positive were now negative. I had a PCR done to determine what undetermined might mean and that came up 'detected'. Curious as to how an apparently diminishing virus was detectable, I followed the PCR with another antibody test. The result was completely negative. My amazing seroconversion then mysteriously reseroconverted to positive on the next visit to the lab.

I wish I could say I find antibody testing an entertaining pastime or that the varying results mean nothing to me. It is, instead, an obnoxious and confusing nightmare no doctor I know can explain. Depending on the week and according to the accepted wisdom, I am or am not dying and may or may not be considered an object of pity and/or fear. The whole thing sucks.

Does your group have any clue as to how tests can vary to such degrees and is there anyone else out there with a similar experience? Thank you again for your continued existence and for allowing me to be cranky about this in a public forum.

What the 'HIV' Test Means

Despite cases like Christine's, the antibody test does tell us something in people who are clearly and repeatedly positive. 'When you are ill, especially when you have an infectious disease, you have a lot of antibodies to a variety of things,' Eleopulos says. 'When a foreign substance comes into your body, and you make antibodies to it, these do not react only with that substance, but with other substances too. So the more antibodies you have in your body, the higher the probability that you will react to a substance to which you have never been exposed. The Aids risk groups – the gay men, the illicit drug users, the haemophiliacs – have millions of antibodies, because they are exposed to so many antigens. So whether or not they have HIV in them, they are more likely to test positive for the antigens in the HIV test. The same is true for Africans. Black people, even the healthy ones, have much higher antibody levels than whites, and on top of that they are often poor, they suffer TB, malaria and many other infectious diseases. But if you test a young American military recruit who has never been exposed to foreign antigens, it is very unlikely that his blood will react. The HIV antibody test can be used as a marker of risk for the development of Aids, but not as proof of HIV infection.'

A year after *Bio/Technology* published Eleopulos's review article, powerful confirmation of its conclusions was provided by a study headed by Dr Max Essex, of the Harvard School of Public Health, one of the originators of the hypothesis linking HIV with Aids and a leading exponent of the theory that the virus originated in Africa. Essex had been working with scientists from the University of Kinshasa and the health ministry in Zaire to see whether leprosy patients, and those in close contact with them, were at increased risk of being infected with HIV.

The results, published in the *Journal of Infectious Diseases*,[15] were remarkable. Out of serum samples from fifty-seven leprosy patients, forty-one tested positive using one Elisa kit, thirty-nine using another, and thirty-seven (65 per cent) by both. Among the sera from thirty-nine contacts, the figures were twelve, ten and nine (23 per cent) respectively. When the sera were tested with western blot (WB) and radioimmunoprecipitation analysis, however – tests which, because of their expense, are never normally performed in Africa – only two of the leprosy patients and none of the contacts were confirmed as positive. Even those two could be considered false positives, because the diagnosis was made on the basis of reactivity with two of the three bands gp160/120 and gp41, and as we have seen, the gp160/120 proteins are normally just multiples of the gp41 band.

Most of the blood samples reacted with proteins on the WB strips. Such reactions were even seen in 85 per cent of patients, and 57 per cent of contacts who were negative with the Elisa tests, whereas in normal individuals used as controls only 2½ per cent gave a positive WB reaction. Although these large numbers of WB reactions were interpreted as 'indeterminate' by Essex *et al.*, in most laboratories around the world they would be considered positive, according to Eleopulos.

Laboratory investigations indicated that proteins from *Mycobacterium leprae,* the microbe responsible for leprosy, were causing many of these cross-reactions and false positives, both with western blot and Elisa. P24 was the most frequently recognised 'HIV' protein in the WB test, but cross-reactivity also occurred with all the others. *M. leprae* might have this potential 'since the disease it causes is associated with an immunodeficiency that resembles HIV-1 in several respects', the researchers said. 'In addition, the immune dysregulation induced by *M. leprae* is often accompanied by the production of autoantibodies to numerous cellular proteins.'

They concluded that leprosy patients and their contacts 'show an unexpectedly high rate of false-positive reactivity of HIV-1 proteins on both WB and Elisa'. Since *M. leprae* shared several antigens with other members of the mycobacterial family, including *M. tuberculosis,* the agent responsible for TB, 'our observations of cross-reactivity... suggest that HIV-1 Elisa and WB results should be interpreted with caution when screening individuals infected with *M. tuberculosis* or other mycobacterial species. Elisa and WB may not be sufficient for HIV diagnosis in Aids- endemic areas of Central Africa where the prevalence of mycobacterial diseases is quite high'.

'Quite high' is an understatement. According to a *WorldAids* briefing paper published by the Panos Institute in September 1992, about one third of the world's population are latently infected with TB, and at any one time between 9 and 11 million people are suffering from the active infection – 95 per cent of them in Asia, Africa and Latin America. 'In Africa, TB has already become the prime cause of death in adults with HIV,' the paper said. 'A recent study in the Ivory Coast showed that 35 per cent of adults with HIV died of TB. "TB is clearly the most important HIV-associated disease in Africa," Dr Sebastian Lucas, author of the Ivory Coast study, told the 8th International Conference on Aids in Amsterdam in July. "Since Africa has 65 per cent of all cases of HIV, that makes TB the most important Aids-associated infection in the world."' According to Panos, 'the established epidemic of TB and the new epidemic of HIV have shown a disturbing tendency to coalesce and to co-infect individuals. It is a dangerous liaison both for those who are co-infected and for those communities in the developing world at risk of TB'.

It seems clear from the Zaire study that this 'epidemic of TB/HIV co-infection', as the WHO has taken to calling it, is another of the tragic errors created by the non-specificity of the 'HIV' test. People with active TB infection are at greatly increased risk of testing positive because of *M. tuberculosis,* not HIV.

When I wrote a news report on the study in May 1994, I tried several times to speak to Max Essex to explore the implications of the research further with him, but he was unwilling to come to the phone. I did, however, quote Professor John Papadimitriou, one of the co-authors of the original *Bio/Technology* paper, as saying that the Zaire research demonstrated the inadequacy of the HIV tests. 'Why condemn a continent to death because of HIV,' he said, 'when you have other explanations for why people are falling sick?'

An HIV diagnosis is potentially lethal in the West as well as in Africa, as the following letter to the *Sunday Times,* written in response to our article on the Eleopulos paper, made clear:

> I read Neville Hodgkinson on the recent report questioning the reliability of the HIV test as a predictor of Aids with the anguish which he accurately predicted. The night before I had learned that yet another of my circle of friends had by virtue of being unwell and gay been subject to and had received an HIV+ result from this iniquitous procedure.
>
> Would he read this article and would it sufficiently impress him that he need not conclude – as so many have during the last 10 years – that HIV spells untimely death?

Your newspaper has been almost alone in this country in reporting the opposition to the orthodox view that HIV causes Aids. There must eventually come a time when this lethal paradigm which has caused untold misery and untimely destruction of lives is demolished.

When I get the opportunity to meet with this friend I shall urge him to resist this dismal view of his future as do a growing number of healthy alleged HIV positives. I hope that during a period when he will be extremely vulnerable his doctor will not be pressuring him to accept medication. Especially not the highly dubious reverse transcriptase inhibitors AZT and DDI/DDC. I shall urge him with the conviction of personal experience, having been 'diagnosed' two years ago and warned that without drugs, I could expect to count life in weeks rather than years. I have since chosen to disregard that bleak counsel and the drugs and continue with my life. The intellectual justification for such obstinacy is expanding thanks to brave souls such as the authors of the report described and Prof. Duesberg, Dr Sonnabend and others who resist the pressure to subscribe to the prevailing views of the Aids industry. The empirical support can be found in the lives I am glad to say of many of my friends and acquaintances. Much much more questioning, challenging and overturning is needed. But thank you for playing your part.

Despite the absence of scientific debate or discussion over the *Bio/Technology* review, it was clear that the *Sunday Times* reports were beginning to have an impact at the grass roots. A freelance illustrator in Yorkshire told us of how he felt life was only just beginning to return to him, four years after an HIV diagnosis had robbed him of his confidence, self-esteem and drive. On the day his HIV-positive partner died of pneumonia, he was told he was positive too and had probably two years to live if he took AZT – eighteen months if he did not. He went home thinking about how conventional treatments had failed to save his partner's life, and of side-effects friends were suffering.

I had lots of friends who were HIV-positive but absolutely fine until they started taking the drugs. Everyone thought I was barmy for refusing medication but time has confirmed my suspicions. I knew the time would come when the validity of the tests themselves would be questioned. Now that has happened, I am so furious I feel like suing the doctors and the drug companies for stealing four years of my life.

When I had to tell people I had tested positive, I was thrown out of the house I had been sharing with my partner; I lost my self-esteem, my sense of direction and my drive and subsequently suffered from depression.

Things got so bad at one time, I thought about suicide. I am angry when I think about the people who have killed themselves because of a so-called positive test.

I realise the doctors have a difficult job to do, but someone has to question the whole empire that has been built up around the industry before even more people are killed through ignorance. There is a growing element of defiance, with more and more people flushing their drugs down the toilets and saying 'Look, I'm still here and I've been so-called HIV-positive for years, so what is going on?'

It would be nice though to hear something like regret or an apology from the medical profession instead of the deafening silence out there now.

We also learned of the difficulties faced by care workers and others in knowing how best to advise those diagnosed HIV-positive. One health adviser specialising in HIV/Aids said:

I would hate to be newly diagnosed as HIV-positive because the whole thing has become horrendously confusing. Five years ago, I would have told clients with a low T-cell count they should take the drugs, now I tell them they have to decide for themselves but that they should question the doctors so they are making an informed choice.

Having said that, there is no independent body to give them the advice and no forum for the wider debate of all the issues raised so how they are supposed to make an informed choice, I don't know.

I am amazed at the increase in the number of people diagnosed as HIV-positive who are questioning mainstream thinking from the start but if I want to keep my job, I cannot be seen to be rocking the boat. I feel I

> am walking on eggshells all the time because there are so many things it is politically not acceptable for me to be telling clients.
>
> There is this terrible fear throughout the field that it will be discovered we have been walking down the wrong route all these years and advising people to do things which will turn out to be the wrong things. I think about quitting all the time.

That was a good reminder, amid the anger that was beginning to be aroused among patients as the inadequacies of the HIV theory became more widely known, that people in the 'Aids industry' were also sometimes suffering greatly from the pathological science affecting their field of employment.

It was and is wrong to tell people they are carrying a deadly new virus on the basis of an unvalidated test, beset with technical problems and pitfalls in interpretation, vulnerable to shipping, climatic and storage conditions, and subject to unmeasured and probably immeasurable cross-reactivities and hence false positive results. It is very hard for doctors, scientists, politicians, the World Health Organization, gay leaders, Aids charities and even journalists to admit to this today, since they have all been instrumental in bringing about the climate of opinion in which this unvalidated test was inflicted on millions. But those are the facts. Regardless of whether or not the test has any relevance to a retrovirus, there are so many other possible causes of a positive result that on present knowledge, no one should be diagnosed as suffering from 'HIV' infection or disease. No one cognisant of these facts will ever wish to allow themselves to be tested. The sooner the error is acknowledged and the test relegated to history, the quicker we may see a return to sanity in Aids science.

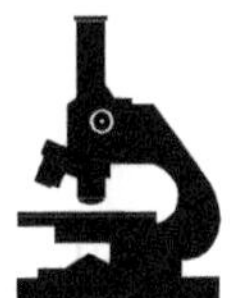

10: THE PLAGUE THAT NEVER WAS*

The lack of any effective response to our story on the non-validity of the 'HIV' test gave me the push I needed to undertake a venture the editor had long since approved: to mount our own investigation of Aids in Africa. Was the situation as described by Harvey Bialy and the Meditel team in Uganda and Ivory Coast also true of other central African countries? On 18 August 1993, armed with the *Bio/ Technology* paper, I flew to Nairobi, Kenya, and began to make inquiries.

It soon became clear to me that because of the idea that HIV was lethal and rampant, there was a consensus belief that one could hardly be too alarmist in public pronouncements about Aids. The *Kenya Times*, for example, earlier that year had reported estimates by the Kenya Medical Research Institute (Kemri) that the country had about 100,000 Aids cases, and about 1 million people 'who have the Aids-causing virus'. It added that 'once a person is infected with the killer disease, his next step is definitely death'. But the figures were impressionistic. They were put out by researchers who had been alarmed to find that about half of the people going to various hospitals for general medical reasons were testing positive. Perhaps the whole edifice of fear and concern sprang from a scientifically unvalidated test, and a misinterpretation of the meaning of a positive test result.

According to Kemri's Dr George Gachihi, 'when you see a young man or woman die after a short illness, chances are that he succumbed to the Aids disease'. It was that perspective which led the *Kenya Times* to report that 'thousands of Kenyans die each year from Aids, though the certificates always

* Some of the material in this chapter has appeared in *Aids: Virus – or Drug Induced?*, a collection of papers and essays edited by Peter Duesberg and published in 1996 by Kluwer Academic Publishers.

indicate that they died from other causes'. When one looked at the figures through the perspective of the *Bio/Technology* critique, however, there was no longer any need to see the deaths as other than from the stated causes. Similarly, despite stories about hospitals being filled to overflowing with Aids victims, when I visited the huge Kenyatta National Hospital in Nairobi I found that although there was immense overcrowding, only a handful of patients had been admitted with an Aids diagnosis.

I also found that political factors were playing a part. Kenya had lost an estimated $300 million in desperately needed foreign currency in November 1991, when the industrialised world tried to force political and economic reform on the country by cutting aid. A recent crisis announcement on Aids by the country's health minister was seen within the international aid community as an attempt to win back donor sympathy and funds, according to the journal *Africa Confidential.* 'A far-from-veiled theory in circulation says figures which show Aids spiralling out of control have been massaged to extract sympathy,' the journal said. 'In stark contrast to the recent past, when Aids was a banned subject to protect the tourist industry, the press has started reporting ever more startling increases in Aids cases and newspapers are competing for horror stories of Aids deaths.'

It did seem to be true that doctors were reporting growing numbers of Aids cases, especially among prostitutes. But in this latter group, the actual cause of death was often unknown. When a prostitute who had tested HIV-positive subsequently disappeared, it was assumed that she had gone back to her home town to die of Aids. I also found that researchers knew nothing of the doubts over the HIV test, and had not established the extent to which the increase in cases of immune system dysfunction was genuinely the result of a new virus, as opposed to a consequence of an intensification in long-established threats to health. According to some observers, poverty had driven millions of women into prostitution, and young African males had also been drawn into the trade. When treatment of the resulting repeated infections was either absent or inadequate, their immune systems could be overwhelmed. Those who harboured a cocktail of infections could also become lethally infective. But a huge gap remained between widely acknowledged threats to health associated with prostitutes and their contacts, and the apocalyptic vision of Africa's future espoused by the WHO on the basis of its HIV statistics. At that time, based on returns from its regional offices, the WHO was saying that the virus had infected 8 million Africans and would be killing 500,000 a year by the end of the century.

I found in Kenya as elsewhere that these statistics were often founded on small clinical surveys, with the results then *writ large* by computer to form an estimate for the country as a whole – and all this using a nonspecific test. One WHO official told me: 'Aids is there. No doubt about it. And it is widespread and increasing. My colleagues in the other countries can tell you the same.' But she added frankly: 'If you come with this postulate that there are a lot of false HIV-positives, it is very difficult to tell.'

The first story I filed back to London focused on the experience of a remarkable doctor whom I met in Nairobi, Father Angelo D'Agostino. Then aged sixty-seven, he was a former surgeon who had trained as a Jesuit priest and become a professor of psychiatry in Washington before going to Africa ten years previously. In 1992 he had founded Nyumbani, a hospice for abandoned and orphaned HIV-positive children, after finding that because of the panic over Aids, nowhere else would take them in. Regardless of HIV, there were good reasons why the foundlings, whose plight he learned of through work with a local Barnardo's home, should often perish. Abandoned by their shocked and stigmatised HIV-positive mothers, the children died of multiple infections, malnutrition and misery.

'People think a positive test means no hope, so the children are relegated to the back wards of hospitals which have no resources, and they die,' D'Agostino said. 'They are very sick when they come to us. Usually they are depressed, withdrawn and silent. Some have been in very poor conditions. But as a result of their care here, they put on weight, recover from their infections, and thrive. Hygiene is excellent, that they wouldn't have in the slums they have usually been living in. Nutrition is very good: they get vitamin supplements, cod liver oil, greens every day, plenty of protein. They are really flourishing. Even one that came in with TB is doing better now.'

A year on from opening the hospice, D'Agostino was puzzled. Elsewhere in Kenya and across sub-Saharan Africa, according to the WHO, tens of thousands of children were dying because of HIV, usually in their first year. The WHO regional office in Brazzaville said infant mortality had increased so much because of Aids that gains made in child-survival programmes of recent years were being eroded. But most of the Nyumbani babies were thriving, as I knew from spending a couple of hours there with several of them crawling all over me. Only one of the first forty-five children had been lost – a six-week-old who was so sick when she came that she had to go to hospital almost immediately, and died two weeks later.

In an extensive interview, D'Agostino told me: 'I'm a physician, and I bought the theory that HIV is the cause of Aids. But there are not a lot of things I would die for, and certainly not a scientific hypothesis. In fact, I would welcome with open arms any proof that these children will be free of disease. It is surprising. We expected more deaths, and a lot more serious illness. According to most predictions, the children should have died within two to three months of coming to us. Instead, we have now had to set up a nursery school, which I didn't think would be needed, and I'm planning to negotiate their entry into primary school.'

He had also been preparing to establish group therapy for the mothers and other care-givers, to deal with their grief at the loss of the children. Instead, the only losses were happy ones: some of the children became HIV-negative, and were taken back by relatives or ordinary children's homes. Even those who persistently tested positive were staying well. 'I don't have any explanation for it. Will they be alive this time next year? I have no reason to doubt it: they are healthy.'

Most of the hands-on work with the Nyumbani children was done by women, usually single mothers, who were quick to bond with the babies in their care. 'They have no money and no husband,' D'Agostino said, 'but they have been mothers – that is their big advantage.' Sister Mary Owens, D'Agostino's assistant, felt that most important to the babies' survival was a big dose of TLC – tender loving care. 'Their whole experience in the home is one that makes them happy children.'

Some of the babies became HIV-negative after a few months, an observation seen with 'HIV' babies worldwide. The usual explanation for this is that they were never truly virus-infected, but instead inherited their mother's antibodies to HIV, which fade with time. This has always seemed an unlikely idea, for a baby that has shared its mother's circulation through the pregnancy, but the HIV hypothesis allowed no other explanation. It makes more sense to see the antibodies as non-specific indications of immune system activation in babies born to mothers who are unwell, which can disappear as the child is restored to health.

Mothers, too, were being misdiagnosed. D'Agostino told of one woman who turned up with her sick baby, begging to be allowed to work for the hospice in return for care for the child. 'She had been to hospital seeking treatment for the baby, and they found among other things that it was HIV-positive as well. The baby's grandmother threw both of them out of her house. We took them in, and three to four months later sent the baby for another test. It was negative. The mother was delighted. The grandmother took them back. The mother kept working for us and some months later, when she was assigned to go with another child who was to be tested, she asked if she could have a test at the same time – and lo and behold, she was negative too.'

The experience at Nyumbani, I wrote, flew in the face of conventional theories about the history of Aids in Africa. After Gallo's 1984 announcement on HIV, western doctors invaded the continent with testing kits and computers to map the extent to which people were infected there. Virus-hunters did succeed in finding large numbers of positive test results, and as far back as 1986 there were said to be 5 million HIV-infected people on the continent. Lurid predictions followed, such as one newspaper claim that within ten years Aids would leave 'vast areas of now-populated land devoid of a single living person'. The tests that led to those estimates were now admitted to be unreliable, producing a high proportion of false positive results. Newer tests were said to be more accurate; but none had been scientifically validated. Instead, as Eleopulos had demonstrated, multiple, non-specific assaults on the immune system might be causing millions to test positive when they were not infected with HIV. Such assaults were extremely common in Africa as a result of poverty, prostitution and a breakdown of medical and social services that had followed years of civil war and economic upheaval in several central African countries.

National hospital out-patient figures for Kenya in 1991 showed malaria as the most common illness, leading to 4,343,000 visits – 23.4 per cent of the total. I learned that across central Africa there had been an upsurge in malaria cases and deaths, especially among young adults, as a consequence of childhood prophylaxis programmes. These had kept alive some children who would otherwise have died, but left them without adequate resistance to future attacks of the disease. The net result was an increase in the sum of human misery, when these half-protected people died after they had started families of their own, so that their children were orphaned. The second most common category of illness was diseases of the respiratory system, including pneumonia. Third came skin diseases, then intestinal worms, followed by diarrhoea. There was clearly a very substantial burden of morbidity, often of a chronic nature. No one was able to tell me to what extent this might be causing people to test positive for 'HIV' antibodies. The only tests used were Elisa. Often a single Elisa was all that could be afforded, although sometimes the test was repeated to 'verify' indeterminate or unexpected results.

I obtained details of two of the tests commonly used. One was Recombigen, made by the Cambridge Biotech Corporation of Worcester, Massachusetts. It employed genetically engineered antigens, and was said to give more consistent results than the previous generation of tests made from cell-line cultures. But who was to say whether or not those results were consistently wrong? The manufacturers warned that the kit was developed as a screening test, and as such was extremely sensitive. 'As a result of this sensitivity, non-specific reactions may be seen in some samples.' Both the degree of risk of infection of the person studied, and the degree of reactivity of their serum, might be of value in interpreting the test, the product leaflet said, but 'these correlations are imperfect. Therefore, in most settings it is appropriate to investigate repeatably reactive specimens by additional more specific, or supplemental tests'. The other kit, Detect-HIV, made by BioChem ImmunoSystems of Montreal, Canada, contained a mixture of synthetic proteins. Its leaflet contained similar warnings, including the frank statement that 'falsely reactive test results can be expected with a test kit of this nature'. Initially reactive specimens must be retested in duplicate, it said, and if the test was to be used for diagnostic purposes, repeatedly reactive specimens should be submitted for additional testing, such as by western blot. As far as I could ascertain, this happened either extremely rarely, or never.

I heard descriptions of cases of immune deficiency involving such symptoms as chronic Candida infection, persistent diarrhoea, severe forms of sexually transmitted diseases, chest infections, weight loss, unexplained fever and general weakness. Because of reports of increasing numbers of people testing HIV-positive, such cases were now being seen as Aids. But as with the promiscuous gay men and drug abusers who had developed such symptoms in the United States, it did not require the postulation of a deadly new virus to explain such health breakdown.

Studies among prostitutes, who often received pitifully small sums for their services, showed that some had up to 2,000 clients annually. In addition, increasing levels of poverty had caused an estimated 30,000 children to be living on the streets in Nairobi. According to the December 1992 issue of the *Voice,* news bulletin of the Child Welfare Society of Kenya, 'many of the street kids in Nairobi and elsewhere in Kenya sniff glue and petrol in a bid to forget their problems and stave off the cold and hunger pangs. This solvent abuse is damaging their future development and health'.

Another article in the bulletin featured a special report by UNICEF on 'Children in Difficult Circumstances'. It stated that in Africa there were children who had suffered as a result of famine, of drought, and especially of war. During the 1980s, two-thirds of the victims of all wars were African, and at the height of these conflicts an estimated 5 million children were struggling for survival as a consequence of deteriorating social services and food scarcity. Even in nations free of conflict, a relatively new phenomenon was the growing number of children – orphaned, abandoned or homeless – who lived on the streets of African capitals, using their wits to survive. 'Victims of economic recession and often suffering from malnutrition and a host of diseases, these children have virtually no access to health care or education.'

A poem about their plight was written by one of these children, Kennedy Mukabahe, for a 'Day of the African Child' event organised by non-governmental organisations at the Nyaya National Stadium in Nairobi on 27 June 1992:

The Cry of the African Child

On the platform I appear to express my cry,
The cry due to problems, I call upon my colleagues
Attention! All that I have suffered hurts my soul.
The problems that I am encountering, drive me to sadness.
It was in nineteen seventy-six that I was brought into being.

After a period of one year my father died.
It was not a good idea for he to die, while the child is young.
The problems I am encountering, drive me to sadness.
My mother being a wise woman brought me up properly,
But after a period of two years, she also died.
I wished for my death also, but it was impossible.
The problems I am encountering, drive me to sadness.
I went to my uncle and was made a houseboy.
Even to my brother I went and was made a doorguard.
I wished for education, but school fees were not available.
The problems I am encountering, drive me to sadness.
My pieces of clothes are torn rags and my skin is diseased.
My food is from dustbins, and my shelter is in terraces.
I therefore pray to God to deliver me from the bondage of problems.
The problems I am encountering, drive me to sadness.

Kennedy's simple expression of sadness, and of his need for clothes, food, shelter and medicine for his skin condition, heightened my own sense of the tragedy that I suspected had befallen Africa as a result of the HIV story. I felt that 'the virus' was not merely causing the displacement of desperately scarce resources, but was displacing people's feelings of compassion too. The fight against HIV was acting as a mythical focus of concern, in the face of unmanageable levels of suffering.

Big Problem with False Positives

As my travels progressed, through Zambia, Zimbabwe and Tanzania, it became more and more obvious that there were great uncertainties over the extent of African Aids. The belief that there was an epidemic had taken root in many people's minds, and unexpected or unexplained deaths tended to be seen in the light of this belief. But was there really a new, clearly identifiable clinical condition?

Everywhere I went, I found that the WHO had a network of representatives, usually sited in large, air-conditioned offices, whose work had increasingly been dominated by Aids, which they saw as an immense problem. They gathered statistics about Aids cases and HIV incidence that were passed to the WHO's Geneva headquarters. They were good people, who received me kindly. They told me of their own perspective – very much in line with the western medical model, seeing HIV and Aids as almost identical, although in Africa many Aids cases were diagnosed on the basis of clinical signs alone – and listened with tolerance as I explained about the problems with the test set out in *Bio/Technology* and the different outlook I was exploring. I also noted that they exerted a lot of power, helping to channel funds from donor agencies, drug companies and the WHO itself, dwarfing local medical spending. They worked closely with national Aids control programme officers, sometimes seeming to be effectively in charge of those programmes.

It was on the basis of their reports that the WHO had formed its estimate of at least 8 million Africans being HIV-infected. Deaths attributed to Aids had remained stubbornly low, however, relative to such huge figures: by the end of 1992, little more than 200,000 cases in ten years for the whole continent, and even that based on disputed data. According to the WHO, most Aids cases were not being reported and the true ten-year figure was much higher, around 1.5 million. But I found that while some scientists, politicians and medical workers agreed with that view, it was being strongly questioned by others.

In Lusaka, Zambia, I was told by Guy Scott, an MP and former cabinet minister, that the disease threatened to orphan 2 million children, and to take the lives of large numbers of staff in companies, public utilities and government. 'It is ripping through the system. It is an absolute disaster,' he said. Screening surveys conducted in late 1992 had found that as many as four out of ten sexually active people were testing HIV-positive, spurring the government into launching a new anti-Aids campaign.

I knew, however, from Eleopulos that the Elisa screening test was capable of throwing up very large numbers of false positives, even in the context of an industrialised country (in Russia in 1991, only sixty-six 'confirmed' western blot positives out of 30,000 Elisa positive results) and I suspected that lack of recognition of this fact was causing politicians to be misled. Several doctors at the University Teaching Hospital in Lusaka responded warmly to the *Bio/Technology* paper, finding that it reflected and helped to explain their own experience. They had been particularly puzzled by an enormous gap between reports of people testing HIV-positive in Zambia, and the number of people reported as falling ill with Aids – fewer than 1,000 a year, in a nation of 8 million people.

Dr Francis Kasolo, head of virology, said work in his department suggested the HIV figures could not be taken at face value. 'We have found a big problem with false positives,' he said. 'When we repeat the tests, there are a lot of disparities in the results. A test kit from one manufacturer behaves differently from another's.' The conclusion was that 'most of our results are more or less compromised'. Most of the country's eighty testing centres were unable to afford confirmatory western blot testing after an initial positive Elisa. And in any case, the western blot produced widely differing results. A third, rapid test had been shown to produce up to 40 per cent false positive results.

Dr Nkandu Luo, head of pathology and microbiology, believed Aids was over-reported rather than under-reported. Because HIV tests were expensive, diagnosis was sometimes on the basis of symptoms alone, and several studies showed clinicians often got it wrong: thousands of such 'Aids' patients were not HIV-positive. She had also observed that even where HIV testing routinely took place, the results could be unreliable because parasitic and other infections common in Africa could trigger false positive results.

Dr Wilfrid Boayue, the WHO representative in Zambia, said the recent surveys had shown such a big increase in positive results compared with six to seven years previously, when the proportion was only about 5 to 8 per cent, that he shared concern that the country was in the grip of an HIV epidemic. Kasolo, however, thought changes in the type of test kit used might contribute to the changing picture. He had a lot of experience of this, because international aid for developing countries is often tied to use of materials provided by the donor nations, and the donors keep changing.

'Most of the kits are supplied by the donors. If one decides not to provide funds any more, we move to another who will, and the kits come from that country instead. So the kits vary a lot: reporting can be high or low, depending on the kit. We have had individuals tested in one laboratory, and told they are positive, who move on to another, where they are negative. It is important that we address the whole issue of HIV in Africa scientifically.

There is something going on that we do not understand.'

Dr Sitali Maswenyeho, a paediatrician at the University Teaching Hospital and former fellow in Aids research at the University of Miami, said he had long argued against the HIV test. 'It's non-specific,' he said. 'The test itself is killing a lot of people here. The stigma is doing the damage. We have malnutrition, bad water, poor sanitation, and when on top of that you are told you have an incurable disease, that really cuts off people's lives.'

Despite concerns over the validity of the HIV test, the presence of a severe form of immune system failure, affecting mainly sexually active people, was widely acknowledged. But there was argument over its causes. Kasolo maintained that a variety of sexually transmitted infections might be responsible, a view shared by many older Zambians. Others felt it might be associated with over-use of aphrodisiac drugs, made from plant sources.

David Chipanta, twenty-two, an HIV-positive man helping with the work of an Aids education and counselling organisation, said: 'People in the villages tell us it is not new, but that it has become worse because of promiscuity.' Despite disagreeing with that view – he argued that promiscuity was itself nothing new – he supported the challenge to HIV testing.

In Zimbabwe, health authorities were convinced that Aids was a real threat, but Dr Timothy Stamps, the minister of health and child welfare, was also concerned that the WHO and the 'Aids industry' had fostered a damaging epidemic of what he called 'HIV-itis' in Africa. 'My basic worry is that it's distracting money and attention and personnel from the known problems such as malaria, tuberculosis, sexually transmitted diseases and safe motherhood,' he said. He was particularly disturbed by WHO advice discouraging women who had tested HIV-positive from breast-feeding their babies if there was a 'safe' alternative. And in Zimbabwe, as elsewhere in Africa, there had been allegations of medical staff telling HIV-positive patients to 'go home and die' – a trend he was vigorously trying to eradicate. 'The HIV industry, which is multi-million-dollar nationwide, is now in my view one of the biggest threats to health,' he told me.

How a Myth Was Born

Despite clear evidence confirming the thesis that the HIV story was gravely flawed, it was hard for me to be sure, when faced with widely differing views among those I met, whether or not some new, epidemic condition was afflicting Africa. But in Tanzania, I met two medically trained charity workers whose dramatic testimony provided the clearest evidence yet that the continent was not engulfed by an epidemic of Aids – and a profound insight into how the story of an epidemic had come about.

In mid-life, after finding they could have no children of their own, Philippe and Evelyne Krynen trained in France as nurses, with a specialist qualification in tropical medicine, in order to be able to dedicate the rest of their lives helping third world orphans. In 1988, they travelled through central Africa looking for a suitable place to set up a branch of the French charity Partage, which had agreed to support them. They heard that the remote Kagera province in northern Tanzania, where Africa's first cases of Aids were diagnosed as far back as 1983, was now an epicentre of the disease, which had orphaned thousands of children.

After a three-day journey to the province in January 1989, a tour of the worst-hit places conducted by a local Lutheran bishop seemed to confirm everything they had been told. Whole villages were being destroyed, people were dying continuously in and around the main township of Bukoba, and HIV testing suggested that up to half the sexually active population was infected.

Philippe, fifty, a former pilot, and Evelyne, forty-two, a teacher, prepared an illustrated report on their findings, *Voyage des Krynen en Tanzanie,* which was to prove a catalyst for world interest in the social impact of Aids in Africa. It presented a dramatic picture: children alone in houses emptied of adults, or abandoned into the care of grandparents; a football team destroyed by the disease; old people sitting alone with their dead; black crosses painted at the entrances of Aids-stricken homes.

'Here, Aids does not choose its victims among marginal groups,' they wrote. 'It touches the entire sexually active population, men and women alike. Extreme sexual liberty, a weak sense of hygiene and a lack of medical and social support have made the populations of these parts a particularly homogeneous risk group.'

As I reported in a two-page feature in the *Sunday Times*, under the headline 'The plague that never was', it was a message that western medical and charitable agencies, urgently wanting to alert people to the perceived dangers of HIV and Aids, were more than ready to hear. US, French and Belgian newspapers, magazines and television stations took up the story, and it had kept being repeated. On 15 March 1992 the *Washington Post*, for example, ran a long 'special' under the headline 'Tanzanian village devastated by Aids deaths; hard-hit region paints grim picture for spread of disease throughout Africa'. The *Post's* correspondent reported:

> Tanzania's remote Kagera region, on the western shore of Lake Victoria bordering Uganda, is one of the places where Aids first appeared on the African continent, and it is now one of the hardest-hit areas in the world. Elsewhere in Africa, health experts say, the worst of the epidemic still lies ahead. But in Kagera, the disease is already showing its full impact...
>
> Because those dying from the effects of Aids are mainly adults in their most productive years, the epidemic has left large numbers of children and old people with no one to support them. 'It would be better if we had an earthquake,' said Philippe Krynen, director of Partage, a French relief organisation working to help orphans in the Kagera region. 'An earthquake kills everybody of all ages. And when you go to rebuild, what you find left is a little bit of everybody. With Aids, you can't rebuild because what is missing are the working adults.'

The Krynens explained to me that in common with many other westerners who had seen the Aids epidemic as a call to arms against the perils of ignorance and promiscuity, they had felt it was almost impossible to overstate the dangers. They helped one young villager write a letter to schoolchildren. It said so many of his team-mates had died that 'we can't play football any more – so behave, and you won't get the disease like we did here'. The letter featured in pamphlets prepared by a European Community Aids prevention project and was distributed widely to schools in west Africa. Even in 1993, aspects of the Krynens' story were still being quoted around the world by Aids organisations.

'When we came here we had the textbook knowledge of Aids in our minds,' Philippe said. 'That it is a sexually transmitted disease; that it would be very easily transmitted in Africa because other STDs are rampant; that many Africans are HIV-positive and would get full-blown Aids after one or two years, faster than in Europe; and that the virus was passed from mother to child, affecting 50 per cent of children. This was what we had learned from our medical studies. And the people who showed me what was happening here reinforced this belief. What I wrote in my journal was with 100 per cent *bonne conscience.*'

Four years on, Partage Tanzanie was now employing some 230 full-time staff, who were helping 7,000 children in fifteen of Kagera's villages. There were twenty nurses, a doctor, a pharmacist, a laboratory technician, office workers and teachers; and scores of field workers who had got to know the children, caring for them at day centres, monitoring their health and ensuring they were well fed. As a result of the increasingly intimate understanding the Krynens acquired of the region and its people, allied to the questions the couple started asking arising from their own scientific training, a very different picture of what was going on started to emerge compared with their first impressions.

The first clue that there might be something wrong with the standard medical model of HIV and Aids came when they started to try to organise help for children in the border villages. 'Our aim was to help the people help their children,' Evelyne said. 'But in some of the villages we found nobody was interested in the future, or in the kids, any more. One reason, we thought, was that they had been told 40-50 per cent were infected and were going to die, and this in a context where people were indeed dying a lot, because of poverty and an upsurge in malaria.' (Anti-malarial drugs had helped more children through to early adulthood, but left them still vulnerable to the disease. Previously, those who survived the illness in childhood were more likely to have lifelong immunity.)

'The young people were convinced they were going to die anyway, so why should they think of the children or the future. We said that even if 50 per cent are infected, 50 per cent are not, so let us find out which are which. Then those who are free of the virus can think about the future again.'

A pilot study offering HIV tests to their own staff produced a shock: only 5 per cent were positive, although almost all were young and sexually active. Perhaps they were unrepresentative, the Krynens thought, because their level of education was above average. So in 1992 they proposed a mass testing programme in Bukwali, a village on the border with Uganda where some of Africa's first Aids cases had been reported nearly ten years previously. Encouraged by the promise that a clinic would be established to give free treatment to anyone testing positive, about 850 people agreed to take part – almost the entire population aged between eighteen and sixty. This time, 13.7 per cent were found to be HIV-positive, still much lower than the villagers had been led to believe. The Krynens found for themselves that a single positive test could not be relied on – repeat testing would frequently show the same patient to be negative. The villagers may have shown a higher rate of HIV-positives simply because they were older, with an average age of about forty-two, compared with twenty-four in the staff study. They had been exposed for longer to 'whatever it is in Africa that can so readily cause the blood to test positive', as Evelyne put it.

'We have noticed that with the women, the more children they have, the more likely they are to be positive. We have five HIV-positive women on our staff, and all have children, but a stable life. It could be because being more in contact with doctors and hospitals, and taking more drugs, or even just giving birth, causes you to accumulate reactivity to the test. It may not have anything to do with a virus.'

The Krynens also found that when appropriate treatment was given to villagers who became ill with complaints such as pneumonia and fungal infections that might have contributed to an Aids diagnosis, they usually recovered.

'All of a sudden you put all you have been told about the disease in the garbage can, and try to reconsider,' Evelyne said. 'The fifteen villages we have looked at are in the most affected area of a region that is supposed to be at the epicentre of Aids in Africa. When you listen to the people, you find they had been shocked by some deaths where the effects on the body were very visual, with fungus infections and skin rashes. But these can be secondary effects of antibiotics, and the people who died with these conditions had all been treated before for conditions such as bronchitis. Nothing is sure; everything is just wind.'

Most of the first deaths reported as Aids were in young men trading in black-market goods in the aftermath of the Ugandan war. It started at the border, where people were dealing in drugs as well as other goods, said Philippe. 'It's true this group had money and was affected with immune suppression and a wasting syndrome. But it was not because they had sex like rabbits that they died. This is what was put in people's minds by missionaries and other people, but whatever killed them was not sexually transmitted, because they have not killed their partners. They have not killed the prostitutes they were using; these girls are still prostitutes in the same place.

'Was it a special booze? Was it an amphetamine or aphrodisiac? It is difficult to give more than hints, but when you listen to the people's descriptions of those first affected, you find they were saying they had been poisoned. If the local people said that, for two or three years before the word Aids came to the region, why don't we believe them a bit, and look at what could have poisoned them?'

I asked the Krynens about studies elsewhere in Africa, in particular one carried out in Uganda that was made much of by Aids experts in London, showing greatly increased death rates among those who tested HIV-positive (although only five 'Aids' deaths were recorded). They thought it might be a consequence of health workers – and patients – giving up hope in the face of an HIV 'death sentence'. Philippe said: 'We have fewer casualties, proportionately, in those who test positive than in those who are negative. That may be because they are able to report to our clinic where they are treated free.' The couple had tried from the start to play down the significance of a positive test result.

The children who were brought to them usually thrived once they were properly fed and cared for, although some were so poorly from birth, regardless of 'HIV', that they remained vulnerable to infections. 'In all the children we have lost there was a very well designated reason, an illness we could not cope with because we hadn't the means to do it: heart failure, TB treated too late, cerebral malaria, acute hepatitis – probably caused by a drug taken for the wrong reasons,' Philippe said. 'You have no right to call any of these deaths Aids. I can't tell you of a single child I have followed who has died of a so-called Aids-related illness.' The Krynens had an adopted

Tanzanian son, Joseph, aged five, whose one-time diarrhoea, coughing and wasting were said at a local hospital to be untreatable because of HIV. Now he was cheerful, and in near-normal health. 'Joseph is what people call an Aids baby, but he is living well,' Philippe told me. 'He is a sample of the manufactured Aids you can have in this region. We put him on anti-fungal drugs for his diarrhoea, and sent him to France in January this year for bronchial washing – and now look at the kid.'

Philippe said that whenever he had been able to follow people reported to have Aids for any length of time, he had seen them to be cured. He went on:

> When you really look into it, they are not Aids cases. So where are these cases? Always in the hands of other people – hospitals, reporters, photographers.
>
> A sixty-five-year-old who tested HIV-positive had been getting sick, suffering stomach troubles and losing weight. I explained to him that HIV and Aids were very different things, that we could not really make a link between them. The other day I heard that the fellow is not sick any more. He doesn't believe he is going to get Aids. He has regained four kilos and is doing very well. This type of resuscitation is very common in our programme.
>
> A woman of about forty, with two daughters, was dying of chronic diarrhoea and chest infections, said to be HIV-related. Her husband was said to have died of Aids, although nobody has been able to tell me precisely what killed him.
>
> We admitted one of the daughters to our day-care centre, supported the other at school with books and meals, and treated the mother with rifampicin, a drug normally reserved for TB which we have found to be very effective in such cases. After a month she did not have diarrhoea any more, she was able to go to the fields again and has started to gain weight. I can swear to you that this woman will not be sick for a long time, as long as she knows we are supporting her. We have stolen another Aids case from the statistics.
>
> It is good to know that this epidemic which was going to wipe out Africa is just a big bubble of soap.

The couple were continuing to use the HIV test, 'just to prove that we have to stop doing this, that it has nothing to do with Aids'. They were training their field workers not to mention HIV or Aids, but instead to deal with any known disease they encountered with the best treatment available, regardless of the patient's HIV status. 'It is not known whether HIV causes Aids,' they said in a pamphlet produced for the team. 'It is time to come back to science and abandon magic thinking.' Philippe declared: 'There is no Aids. It is something that has been invented. There are no epidemiological grounds for it; it doesn't exist for us.'

If Kagera is not, after all, in the grip of an epidemic of 'HIV disease', and if there is no Aids, where have the thousands of orphans come from? The answer, say the Krynens, is that most of the children are not orphans at all. Their final disillusionment was to discover that although many children were raised by their grandparents, that was a long-standing cultural feature of the region.

'The parents expatriate themselves a lot,' Philippe explained. 'They move away from the region, sending a little money, returning little or never, but still have many children in the village. They are outwardly orphans, but raised by the grandmother or grandfather. It has always been like this here; they may need help, but it has nothing to do with Aids. Polygamy is also rampant here and they don't raise all the children. They select very few and the others are just made and abandoned.' Other children are born to prostitutes, who may spend much of the year away from the region, working in the cities.

'You come as a European and ask: "Who has no mother or father?" They produce all these children, even though they have a mother or father in another place. We have been shown false orphans since the beginning – children who have parents who never died, but who will not show up any more. And when the parent has died, nobody has been asking why. It has nothing to do with an epidemic. Families just bring them as orphans, and if you ask how the parents died they will say Aids. It is fashionable nowadays to say that, because it brings money and support.

'If you say your father has died in a car accident it is bad luck, but if he has died from Aids there is an agency to help you. The local people have seen so many agencies coming, called Aids support programmes, that they want to join this group of victims. Everybody claims to be a victim of Aids nowadays.'

Posters warning of the dangers of *ukimwi* (Aids) adorn the cabins of the Victoria, a steamer that ferries passengers on the nine-hour journey from Mwanza, on the southern shore of Lake Victoria, to Bukoba. When the Krynens first made the journey, they found a small town with only a handful of foreigners and few cars. Today, as the ferry arrives, the tiny port seizes up with vehicles, including the white Land Rovers and Toyotas characteristic of the numerous Aids agencies that have flourished in much of central Africa.

'We have everybody coming here now – the World Bank, the churches, the Red Cross, the UN Development Programme, the African Medical Research Foundation – about seventeen organisations reportedly doing something for Aids in Kagera,' Philippe said. 'It brings jobs, cars – the day there is no more Aids, a lot of development is going to go away.'

The Krynens were working hard. They kept files on all their donor families and careful records of how the money was spent. Their home, a modest bungalow on a hillside overlooking Lake Victoria, was the hub of the project, with its own HIV-testing laboratory. All day a stream of workers came by to give feedback and take directions. A few children who had nowhere else to go lived in an adjoining building. With such direct, practical help being given to suffering people, perhaps it did not matter too much whether the children were Aids orphans or not. But the Krynens were angry because false information continued to be spread to Africa and the world.

'Africa is a market for many things, an experimental ground for many organisations and a "good conscience" ground for many charities,' Philippe said. 'It is very easy to "do good" in Africa. It is so disorganised that the one who is doing the good is also the one reporting the good he is doing. So it is a perfect field for charity – the fake charity which is 99 per cent of the charity in Africa, charity which benefits the benefactors.' The Krynens felt strongly about this because of their own involvement in triggering an invasion of Aids agencies to Kagera. They now knew that the stories they told, of houses and villages abandoned because of Aids, were untrue.

'The houses that were empty were closed because they were the second or third homes of someone in Dar es Salaam,' said Philippe. And the black crosses painted outside homes were leftovers from a population census, not a warning of Aids:

I learned this later. I have never seen a village with no adults, where children are like wolves in the forest. You know who is responsible for these stories? Partly, Partage. We said that if we did not do something very quickly, these villages would be emptied of adults and children would be like wild animals. The stories have been printed and reprinted, without the 'if'.

My medical studies led me to believe that Aids was devastating and the people who showed me the situation here reinforced this belief. I jumped into this, and made others believe it. And now I know it was not true. But I know many more things that were not true. Nothing was true.

It is terrible to consider you have done so many things you thought worthwhile, when in fact you were misled. It is difficult to adjust afterwards. Nobody knows who is responsible for the first misinterpretation, but as time passes it gets bigger and bigger. These ideas were not based on any studies; they were just fashion. But when you are here, and you have to witness the reality of what happens in the field, you cannot agree with any of the statements they are making in Europe about Aids in Africa. We discovered we were in a full-blown lie about Aids. Everybody participates in this lie, willingly or not. No individual is responsible, but it is a big scandal.

The world has been brainwashed about Aids. It has become a disease in itself, without the necessity of having sick people any more. You don't need Aids patients to have an Aids epidemic nowadays, because what is wrong doesn't need to be proved. Nobody checks; Aids exists by itself.

We came here to help orphans of Aids. Now we are facing a situation where there are no orphans and no Aids. We are in the heart of Aids country. You are talking to people who 'discovered' Aids here, and who now say it is a lie. The figures are not real. We have been making Aids. Now we have to witness how we can de-make it again. We expect to have to pay for what we say. It will be the price of truth.

Father D'Agostino Reaffirms Belief in HIV

Articles I filed from Africa were sometimes followed up or reprinted in regional and national newspapers there, after they had appeared in the *Sunday Times*. With the issue being such an emotional one, and with money and prestige as well as lives at stake, this caused some of the people I had interviewed to come under great pressure to recant. They responded differently to these pressures.

Father D'Agostino was upset to see the puzzlement and hope he had expressed in relation to the survival of his 'Aids babies' put in the context of the wider critique of the HIV theory of Aids that the *Sunday Times* had been airing. To the medical profession, this is a heresy, not just a different interpretation of the facts, and a press release he issued on 17 September on behalf of the Children of God Relief Institute, which runs Nyumbani, read more like a religious creed than a comment from a scientist. It stated:

> Recently, the 'London Sunday Times' ran a long front-page story and the Nairobi 'Nation' an editorial page 'special report'. Both papers misconstrued the facts of the unfortunate life circumstances of the children at 'Nyumbani' in order to prove an erroneous thesis. While this does no harm to the children themselves, it does a grave disservice to the larger community because it panders to the all too prevalent mental process of denial. This denial only increases the universal and deadly threat of HIV/Aids. In order to correct these errors, we must assert:
>
> 1. We do believe in the 'germ' theory of disease as proposed by Louis Pasteur. This universally proven theory is accepted by compassionate and credible scientists world-wide.
> 2. We believe that there is a virus designated 'HIV' which has been isolated and is responsible for the fatal disease called Aids.
> 3. Since there is no cure for the ravages of the HIV virus, we believe that the only strategy to contain and prevent spreading of the disease Aids is for all sectors of society to -
>   i. join hands in creating awareness and,
>   ii. urging action in an appropriate manner.
> 4. Compassion, understanding, care and respect for human dignity must fashion any programme to help those suffering from HIV/Aids.
> 5. We invite any party so inclined to help our efforts to assist in alleviating the tragic plight of those voiceless HIV/Aids sufferers – the abandoned child.

6. We totally disagree with any scientifically unsubstantiable theory that denies the reality of the causation of the disease HIV/Aids.

The uncertainties Father D'Agostino had clearly expressed in a recorded interview, as he pondered the surprising good health of his foundlings, were now gone, replaced by a reaffirmation of belief in the HIV doctrine of Aids. I knew nothing of this press release at the time – I was still travelling through Africa, and had not even seen the *Sunday Times* article – and although Father D'Agostino says he faxed a response to the article to the newspaper's office, it was never received there.

In fact, the first I knew of his dissatisfaction was when I received the following letter, dated 22 October, after I had written to him on my return to London enclosing cuttings of my Africa articles.

Dear Neville,

I want to thank you for the courtesy of sending the article appearing in the 3rd October edition and also for the pleasant experience that we all had when you visited Nyumbani. That being said, I must confess to some reservations.

You and I look at the world with quite different perspectives. You, from that of a journalist and myself, as a committed medical man. Our goals are quite different. I, after having spent at least fourteen full years in the pursuit of medical knowledge, am committed to using that eclectic knowledge for the good of mankind. I am not espousing any particular philosophy or theory when I attempt to enhance the body's (and mind's) natural healing powers. That being said then, I quite disagree with your point of view. I am trying to be charitable in assuming that you have taken this task for humanitarian reasons, but I must say there is a question about that at times.

I certainly question the *Sunday Times* approach to the problem because it is quite evident that they are more interested in selling copies rather than the pursuit of truth. They have no care for the terrible consequences to people when they are permanently and fatally injured by believing the misinformation that is being peddled. A primary principle in the practice of conventional medicine is that if one cannot do any good, at least do not do any harm. This principle is observed only in the breach by the *Sunday Times* because they are doing great harm without even considering the possibility... and for mere gold.

Another point: I was able to fax a response to the article but never got any sort of admission of reception or acknowledgement. Would it be possible for you to inquire as to whether or not they did receive my fax and what they plan to do about it, if anything?

Finally, I want to state that this is not a personal issue and I would look forward to your visiting us once again, but this time, being quite open about our stand with regard to the terrible consequences of the infection by the HIV virus.

With all best wishes,
A. D'Agostino, SJ, MD

On 29 October I replied as follows:

Dear Father D'Agostino,

I was greatly distressed to receive your letter of October 22 today. Firstly, because neither I nor the Letters Editor had known anything of your sending a response to my article of October 3; and secondly, because of your evident distress over what you call the *Sunday Times* approach to the issue of HIV and Aids. I had felt that my article was a straightforward description of what you had told me and what I had observed for myself. I also know how much both the Editor and myself have wanted to contribute to understanding about HIV and Aids, and how wrong you are to allege that we are doing harm 'for mere gold'. Have you seen the other articles I filed? Some of the people involved in those have subsequently come under bitter attack from parties who feel both the truth and their own interests have been threatened, but perhaps the difference is that they were aware of what a contentious issue this is. It is not possible to back away from these issues: the point of view to which the newspaper has been giving an airing is that immeasurable harm, including much loss of life resulting from panic and false diagnosis, is being done by the blind pursuit of the HIV hypothesis against much evidence of its inadequacies. Indeed, we quoted – accurately – Dr Timothy Stamps, Minister for Health and Child

> Welfare in Zimbabwe, as saying 'the HIV industry ... is now in my view one of the biggest threats to health'.
>
> Your own uncertainty was very clear when we met. What has happened to make you write as you did? I do apologise if you have been embroiled in a controversy against your wishes, but the strength of feeling on this issue should help to indicate to you that something may be terribly wrong in the view that your profession has currently espoused so dogmatically about the cause of Aids.
>
> I thank you for your kindness in emphasising that you do not see this as a personal issue. Please do send a copy of your original fax to the Letters Editor, with a copy in the post in case of further problems. Mark the letter clearly for the Letters Editor. I should also be grateful to receive a copy: the news desk fax, which is nearest to me, is —.

Neither I nor the newspaper ever received that fax from Father D'Agostino. He told me by phone, when the issue flared up again months later, that he had decided against sending it, after receiving my letter, feeling it was by then too late. He added that he had seen some of the letters published in the *Sunday Times* about the controversy, and felt that 'they just went along with the same views. It was obvious they weren't interested in the scientific truth of the matter ... I just gave up'.

That did not stop him making a statement to the *Independent on Sunday*, a newspaper which has been most vociferous in Britain in promoting the official view on HIV and Aids and in attacking my own reporting. In it, he condemned the 'gross distortions and quite incorrect implication' made as a result of my interviewing him, and declared that he had received no acknowledgement of his original fax.

I like and admire Father D'Agostino and am sad that I caused him distress, but I feel sure we were right to run the article. The quotes directly attributed to him were taken verbatim and expressed his observations as a human being and a doctor, as opposed to a politician and defender of the HIV faith.

I can understand his discomfort at the sweeping front-page headline used on the story, 'Babies give lie to African Aids'. There was also an unfortunate piece of editing that attributed more uncertainty to him than he had expressed. The article I filed from Nairobi included a paragraph in which I wrote: 'The suspicion is growing that many "Aids" cases are really old diseases given a new name, though sometimes made worse by civil war and economic and social decline, and that people who test HIV-positive are not, as most have been led to believe, the victims of a new, inevitably lethal disease.' The edited version correctly stated that in common with growing numbers of scientists and doctors around the world, D'Agostino was beginning to question whether HIV really was the killer it had been made out to be. That was the purport of the entire interview, during which I had told him about the *Bio/Technology* paper and the reappraisal of the HIV theory of Aids being sought by those doctors and scientists. But the article then went on to state that 'He, like them, suspects that many "Aids" cases are really old diseases given a new name...' etc., a suspicion I had not attributed to him.

His statement to the *Independent on Sunday,* however, made it plain that he was now putting *all* his doubts behind him. He said four children in his care had since died of Aids out of a total of fifty-five with HIV, and that two or three others had Aids. He had no doubt, the paper reported, that children infected with HIV would eventually succumb to Aids.

Since my work in this field has so often shown me how that very expectation among doctors tends to become a self-fulfilling prophecy, I rang D'Agostino in disbelief to ask him if that was really what he now thought. Yes, he said, 'I never questioned the medical model; the only thing I questioned was why they didn't die at three; why they were still alive at seven. I never questioned that they would die. I know they will succumb.' There was 'no question' in his mind that the four had died of Aids. In one, it had been 'mild' carditis that refused to clear up with the most up-to-date antibiotics. When I questioned whether that was an Aids-defining illness, and asked him about the other deaths, Father D'Agostino grew angry and told me they died of HIV, and he was a doctor, and I had no right to question his clinical judgement. He told me he had come under a lot of pressure locally, in particular through medical channels, and I do not know what other pressures he had to bear. It still hurts that he spoke as he did, but I have to remind myself that he did not choose to become embroiled in controversy and must have felt equally hurt over the outcome of my visit to Nyumbani. I hope that time will show him that the issue we were exploring was a genuine one, and not a controversy trumped up 'for mere gold'.

Krynens Lose £350,000 EC Grant

Philippe Krynen, by contrast, had resolved in his heart that he had to try to counter the disinformation about African Aids that had been fed to the world, and to which he had contributed significantly. This was fortunate, because the pressures he and Evelyne faced, after a two-page article about their changed vision of Aids in Africa was published on 3 October, could hardly have been greater. At one point, they were nearly evicted from the country.

The European Community's Aids Task Force immediately threatened to cancel a Fr3 million (£350,000) grant agreed for the Partage operation. It remains suspended to this day, and is unlikely to be forthcoming. Yet previously, the task force had made a star of Philippe Krynen. Its most recent strategy review, 'The European Commission in the Global Fight Against Aids', cited the Tanzania orphan care project, which it described as 'the human face of EC funding'. A video that included twenty-two minutes on work in Tanzania was sent to Aids control units throughout Africa. The task force had paid for Krynen to fly to three international Aids conferences, where he was invited to present scientific papers and was brought into an inner circle of Aids activists. Now, it disowned him.

In view of all that they believed, it wasn't surprising that instead of examining the Krynens' arguments, the reaction of Aids activists at the European parliament in Brussels, where the task force was based, was anger and abuse. A press statement issued by the Socialist Press Office at the parliament declared that the *Sunday Times* report 'sparked outrage' at a meeting of the EC's joint assembly. It quoted Dr Lieve Fransen, head of the Aids task force, as warning that if people accepted claims that the Aids epidemic in Africa was a myth, computer predictions of 40 million HIV-positive people by the year 2000 could soar to 100 million. The statement also said that Janey Buchan, Labour Member of the European parliament for Glasgow, had circulated the assembly with a dossier of 'world-wide scientific condemnation' of the newspaper's reports.

Philippe Krynen was unrepentant when told of this angry response, and the threat to Partage's EC grant. He recalled that at a meeting preceding the International Aids Conference in Amsterdam in 1992, which ended with dinner at the Holiday Inn, Buchan was helping Fransen fight a threat to disband the task force. 'It is a little family,' he said. 'They have a lot of money, and they make a lot of noise. It is incredible: five people can make you believe the European parliament is behind them, when it may just be a little private affair.' He was resigned about the funding threat. 'I am not afraid at all,' he said. 'Missing money doesn't mean you are missing the point. The "Aids makers" know that the figures have been inflated. They have their backs to a wall that is crumbling down.'

In a follow-up article on 17 October reporting these and other developments, I said that after meeting scientists, doctors, politicians and patients in four African countries, my own view was that there was no good evidence of a new, epidemic condition in Africa. This did not mean, however, that there had been a plot to mislead. Aids workers genuinely believed HIV presented a huge threat which would destroy millions of lives tomorrow, even if it had not done so today. 'This belief has been sustained by a lack of good science. Aids workers simply do not know that the HIV test has never been properly validated, nor that there are indications that it is probably useless in Africa, where numerous parasitic and other conditions cause cross-reactions. Because they believe there is an epidemic, they think they are doing the right thing in multiplying HIV and Aids statistics out of proportion to the facts. Estimates for whole countries are based on small, scientifically uncontrolled studies using questionable diagnostic criteria. People tell you that their hospitals are bursting with HIV-positive patients; but these patients are not dying of Aids in the sense that we know it in the west. They are dying of diseases long known to Africa, such as tuberculosis, malaria and chronic intestinal infections.' The article also stated:

> Numerous interests – commercial, financial, political and even religious – are served by the idea that an epidemic of a new sexually transmitted disease is ripping through Africa. It distracts attention from rising death rates caused by economic exploitation and decline following periods of unsustainable population growth. It keeps the Aids industry alive in the wake of the collapse of its predictions of an epidemic in Europe. It provides a marketplace for test kits, condoms and vaccine trials, a breeding ground for charities, a field of action for researchers and a vehicle for the projection of western fears about the consequences of sexual promiscuity.

> It may also distract attention from illegal alcohol manufacture or drug abuse, a growing problem in some African countries.

The stories from Africa provoked a flood of correspondence, including condemnation from the highest level. A letter from Baroness Chalker, the UK's Minister for Overseas Development, which was also signed by Sir David Steel, the Liberal Democrat spokesman for foreign affairs, and Tony Worthington, the Labour Party's foreign affairs spokesman for Africa, accused me of writing nonsense. They wrote:

> Mr Hodgkinson says that the scientific community have collectively failed to validate their tests for HIV and have deliberately inflated statistics. If we are to believe him, these scientists have fooled the World Health Organization, governments in developed and developing countries alike, international development organisations like the Save the Children Fund, ActionAid and Oxfam, institutes of public health, journalists and the general public.
>
> The sad fact is that Africa is in the grip of a major HIV epidemic. Tens or hundreds of thousands have already lost their lives: tens of millions are at risk. Mr Hodgkinson has got it badly wrong, and you do your readers a grave disservice in giving credence to his nonsense.

The letter had also been seen and agreed by heads of voluntary organisations and medical establishments concerned with Aids, although their names were not published as it was not the newspaper's policy to do so without the actual signatures. They were Sir Donald Acheson, former chief medical officer for the UK, now with the London School of Hygiene and Tropical Medicine; Professor Michael Adler, head of genitourinary medicine at the Middlesex Hospital in London; Professor Roy Anderson, of Oxford University; Dr Kenneth Calman, the current chief medical officer; Dr Ian Campbell, chair of the UK NGO Aids Consortium; Professor Richard Feachem, dean of the London School of Hygiene and Tropical Medicine; Martin Griffiths, director of ActionAid; Professor David Molyneux, director of the Liverpool School of Tropical Medicine; Sir Dai Rees, director of the Medical Research Council; Dr Les Rudd, director of the National Aids Trust; Stewart Wallis, deputy director of Oxfam; and Professor Sir David

Weatherall, also of Oxford University.

Most editors, I suspect, would have wilted under an all-party, allprofessional onslaught of this kind, but I was fortunate in that Andrew Neil had followed the arguments closely and continued to believe the issue was of genuine concern, and that I was reporting it as straightforwardly as I could. He published many critical letters that contributed to the debate, but tended not to use those that were merely abusive, or that contained demonstrable misunderstandings or untruths. There were also some good letters that did not get used, either because other correspondents had made the same point or, particularly in the case of some that could not be cut, because of lack of space. The choice of which letters went into the paper rested with the letters page editor and the editor himself, but I was usually sent copies for reference and sometimes asked to comment.

The 'dossier' circulated by Janey Buchan comprised five unpublished letters that had been sent to the *Sunday Times* in response to my report from Nairobi. Three other letters on the issue, two of them covering similar ground to those rejected, had appeared in the paper at that time.

Three of the unused letters were from religious-based development agencies whose primary fear was that the article could threaten the flow of aid to Africa, a legitimate concern although not relevant to the scientific argument, nor taking into account the social damage 'HIV-itis' was causing.

A fourth letter was from Fransen. It carried twenty-two other signatures from Aids workers, who had evidently been attending an EC meeting. It claimed my conclusions were based on a 'gross misunderstanding' of the facts. The letter stated: 'It is well established that many children infected with the Aids virus may have a long period without any signs of disease and only a small proportion become ill very early and die in infancy.'

That was very different from a WHO statement I had quoted in my report, that tens of thousands of children were dying because of HIV, usually in their first year, and that infant mortality had increased so much because of Aids that gains made in child-survival programmes were being eroded. It also conflicted with a claim by UK Aids specialists Geoff Garnett and Roy Anderson the previous March, that 'infected children have a short life expectancy in developing countries (a conservative estimate is four years from birth)'. This statement was made in an effort to undermine an observation by

Professor Beverley Griffin, of London's Hammersmith Hospital, concerning blood samples she had received from hundreds of children in Malawi: the HIV-positive proportion had remained unchanged, at around 1-2 per cent, for seven years, in contrast to claims elsewhere that about a fifth of Malawi's population were infected. Garnett and Anderson suggested that most of the HIV-positive children had died before they could reach the age group – five to eight – being studied by Griffin. It seemed that in Africa, so little was known for sure that you could find statistics to support almost completely opposing points of view.

Fransen also repeated a point I had made in my article, that a positive test for HIV antibodies in babies under fifteen months did not necessarily indicate infection. The letter concluded: 'Prevention of HIV/Aids transmission should be a high priority in all countries in order to save lives. Also, the recognition of Aids in children has led to improved management and support for their families. It is damaging, counter-productive and irresponsible to deny that Aids is a problem.'

The fifth letter in the 'dossier' was from James Neil, a professor of veterinary pathology at Glasgow University and member of the Medical Research Council's Aids directed programme steering committee. He contested my assertion that growing numbers of scientists and doctors doubted the view that HIV causes Aids, saying that 'in my experience this sceptical view is now no more than a fashion followed by a very small number of eccentrics and publicity seekers, none of whom are held in respect by mainstream scientists'. He regarded my article from Nairobi as 'no more than the usual cocktail of incomplete anecdotes and defective logic', and added: 'I fail to understand why the *Sunday Times* continues to support a campaign of misinformation which is undermining all responsible public health information sources.' In a further letter he said my coverage was upsetting many people who were well qualified to comment on the subject. 'The strength of feeling is understandable given the importance of the issue for public health and the feeling that Mr Hodgkinson is wilfully manufacturing controversy to gain a higher profile for himself and for your newspaper.' He called for 'balance' with contributions from a journalist prepared to present the mainstream view.

Andrew Neil had replied that the newspaper's policy was 'to publish reasoned argument and rebuttal concerning the ideas, opinions, and facts reported in the paper, rather than simply to reflect the weight of opinion hostile to a particular reporter's efforts to shed light on a controversial field'. To Janey Buchan, that smacked of 'McCarthyite tactics and language'. No editor should write like that, she said at a World Aids Day news conference on 1 December. The *Sunday Times* coverage was immensely damaging to the fight against Aids and the spread of HIV, particularly in Africa, because of its reputation. 'A newspaper with Rupert Murdoch, a born-again Christian, as owner should have a sense of duty. We cannot get fair treatment from the paper.'

The editor's reply seemed reasonable to me. The newspaper's readers, and probably most of the world, knew what the mainstream view of Aids was. There was a limit to how many times we could repeat it. Now some clear light needed to be shed on the issues we had raised – the non-specificity of the test, the uncertainty over what 'Aids' meant in Africa, whether or not it was transmissible through 'normal' sex, how far it could be countered by proper medical care and good nutrition, the enormous gap between the millions testing positive and actual Aids cases. I was also grateful for Andrew Neil's support for this 'particular reporter's efforts'. The Africa mission had involved five weeks of intensive and often uncomfortable work, and coping with the barrage of abuse that had for months accompanied my Aids reporting sometimes proved an exhausting task.

It wasn't as if the paper neglected to carry critical comment. Throughout the controversy, the letters used tended to be in a ratio of roughly two against for each one that was supportive. A selection published on 17 October, two weeks after we had told the Krynens' story, included the following:

- The Krynens are neither doctors nor trained social scientists, but well-meaning philanthropists. Their conclusions were reached from personal experience in a small area of Tanzania. It is generally believed that adequate nutrition and health care do prolong the wellbeing of an individual infected with HIV/Aids; thus it is not surprising that those cared for in Kagera responded in such a way. Why is it that people with a high social status who can afford good food and health care

are victims also? More than sixty of the 1,000 students who graduated with me from Makerere University, Kampala, in 1985 have died of Aids.

Symons W. Khalokho
Aids Relief Uganda

- If there is no Aids epidemic in Africa, why is it that African men and women arriving here are increasingly found in hospitals dying of an illness identical to western Aids? Most of the women dying with Aids in London are African, infected with HIV before arrival. They are a small but vitally important indicator of the terrible effects of Aids overseas.

Maurice Adams
Aids Care Education and Training

- A seroprevalence rate of 13.7 per cent is serious – equivalent to that noted at the Chikanta hospital in the Mazabuka district of Zambia, where in 1989 I noted a hospital seroprevalence in sexually active males at 43 per cent. HIV does have an impact on the level of illness and the number of deaths. In May 1993, I returned to find that virtually all families in the district served by the hospital (100,000 people) have a family member who died or who is ill and seropositive.

Captain Dr Ian D. Campbell
The Salvation Army

- Neville Hodgkinson's article reinforces the attitudes of many people who are looking for justification for their own behaviour so they can ignore the evidence and continue spreading the Aids virus.

Dr Ian Clarke
High Wycombe

Maurice Adams's letter produced a fierce response the following week from Jody Wells, director of the health activist group Continuum. The answer to his question was quite simple, Wells said:

> The Africans he sees dying in Aids wards in Britain are dying from the very same thing as British Aids patients – Aids medication and medical incompetence.
>
> The drugs that are supposed to destroy HIV in people who respond positively to an HIV antibody test (not a test for live virus) produce destruction of gut bacteria, muscle wastage, hair loss, weight loss, peripheral nerve damage, central nervous system damage and eventual death. These are exactly the symptoms that doctors who have brainwashed themselves into believing that HIV is the sole cause of Aids *expect* to see in people they diagnose as having Aids.

A similarly supportive letter came from Wilmette Brown, of the Black Women for Wages for Housework campaign, responding to the all-party attack on our coverage. Lady Chalker and others had cited the support of governments and international development agencies 'for the twin theories that HIV leads to Aids and that there is an HIV/Aids epidemic in Africa. But all that this confirms is that is that there is a lot of money and political capital at stake,' Brown wrote. 'Investment in the myth of Aids in Africa enables disinvestment in overcoming genuinely epidemic diseases of poverty…As a Black women's group we consider the Sunday Times articles on the myth of Aids in Africa a public service.'

Five Aids Deaths Condemn a Continent

In a commentary published on the same page as my 17 October review of the controversy, Lady Chalker explained 'Why we must keep up the war on Aids'. She acknowledged that predictions of drastic population decline across Africa resulting from HIV 'were not only misguided, but they also undermined the efforts of African governments to restore both public and external confidence'. (Dr David Nabarro, the ODA's chief medical adviser, who used to work in Nairobi, has struggled for several years to counter such ill-founded predictions.) But she also cited as 'clear' evidence against the Krynens' challenge to conventional wisdom the results of a study in Uganda by the British Medical Research Council, demonstrating that people who are HIV-positive are more likely to die. The study involved fifteen villages in rural Masaka, southern Uganda – about 10,000 people in all. Adolescents and young adults infected with HIV-1 were sixty times more likely to die in the next year than those who were not infected. More than half of all adult deaths, and more than 80 per cent of deaths in young adults, were associated with HIV-1.

This same study has been cited several times by those wishing to give scientific support to the idea that Africa is in the grip of a new infectious disease. The first time I saw it mentioned was in an article by Peter Smith, professor of tropical epidemiology at the London School of Hygiene and Tropical Medicine (LSH), published by the *Observer* in March 1993. Headlined 'Half-truths and misconceptions', the article was written as a response to the Meditel documentary on Aids and Africa made for Channel 4's 'Dispatches' programme. Smith said the survey found that 8 per cent of adults were infected with HIV, and 11 per cent of those died in the next year, compared to 0.6 per cent among those not infected. He went on:

> HIV infection increases susceptibility to a range of other infections, most notably tuberculosis. Thus many deaths from tuberculosis in Africa are now directly due to HIV infection. For the presenters to claim that 'it is hard to find evidence that HIV increases susceptibility to tuberculosis' displays crass ignorance of the many studies demonstrating this, both in Africa and in the United States.

In fact, there have been studies showing that TB responds to treatment just as well in 'HIV-infected' people as in those who test negative for HIV antibodies, which may have been the point the television programme was making. One of these studies, cited in 1992 by the LSH's Dr Paul Nunn, measured the concentration of TB bacilli before and after drug treatment. He reported that 'surprisingly, the rate of decline of the concentration is faster in HIV-positive than negative patients. So the early bactericidal effect of anti-tuberculous therapy is not adversely affected by HIV and possibly the reverse. Nor is the rate of persistently positive cultures at six months of therapy increased by HIV'. Deaths were clearly greater among the HIV-positive group, but the research suggested this was 'partly due to tuberculosis itself, but more important are non-tuberculous, non Aids-defining, bacterial infections... the main contribution to this excess mortality is from curable infections'.

The link between 'HIV' and 'susceptibility to TB' is almost certainly artificial. As we saw in the last chapter, the 'HIV' test has never been validated by the only certain gold standard for a diagnostic test of this type, which is to isolate the virus. Scientists have not been able to take a group of people in whom the virus has been isolated and compare the results they give on the antibody test with those given by a group of people who do not have the virus. As a result of this failure to validate, no one knows precisely what 'HIV-positivity' really represents, other than some kind of immune system activation. It is not known whether people who test positive really are infected with HIV, as opposed to some other microbe or microbes, or environmental assaults, that activate the immune system in such a way as to produce the proteins attributed to 'HIV'.

What we do know, however, as a result of the leprosy study in Zaire, is that the test detects the presence of antibodies to antigens associated with infection by *Mycobacterium leprae;* and that *M. leprae* shares several antigens with other members of the mycobacterial family, including *M. tuberculosis,* the agent responsible for TB. People with active TB infection are therefore liable to be at greatly increased risk of testing positive because of *M. tuberculosis,* not HIV, and in fact 30-50 per cent of African 'Aids' deaths involve TB. Of the 660 million people in sub-Saharan Africa, an estimated 2-3 million have active TB, with an annual mortality of 790,000. The 'range of other infections' cited by Smith as associated with HIV-positivity are probably also ones we should look to as causing false positive reactions with the test, rather than thinking that they indicate increased susceptibility arising from HIV.

If Smith and others at the LSH had been more open towards the dissident views aired by Meditel and the *Sunday Times,* they might have spared themselves – and Africa – from repeatedly drawing the same mistaken conclusions from the Uganda research. As it was, the mistakes came up time and again.

In May 1993, the LSH organised a special public lecture/press conference 'to counter the misleading and incorrect information' contained in 'recent reports in the press and on television' suggesting that the problem of Aids in Africa might have been greatly exaggerated. I attended this event, ready to report any developments that moved the story on, but it was a disappointment.

On the HIV test, for example, it was stated that these were now 'highly sensitive and specific', and had been so for about five years, although it was admitted that there had been problems with cross-reactions and false positives in the early 1980s. No evidence was offered to back up the assertion of specificity, however, other than that there was a virtual absence of positive results in children aged five to fourteen years. If there were widespread cross-reactions with other pathogens, it was argued, you would expect to see many more testing positive in that age group. That was an interesting observation, but hardly an adequate counter to the *Bio/ Technology* review article's fundamental critique of the HIV test.

The Zaire study, although I did not know about it at the time, suggests a possible explanation for this observation. As its authors stated, *M. leprae* might have the potential to trigger reactivity with 'HIV' proteins 'since the disease it causes is associated with an immunodeficiency that resembles HIV-1 in several respects', and since 'the immune dysregulation induced by *M. leprae* is often accompanied by the production of autoantibodies to numerous cellular proteins'. Perhaps it took a few years, as well as exposure to the stresses of adulthood, before these reactions occurred. The association was supported by another observation at the LSH press conference, that there was a 'sixteen-fold greater morbidity in HIVpositive patients from TB'. In any case, a test capable of producing almost 100 per cent false positives in leprosy patients and their contacts – and by implication, in TB patients as well – can hardly be said to be specific for HIV.

The Uganda study data were presented by Dr Daan Mulder, director of the Medical Research Council/Overseas Development Administration research programme on Aids in that country. Over a two-year period, 23 per cent of HIV-positive adults died. This was a much higher death rate than among non-HIV-positive adults, and it was concluded that the excess, which resulted in a doubling of the overall death rate, was attributable to HIV. Deaths in the thirteen to forty-four age group totalled fifty-one among those who were HIV-positive, and eighteen among those who were HIV-negative. On the basis of those figures (and because there were far more HIV-negative than HIV-positive villagers), young HIV-positive adults were calculated to have a sixty-fold greater risk of dying than the 'non-infected'.

But dying of what? We had no details, other than that the poor were the most seriously affected. Was it an area rife with TB or leprosy? At the press conference, I asked Mulder how many of the deaths were from Aids. The answer was... five! That was the number who had clinical Aids on their last medical examination, he said. 'Of those who died who were HIV-positive, where we have the information, five of those had Aids.' So on the basis of a study involving five cases of Aids, we were being asked to believe that the African Aids epidemic had now been established scientifically as a reality.

I did not write a report on this press conference for the *Sunday Times*. The newspaper was not interested in knocking down Aunt Sallies. It wanted evidence on what was actually going on; it could not inflict too much scientific disputation on a lay audience. In retrospect, however, I have wondered whether I should have made the effort. It might have helped to preclude subsequent repetitions of claims which have seemed to me to indicate the contorted reasoning which those defending the HIV story have been driven to adopt.

On 14 November, following publication in the *Sunday Times* of our series of reports from Africa on the doubts and uncertainties being expressed there, Mulder's statistics were revived by Steve Connor in the *Independent on Sunday*. According to Connor, this 'latest and most comprehensive study of Aids in Africa' provided 'conclusive evidence that HIV has become a major killer on the continent', contrary to claims that the African epidemic was a myth. The research provided an unambiguous link between HIV and death. It also clearly demonstrated that HIV was transmitted between the sexes. 'Both findings contradict a long-running campaign by the *Sunday Times* newspaper, which has been trying to prove that HIV is not lethal and heterosexual Aids largely a myth.'

Connor, whose five-column story was headlined 'HIV is Africa's big killer — the latest study refutes the claim that the Aids epidemic is a myth', did not mention that only five Aids cases had been identified. Instead, he picked from the study data the horrific-sounding statistic that 'young adults with HIV were eighty-seven times more likely to die prematurely than their uninfected contemporaries'. This referred to the thirteen to twenty-four age group, among whom fourteen people died who tested HIV-positive, and only three out of a much larger group who tested HIV- negative, producing a relative mortality ratio of eighty-seven. I suspect that few people reading of an eighty-seven-fold increase in risk would suspect that such a statistic was based on fourteen deaths. But regardless of such statistical shenanigans, one only has to postulate that a few of those deaths were from TB or leprosy, which as we have seen produce antigens that can trigger HIV-positivity, and the bottom falls out of the whole argument.

Connor quoted Professor Richard Feachem, the school's dean, as protesting that there was 'complete zero' mention of the study in subsequent articles. 'The failure of the *Sunday Times* to make any reference to this briefing, or to make any use of the new and extensive information provided, is a flagrant example of the selective nature of its reporting,' he said. 'The *Sunday Times* repeatedly presents at length the opinions of a tiny fringe group, while failing to provide their readers with a full, balanced account.' Connor's report continued:

> Asked why he had not published the research, Mr Hodgkinson said there were only a 'tiny handful' of Aids cases reported in the study which made it problematical. He also questioned the reliability of the blood tests used. 'HIV-positivity does not necessarily mean infection with HIV,' he said. But Mr Nunn [the statistician on the study], in common with the overwhelming majority of Aids scientists, dismisses suggestions that the two blood tests for HIV antibodies used are inaccurate.
>
> Scientists, doctors and health organisations working in Africa are incensed with what they see as distorted reporting on Aids in an influential newspaper. They claim scientific facts and the opinions of field workers in Africa are being deliberately ignored in favour of a 'fringe minority' who are presented as representing a 'growing body' of scientific opinion.

Connor went on to report further criticisms of the *Sunday Times* by scientists and aid organisations whose letters on the issue had been cut or not used. He concluded with a comment from Dr Spencer Hagard, chief executive of the UK Health Education Authority, who he said was exasperated with the *Sunday Times's* view on HIV and Aids: 'It is quite clear that it's been tremendously difficult to get the *Sunday Times* to carry and properly assess the overwhelmingly accepted view about HIV transmission and the causation of Aids. Its approach is akin to believing in medieval alchemy.'

Aids is a very emotional subject, and I am sure that Connor was doing what he believed to be right. Perhaps he felt the *Sunday Times,* was pursuing the issue in the way it did for ideological reasons, or for purposes of sensationalism. I cannot help feeling, however, that if that is really how he saw the issue, he had never done me the justice of reading the articles I was writing with an open mind. I had not been 'trying to prove' anything. After reporting Aids conventionally for many years, I had come across facts and arguments that gradually gave me a different perspective, and I was doing my best to report in a way that was true to that different view. At least *Sunday Times* readers had been given a chance to learn of both points of view, the conventional and the 'dissident', which was more than could be said for readers of most other newspapers.

I feel it is dangerous for a science correspondent repeatedly to write in such a way as to imply that disagreement with 'overwhelmingly accepted views' is irresponsible. Connor's dismissal of the case against the HIV test, without any examination of the *Bio/Technology* critique or other arguments, on the basis that 'the overwhelming majority of Aids scientists' said the test was sound showed a faith in authority that betrayed the name of his newspaper.

I wrote to the *Independent on Sunday* to point out that the study had only identified five Aids deaths, that the HIV test had not been properly validated, and that although widespread testing by researchers in Tanzania had confirmed the link between HIV-positivity and risk of illness, most of the HIV-positive patients thrived when they were treated for their various infections. That produced the following letter from Dr Alan Stone, head of the Aids secretariat at the Medical Research Council in London:

> Neville Hodgkinson's letter ('HIV is not a death sentence', 21 November) grossly misrepresented the recent findings of a study in Uganda supported jointly by the Medical Research Council and the Overseas Development Administration.
>
> The letter failed to point out – even though this was highlighted at the London press conference – that within the adult population aged thirteen to forty-four the annual risk of death in HIV-positive people was sixty times the risk in HIV-negatives.

> The letter states that only five out of sixty-four deaths in HIV-positive people were diagnosed as Aids-related, implying that the remaining fifty-nine died from other causes. In fact, at the time of the medical assessments, in addition to the five cases of clinical Aids, thirty-one others had one or more major disease symptoms; twenty-eight had no major symptoms. Nevertheless, all, including those who had been asymptomatic, died within twelve months of examination.
>
> Mr Hodgkinson's assertion that the HIV test used by the study team has not been properly validated is simply untrue. The team participates in a World Health Organization international quality control network and the accuracy of their HIV test is close to 100 per cent.
>
> Finally, I was astonished by Mr Hodgkinson's implication that the team in Uganda do not treat HIV-positive patients. Both HIV-positive and HIV-negative study participants regularly attend the team's clinics and those who are ill receive appropriate medical treatment.

I was beginning to feel as if I was caught up in some Orwellian nightmare. How could Stone accuse me of gross misrepresentation for not repeating the figures in Connor's article to which my own letter had been responding? He had highlighted the huge excess ratio of deaths associated with HIV-positivity, but had not mentioned that only five had been diagnosed as from Aids.

Stone's point about there being 'one or more major symptoms' in thirty-one of the deaths, implying that these almost qualified as Aids, was also shockingly misleading. Because of the cost of HIV testing, the WHO has drawn up a 'clinical case definition' of Aids for use in Africa. The guidelines state that 'Aids in an adult is defined by the existence of at least two major signs associated with at least one minor sign in the absence of known causes of immunosuppression such as cancer or severe malnutrition or other recognised aetiologies'. The major signs listed are weight loss of more than 10 per cent, chronic diarrhoea lasting more than a month, and prolonged fever (intermittent or constant) lasting more than a month. The minor signs are persistent cough, generalised dermatitis, recurrent herpes, Candida infection, chronic and progressive herpes and swollen lymph glands.

It is obvious that those 'major signs' of weight loss, diarrhoea and fever could have a multiplicity of causes in Africa, and the clinical case definition has been criticised for exactly that reason by some scientists. TB in particular could be misinterpreted as Aids, which is probably exactly what has happened all over central Africa. One group of authors, calling for more widespread HIV testing in Africa, stated in the *British Medical Journal*:1 'Many patients with tuberculosis, irrespective of HIV state, have weight loss, fever, and cough, and the WHO clinical case definition for Aids therefore has a low specificity in this population... Unless the results of HIV tests are known many patients with tuberculosis who have no HIV infection might be reported as having Aids.'

Another article in the same issue of the *BMJ*,[2] headed 'What Use is a Clinical Case Definition for Aids in Africa', argued that despite having become widely accepted and used in sub-Saharan Africa, the definition might be so inaccurate as to be unworkable. The author, Dr Charles Gilks, a visiting scientist at the Kenya Medical Research Institute in Nairobi, pointed out that pulmonary TB (TB of the lung, the most common form of the disease) had never been an Aids-defining condition in the US, adding: 'If different ways are used to define a case it is a fundamental epidemiological principle that they must be standardised and identify the same conditions. It is surprising that such an important inconsistency exists between the clinical case definition and the Centers for Disease Control definitions for Aids. In those countries where the incidence of tuberculosis is high and which are using the unmodified clinical case definition for surveillance substantial numbers of people reported as having Aids may in fact not have Aids.'

The American journalist Celia Farber had identified this problem in 'Out of Africa', a brilliant two-part series in *Spin* magazine. It demonstrated how in Uganda, where 60 per cent of the children were stated in the *Lancet* in 1986 to be HIV-infected (the figure was later revised to 5-7 per cent), almost all illness had come to be seen as Aids. Farber had accompanied Harvey Bialy and Joan Shenton on their travels through central Africa.

> 'The symptoms are the same by and large,' said Dr Okot Nwang, a TB specialist working at Old Mulago Hospital in Kampala, Uganda. 'Prolonged fever? The same. Loss of weight, the same; loss of appetite, the same. Blood

count? A little confusing, CD4 count, both low. So what's the difference? Maybe diarrhoea.' From 1985 to 1989, the number of TB patients at Mulago Hospital practically doubled. Most of these were cases of pulmonary TB. It is estimated that there are 4 to 5 million cases of highly infectious TB per year world-wide. Annually, 3 million people die of the disease. According to a study by Nwang, pulmonary TB is most common in the age group of fifteen- to forty-four-year-olds, who comprise 70 to 80 per cent of all cases. In light of this, it seems odd that so many doctors make the point that Aids in Africa is 'new' because it is a disease that is killing young people. TB is also killing young people. The ratio of male to female cases with TB is also similar to that of slim [Aids], two males to one female. How much of what is called Aids in Africa is really TB?

We see here again what a mental tangle the HIV story had created. Tuberculosis on its own was sometimes tuberculosis, or, if it produced symptoms judged to meet the clinical definition of Aids, it was Aids. Tuberculosis plus a positive HIV test result was Aids in Africa, but not in America. And as the Zaire paper has warned, tuberculosis triggers the production of antigens which can cause a person to test HIV-positive.

Stone's assertion that the accuracy of the test used by the Uganda team was close to 100 per cent might have had some credibility if the MRC or London School of Hygiene had responded to the *Bio/Technology* indictment of the Elisa and western blot tests, both used in the project (the testing procedure was two different Elisas, followed by western blot in doubtful cases). They had not done so, even though the school had more than forty Aids-related projects in progress, the majority of them taking place in Africa.

Finally, I wondered what kind of treatment it was that was allowing these African people to die, on average, within six months of examination, when the Krynens were finding that most of their HIV-positive patients responded well to treatment for the specific conditions with which they presented. Were the Uganda researchers leaving diseases such as TB and leprosy untreated, because of mistaking them for 'HIV disease'? Were they giving them nutritional and social support, as the Krynens had done? We had no information. And what proportion of these poor people were being told they were HIV-positive? Some certainly were; a counselling service had been made available for those who wished to be informed. We had been told that few of those tested took up this option, but did others get to know informally? I knew that in the African context, where western doctors were like gods, the diagnosis alone could be even more lethal than in Europe and America.

A problem with divergence of goals between African and western researchers had been identified in the *Lancet*[3] in 1990. Two African doctors from Makerere University Medical School in Kampala wrote to complain that although perhaps from good intentions, such as a desire to understand HIV and to find novel treatments as soon as possible, 'several western-financed studies have not included a service commitment to the local population, and there is a tendency to address problems more relevant to western populations rather than those felt most appropriate by local workers'.

Farber had also picked up on this tendency in her report:

> We were the only car on the road. Joan and I, seated in the back, stared out the car windows, silenced by the sight. It was as if the whole place had been shredded – a chaos of dust and debris, rotting wood shacks, garbage, people in rags, children in rags. The poverty in Uganda was crushing, total, and unrelenting. As we drove deeper and deeper into the Rakai district, the 'Aids epicentre of the world', all this talk of HIV and T-cells and safer sex started to seem a little absurd. We got out of the car and surveyed what looked like a swamp, with a pipe emerging from it. This was, it turned out, the surrounding villages' water supply. It was also where the sewage was deposited. People looked listless, malnourished. Many of the children had swollen bellies, the telltale sign of malnutrition.
>
> 'Don't ask them what they eat,' advised one doctor we spoke to, 'ask them how *often* they eat.'
>
> The nearest hospital was miles away. There were no cars; the only means of transportation were donkeys and the occasional bicycle. The Ugandan government sets and enforces fees for medication, which most people can't afford. It became clear to us that most people living in the Rakai district had no access to health care whatsoever. Malnutrition, filthy water, diseases left untreated – and the WHO had come in with 'Aids educational programmes', instructing people how to use condoms?

They went back to the main road and drove on to another village. Farber had asked a Ugandan radio journalist, Samuel Mulondo, to come with her to interpret, although some of the villagers spoke English quite well. She introduced herself and started asking about Aids, called slim disease in Africa because it is characterised primarily by extreme wasting.

> 'Terrible,' said one of them. 'I have had two brothers and one sister die of Aids already.'
>
> 'I'm sorry,' I said. 'What did they die of?'
>
> 'Slim. Aids.'
>
> 'I mean what was the cause of death?'
>
> 'Ahh. Well, my brother, for instance, he had malaria and we couldn't afford to get him treatment, so he died.'
>
> 'So he died of untreated malaria,' I offered.
>
> 'Yes, malaria.'
>
> 'Why did you say he died of Aids?' I asked.
>
> He shrugged. 'Slim is a formula for everything,' he said. 'When somebody dies, we call it slim.'

The Mulder team's study was featured as part of a five-page article, 'HIV: Beyond Reasonable Doubt', published by the *New Scientist* in January 1994 as a response to the *Sunday Times* articles. The authors were Dr Angus Nicoll, consultant epidemiologist with Britain's Public Health Laboratory Service, and Phyllida Brown. Again, the 'sixty times more likely to die' figure was quoted, without reference to the numbers of deaths involved. Nor was there any mention of the fact that only five Aids cases were diagnosed. Instead, it was stated that 'nearly half the community's adult deaths were attributable to Aids, even though only 5 per cent of living adults were infected with HIV'. This equivalence in the minds of the authors between HIV-positivity and Aids, no matter what a person dies of, provided a clear example of the muddle that had terrorised Africa, and which is still confounding thinking on Aids internationally.

Unfortunately, the whole issue flared up yet again when the Uganda study was published in the *Lancet* the following April. This time, it was at least acknowledged that the rapid progression of illness and high death rate might have had something to do with lack of medical care, and an accompanying commentary from Dr Timothy Dondero and Dr James Curran of the US Centers for Disease Control also emphasised that 'more information is needed to clarify how many of the excess deaths could have been delayed through optimum medical prevention and therapy of such HIV-associated illnesses as tuberculosis, other pneumonias, and diarrhoeal disease'. Notice that tendentious use of the word 'delayed', however. Dondero and Curran concluded that the study 'squelches the mischievous claim of some that HIV on that continent and the Aids that results from it are unimportant. The overwhelming data on the impact of HIV in Africa should now reinforce the conscience for a world-wide prevention effort'. The *Lancet* put out a press release including this quotation, and referring to 'a few maverick researchers and journalists' who took the minority view that HIV does not cause death or even Aids in Africa.

The story was taken up in the UK, and around the world. Chris Mihill, the *Guardian's* medical correspondent, wrote: 'The study is being hailed as final refutation of claims that HIV does not cause Aids, and that Aids has not increased death rates in Africa. A series of articles in the *Sunday Times* – dismissed by reputable researchers – helped to foster the belief among some politicians and members of the public that Aids is a trivial disease and that warnings against it are merely hype.' In the *New Statesman & Society*, diarist Sean French awaited 'a grovelling apology on Aids' from the *Sunday Times*. Nowhere was it mentioned that the number of Aids cases identified in this earth-shattering study, now seen as the best-ever evidence that HIV really was behind an epidemic of Aids in Africa, was *five*.

Journalists Pulled into Propaganda War

It felt strange that some of the fiercest attacks on our efforts came from fellow journalists. Britain's Health Education Authority (HEA) even sought to encourage this trend. In November 1993 it created the first 'Aids journalism' awards as a direct response to the row. Winners would be those whose coverage of the issue was least like that of the *Sunday Times*, as Dr Jacky Chambers, HEA deputy chief executive, made clear in a letter to the editor, responding to an acerbic comment about the launch of the awards by *ST* columnist Jonathan

Miller. Our 'wilful misrepresentation' of Aids in Africa, Chambers wrote, did no credit to a once respectable Sunday newspaper. It was 'precisely such articles as these which have prompted the Health Education Authority to create its new awards for excellence in HIV, Aids and sexual health journalism'.

The HEA had teamed up with the National Union of Journalists to produce an HIV and Aids reporting guide. This contained some useful guidance to help protect HIV-positive people against hurtful reporting, but was itself fundamentally prejudiced – and, ultimately, hurtful – in its complete acceptance of the official view on several contentious issues. These included heterosexual spread – 'the World Health Organization estimates that 80-90 per cent of people with HIV have contracted the virus as a result of heterosexual intercourse'; the deadly role of the virus – 'almost all people with HIV will eventually develop Aids'; and AZT as 'the most widely available treatment for HIV-related illness'. 'Safer sex' guidance was also included, and injecting drug users were advised that they 'should always use their own needles and syringes, but if they do share, can lessen the risk of infection by cleaning equipment with bleach after each use'. There was no mention of the immune-suppressing effects of the drugs themselves. Journalists were advised always to check anecdotal 'evidence' or 'expert' views with an official body, 'such as the Department of Health or the Health Education Authority'.

What was the NUJ doing, putting its name to such a document? Phillip Johnson, Jefferson E. Peyser professor of law at the University of California at Berkeley, has pondered on the phenomenon of 'the uncharacteristic reluctance of journalists to challenge official claims about Aids'. He feels it has been motivated by a genuine desire to save lives, 'but it is nonetheless unprofessional. The job of journalists is to tell the public the truth, not what government officials think the public ought to believe. In any event, an unquestioned official story may itself be a danger to life and health. A diagnosis of HIV positivity ruins lives, by destroying marriages, by making people unemployable, and by leading to the use of harmful and ineffective drugs such as AZT'.

I remembered the criticism encountered by Meditel and Channel 4 after their Aids and Africa programme. Angus Nicoll complained in the *British Medical Journal* that the authorities in Uganda were not given the chance to review the script, prompting a response from Channel 4 spokeswoman Francesca O'Brien: 'Would he not be appalled if he learnt that politicians in this country were given the opportunity to vet scripts, or indeed his own articles, before publication?'

Governments everywhere have their own agendas, and if journalists become identified with those agendas the truth is liable to suffer. Farber had described in *Spin* the obstacles the team had met in obtaining government permission to make their own investigations in Uganda, obstacles which were overcome when she said she wanted to tell her young American readers what a terrible toll Aids was taking. She gave an idea of why officials were uneasy about letting journalists loose: Aids generated far more money in the third world from western organisations than any other infectious disease. Foreign funding for Aids totalled $6 million in Uganda in a single year, while the country could afford to spend only $57,000 on malaria prevention. When doctors from some African countries were sent to Aids conferences around the world, their allowances could equal what they earned in a whole year at home. Added to that, 'blame falls squarely at the feet of the Aids patient, while the socioeconomic setting is ignored – a scenario that is unsettlingly convenient for the establishment'. The poverty-stricken conditions of life in a country such as Uganda, 'subject to two decades of turmoil, war, decay, and the unparalleled dictatorship and wreckage of General Idi Amin', were discounted as a health factor, and momentum given 'to the politically correct, simplistic and unproven party line that Aids is going to get everyone, and that sex is the primary cause'.

Were journalists like Farber, Shenton and myself indeed mavericks, out on a limb on this issue not because the rest of the world had been misled by bad science, as we thought, but because we ourselves were, quite simply, wrong? One hoped all along that that was not the case, but the possibility had to be kept in mind as the attacks continued. It was therefore encouraging to find the occasional authoritative medical voice raised in support of a reappraisal of what was happening in Africa.

Dr Felix Konotey-Ahulu, a highly qualified and experienced physician and medical researcher, born in Ghana and now based at the Cromwell Hospital in London, says: 'Today, because of Aids, it seems that Africans are not allowed to die from these conditions [pre-Aids diseases] any longer. If tens of thousands are dying from Aids (and Africans do not cremate their dead) where are the graves?' He says the question uppermost in the minds of intelligent Africans and Europeans in that continent is: 'Why do the world's media appear to have conspired with some scientists to become so gratuitously extravagant with the untruth?'

In 1992 Konotey-Ahulu wrote in the *International Pharmacy Journal* of the fruits of his own researches into Aids in sub-Saharan Africa. Beginning with an investigation lasting several weeks in 1987, he had visited the continent at least once a year since to review the Aids situation. His inquiries took him to more than twenty-six towns and cities in sixteen African countries.

He believed Aids existed, as a syndrome similar to what was first described among gay men in the US, but that it was often related to anal intercourse and particularly to the international sex industry that operates in several African countries. He learned from prostitutes that in their profession they recognised only two kinds of sexual intercourse, 'normal' and 'abnormal', and they charged more for the latter, which they defined as 'anything other than penovaginal'. The girls disputed a statement by Aids researchers in Nairobi in 1986 that 'these prostitutes performed only vaginal intercourse, without oral or anal sex'. According to Konotey-Ahulu, they said they had no choice in the matter. The mode of sex was not offered, it was 'demanded' by the client, who also often refused to wear a condom. But because anal intercourse was a taboo of enormous proportions in traditional African mores, foreign researchers were unlikely to get honest answers to their questionnaires.

Konotey-Ahulu's investigations led him to the conclusion that 'the best hope of Aids prevention and curtailment in Africa lies less with condoms and vaccines than with jobs, economic uplift, political stability and sensible education'. For his own Krobo tribe in Ghana, for instance, the aim must be to prevent international prostitution in which girls migrated to neighbouring countries with favourable currency conditions to earn money in the tourist sex industry, sometimes returning home desperately ill. But he added:

> Suppose this kind of education in my tribe succeeds in dampening down the exodus for prostitution abroad. 'How,' the tribal chief asks, 'are they going to feed and clothe themselves?' The answer to this question depends, in large measure, on the goodwill of the powerful nations. Africa needs their goodwill not to halve the world cocoa price, as soon as Ghana begins to see the light at the end of a long dark tunnel, and not to pitch the price of copper so low that Zambia is forever indebted. These two

> measures alone will help keep Ghanaian women and Zambian girls off the streets ... A bird's-eye-view of Aids in Africa leads one to the impression that the 600 million people distributed in 2,300 tribes are at the mercy of socioeconomic and sociopolitical factors, not to mention natural disasters and famines, which lift the Aids problem from merely being a question of promiscuity, blood transfusion and unsterilised needles. For many women, international prostitution for foreign exchange is a question of survival, and tackling Aids adequately means finding practical ways to help them.

In a 1989 book about his experiences, *What is Aids?* [4] Konotey-Ahulu quoted one tribal chief as saying to him:

> But *Dorkitah,* we have heard a lot on the radio about promiscuity, robbah (condoms), promiscuity, robbah. Now, as everybody knows, promiscuity has not yet caused Aids in Kroboland. So far all the Aids patients we have had have come from Ivory Coast where they went into prostitution to bring home some money. Our women folk have not once been urged by radio and television not to send their daughters to Abidjan any more. All we hear is robbah, robbah, robbah! The women themselves know that they should stop going in for prostitution, but then income will stop flowing. There are no jobs. It is hard...

Africa needs powerful friends with a conscience, Konotey-Ahulu says. My own impression is that rather than allow cocoa and copper prices to rise, those friends prefer to salve their consciences with condom campaigns, HIV test kits and experimental vaccines of such doubtful value that no one wants to try them elsewhere.*

* A review of the ethics of Aids studies in Africa by Rachel Nowak for *Science* (8 September 1995, pp. 1332-5) found that most researchers 'lamented privately that despite a decade of experience in the field, HIV-related studies frequently violate internationally accepted norms'. Scientifically, however, sub-Saharan Africa was one of the best locales to stage large-scale tests of Aids vaccines and drugs, study the interaction between other infections and HIV, and evaluate ways to block transmission of HIV between mothers and infants. 'Why? Because the sheer density of HIV infection turbo-charges clinical trials, amplifying the statistical power of the results and providing massive savings in time and money.'

Another doctor who has made a genuine attempt to see for himself what is happening with regard to Aids in Africa is Riccardo Leschot, an Aids physician from Buenos Aires, Argentina. I met him at the 'alternative' Aids conference in Amsterdam in 1992, when he had just completed a four-week investigation in Uganda. 'I returned with more questions than answers,' he said, 'but my impression was that malnutrition, and repeated infection with malarial parasites, could be more important factors than generally considered in Africa in the context of Aids. Malaria depletes the same subset of lymphocytes, and in people who have malaria perhaps eighty times in a year it can't be ignored as a factor.' He believed repeated exposure to syphilis was also a prominent factor, in combination with other infectious assaults on the immune system arising from appalling living conditions: 'There was one thing that frankly disgusted me. In one of the "Aids capitals", a town called Kyotera in the Rakai district, a town criss-crossed by the white Toyotas characteristic of North American and European Aids researchers, there had been so many cases of Aids – or so-called Aids – involving hepatitis and meningitis that I couldn't resist asking what water they were drinking. My informer pointed at the gutter on the main street, and said, "Follow the gutter." I did – it took me to an open, swampy pool. It wasn't surprising so many were dying from hepatitis. My colleagues, who had tremendous funding for studying HIV, hadn't found time to sink a well to provide clean water. They had been there for up to four years.'

Leschot had been surprised at how little Aids he saw, in the form of the syndrome as known in Europe and the Americas, though in some villages there was an enormous burden of illness. 'I was expecting to see hospitals full of Aids patients,' he said. 'I had an uncomfortable feeling when I spoke to many of the African and European virologists or physicians that they didn't like my questions. I think they were more cautious than frank. My investigation was a bit uncomfortable occasionally. The Ugandans are friendly, wonderful people, but with undertones of an absolutely terrifying and tragic recent history – it is not an open society. The Europeans didn't convince me; I really felt they were "HIV establishment", though I was very pleased to learn that one of them had in mind to study the possibility that malaria could be one of the causes of the depressed immunity seen in patients with Aids, along with extreme malnutrition.

'I believe Aids investigators ought to have better training in human sexuality. Most are ignorant of this chapter of medicine. I learned that many men in Uganda practise dry sex, in fact they despise women with genital lubrication. There is no erotic participation on the part of the women. The men feel this enables them to assert their machismo. It allows for a violent form of intercourse, which also brings frequent rupture of the vaginal mucosa and damage to the glans of the penis. This may be a co-factor or causal factor in a very high incidence of penile carcinoma in Uganda. Sexually transmitted diseases of all kinds are multiplied in this type of intercourse, and there is an extraordinarily high incidence among Ugandans generally of seropositivity for syphilis.

'The schism between HIV investigators and patients was extraordinary. I did meet some wonderful European physicians, but I was surprised that European virologists who had lived in Uganda for three years or more had not considered it worthwhile learning the language of the tribe they were working with, as though that were irrelevant to the practice of medicine.

'I didn't discount, or accept, HIV as a cause of Aids. It may play a part. I honestly did not know. I was saddened by the experience. I thought I would come back with a clear answer, but instead I felt thrown from one hypothesis to another from day to day. At one point, I would feel this was a rabid viral epidemic; twenty-four hours later, in the next town, I would have a completely opposite impression.

'Looking back, I feel I am starting to understand the experience. I think we have been a bit naive about the triumph of medicine over infectious diseases; that we have swept them under the carpet, rendered them invisible, but that there may be an important immunological disturbance in the bodies of people who have sexually transmitted diseases, malaria, or other infections, on many occasions.'

Leschot was surprised on his return to Argentina to see in the latest WHO returns a figure for Aids cases in Uganda that was 25 per cent higher than the highest reliable estimate he had been given during his stay. Other doctors have also commented on this phenomenon: after Angus Nicoll criticised Joan Shenton's film on Aids in Africa, Dr Mark Mattah, of the Midland Centre for Neurosurgery and Neurology, came to its defence in the *British Medical Journal*, protesting that Nicoll had completely ignored recent concern over the unreliability of predictions about the spread of Aids arising mainly from faulty data and methodology. 'Most of us who have practised in Africa are surprised at discrepancies between the magnitude of the problem actually encountered and the large figures often quoted.'

It is now exactly two years since I arrived at the Krynens' bungalow, which adjoined and partly served as the Partage Tanzanie headquarters, on a hillside outside the town of Bukoba above Lake Victoria. It was seven o'clock in the morning, and there had been no prior contact – I had no phone or fax numbers, nor even much of an address, but a taxi driver in the town had known where to take me. It was too early for a stranger to disturb the household, so I sat outside for ninety minutes, in the cool of the morning, gazing at the lake in the distance far below and wondering what the day held in store. I wanted to find Philippe because I had heard he had begun to question the HIV/Aids hypothesis, but I had no idea the couple had played such a central part in 'making' Aids in Africa, as Philippe put it, nor that they would gradually open their hearts about their radical change in perspective. As they did so, I realised I was witnessing a remarkable story unfolding.

What has happened since, and how does the account they gave me stand up today?

Philippe took in his stride the news that the European Community's Aids task force was threatening to cancel a long-standing promise of funding. The grant had been talked about since 1989, but he had managed without it for three years and was confident he could continue to do so. As the storm of criticism raged around me in London, it was encouraging to receive a fax from him on 5 October that was full of optimism:

> After reading the article, forwarded to us by the Aids Task Force (EEC Brussels) and learning that it would make our programme be cut off from EEC support, I am very keen to tell you my *total satisfaction.* You have reported very exactly what we have told you and you have managed to channel to the reader the feelings that are ours. It is a great, honest, professional job and too rarely witnessed in the media not to be applauded loud!

> A myth is starting to die... you are doing more to resuscitate hope than any of our visitors has ever done in Kagera. Dear Neville, seven thousand times 'merci de tout coeur'.
>
> Our 7,000 kids and Jojo and Evelyne - Philippe

After I had telephoned him to update myself on events, he faxed back several papers demonstrating his previous close association with the task force, including correspondence with Lieve Fransen in September 1992 concerning Partage's HIV-testing programme. In this exchange of letters, he had stressed that there was now a demand from villagers throughout the region for such testing, after a preliminary survey had produced good news for most of them; to their enormous relief, far fewer were testing positive than in previous documented screenings in the region. With these papers came a further letter of encouragement:

> After your long call and all the information you fed me back, I have the feeling that the 'Aids makers' are firing back violently... and that they over-react because they are afraid. The Truth is making its way steadily but surely.
>
> This time, somebody has come to the heart of African Aids. Neville, you have come to the heart of it, not only in the field but also in the group I call the African Aids makers. I am one of them. As you have reported already in your last article, I have contributed to create Aids in Africa. I have been at the same time victim of a fashion and exploited by epidemic makers: since 1989, on my programme, a film has been made, which has been distributed to all the African countries as a proof of the 'plague' to come, articles and pamphlets have been written, newsmen and photographers have been fed with stories and NACPs [national Aids control programmes] with figures.
>
> I have received promises of a lot of money (3 million French francs) since 1989, since the very beginning, by people who have seen me as their field promoter! I have been invited to international conferences and given round tables to chair.
>
> If I had accepted the offers, I would be today an EEC consultant at ten thousand dollars a month plus per diem... Bad luck: I love my children, and came across the truth about the disease by accident.

> My friends of yesterday are the ones who try to disqualify me today. Would it be wrong to use Aids money to prove there is no Aids in Africa? Would it be wrong, if this money was given to fight Aids?
>
> No.
>
> But this money was never intended to fight Aids. It has been made available to *create Aids.* That's the point. That's why 'The Empire Fires Back' today. You have thrown a stone in its private garden, Neville, by questioning Kagera orphans. Fortunately for us, and the rest of the world, the Aids empire is a small family... *Magic thinking* is their power. But not facts! Against the truth of facts they will go back one after the other to the shadows where they come from...
>
> AIDS WILL BE KNOWN AS THE MOST TRAGIC JOKE OF THE HUMAN HISTORY. IT WILL HAVE HAPPENED AT THE END OF OUR TWENTIETH CENTURY, AT A TIME WHEN THE TRUTH WAS CONFISCATED TO HUMANS BY A CHURCH CALLED THE WHO.
>
> Well... enough dreaming.

On 7 October, to Philippe's delight, the Tanzanian magazine *Heko* reprinted the story of the Krynens' change of heart in Swahili. At the end of the month, government officials and non-governmental organisations in Tanzania reacted by saying that the Krynens' statements were 'almost criminal'. However, on 26 November a group of NGOs working in the Kagera region met in Bukoba, under the chairmanship of the regional medical officer, to listen to Philippe Krynen himself. A statement issued after the meeting, although critical of him, showed an openness to new ideas about Aids that indicated more genuineness of purpose among them than Philippe, in his disillusionment, had previously acknowledged:

> After listening to Mr Philippe Krynen himself it was confirmed that magazine and newspaper publications in the *Sunday Times* and the *Heko* respectively were a result of interviews with Mr Krynen himself and whose content was a true reflection of the interviews. Mr Krynen however confessed that the publication, especially the one in the *Sunday Times,* came out too soon before he had time to communicate the information through the normal channels to the National Aids Control Programme.

> We agree with Partage that the HIV theory may not be sufficient in the causation of Aids as many manifestations of both HIV infection and Aids were still unclear to scientists. So there is need for scientists to look into alternative explanation and/or other factors associated with development of Aids in children and young adults.
>
> All NGOs in Kagera are concerned that Mr Krynen has been publicising to the World that there is no Aids in Kagera, that HIV is not sexually transmitted and that Aids is not infectious. We feel his theories need a base and have to have sufficient scientific backup before being consumed by the general public. Mr Krynen is therefore asked to refrain from this dangerous practice which might confuse the public and retard any progress made so far in efforts to control HIV transmission.
>
> We recommend that Mr Krynen should leave this kind of debate to scientists to carefully work out factors or alternative explanations for the cause of Aids which can be beneficial in furthering the control of HIV transmission. Until then current Aids intervention programmes should continue with appropriate evaluation and all useful interventions should be encouraged and promoted. If contrary, scientific evidence becomes available, then appropriate steps and channels should be used to propagate such information to the public.

Although I felt from my close acquaintance with the issue that the Krynens were behaving more as scientists than most of the rest of the Aids establishment put together, the NGOs were not to know that. In the circumstances, their statement seemed to me to be dignified and restrained.

The Krynens were invited to recant, and condemn the *Sunday Times,* by Dr Angus Nicoll, the British epidemiologist who had taken it upon himself to attack journalistic efforts questioning the African Aids story. He inquired through Partage's headquarters in France:

> Further to my communication of December 20th I have been sent the attached letter and press release by Father D'Agostino in Kenya. As you will read they are complaining of some misrepresentation by the *Sunday Times* and are asking that the newspaper convey Dr D'Agostino's views. I also attach a copy of the original article.

> I know that the newspaper never reported this point of view though they have continued to cover the issue. After reading these letters I wondered whether Mr and Mrs Krynen had been fully happy with their coverage and had had any experience like Dr D'Agostino in trying to make a correction?

Philippe Krynen told me that he received the same letter again in January 1994. The answer suggested by such an amazing approach, he said – though he did not actually send it – was 'questions put by the police are only answered in the presence of our lawyer'.

Tanzanian scientists showed commendable tolerance. The National Institute for Medical Research invited Philippe Krynen to attend an annual scientific conference in Arusha in February 1994. Although his subject, 'Rethinking Aids: Africa's Answer to Western-Controlled Health Programmes', was refused clearance for oral delivery at the last moment, he was allowed to make a poster presentation that attracted much interest.

In it, he stated the central problems with the HIV hypothesis, and declared that while predictions of catastrophe had been falsified in America and Europe they were still being maintained in Africa. He warned that as a result of Aids being re-labelled 'HIV disease', despite a non-specific, non-standardised antibody test, millions of Africans were being made eligible for experimental vaccines and medicines. He also claimed that Aids control programmes were diverting human and financial resources away from more important public health needs, and triggering discrimination, discouragement and panic. He concluded: 'Instead of repeating "We are still waiting for a cure, for a vaccine", couldn't we say "We are still waiting to discover what causes Aids"? ... Rethinking Aids may be enough, in itself, to discover that there is no Aids in Africa – only victims.'

Krynen wrote to the conference chairman, Professor W. L. Kilama, to thank him for the opportunity to participate. The move, he said, 'shows how open-minded Tanzanian research can be and justifies my personal belief that we are here most able, among African nations, to rethink the present drama'. He sent copies of both the letter and his poster display to the Prime Minister, Dr John Malecela, who had opened the conference, and to the Minister of Health. He also printed 1,000 booklets of articles from Peter Duesberg, Celia

Farber and myself, translated into Swahili for distribution in Dar es Salaam and elsewhere.

The EC Aids task force, however, wanted Philippe silenced once and for all. As well as postponing 'until further notice' the support that had been promised, the EC sent a consultant, Maria Paalman, on an 'evaluation mission' for the Partage orphan project, known locally as the Victoria Programme. Working through the Ministry of Health, her visit to Kagera took place between 5-12 April 1994. According to Philippe, during the visit the inquiry team were heard by many witnesses as saying 'we come to close this programme' and 'Philippe is given forty-eight hours' notice to leave the country'.

On 28 April, he was served by the regional immigration officer with a notice that he was now a prohibited immigrant, and ordered to leave Tanzania within fourteen days. Defiant to the last, on the same day he sent the following 'personal statement' to the regional authorities:

I came here to defend children,
not to feed politics and politicians.
What I say and do is what I believe is best
for the future of Tanzania and Africa.
My action and my message can only be understood
by people who have concern in children.
As long as those are the policy makers
I shall be fighting for a programme called

VICTORIA

Miraculously, on 4 May he received notice from the immigration officer that the prohibition order had been suspended indefinitely, and that he was therefore allowed to go on with his normal duties in Kagera. He was also sent a message in Swahili, forwarded to him by Mr A. M. Omari, the regional development director, with a covering letter as follows:

> The message above is from the Prime Minister and First Vice President himself, Hon. J. S. Malecela, MP, declaring that the *ORDER* given to you to

> leave the country as soon as possible has been suspended for the time being pending other directives from himself. He has further directed that you continue with your normal activities as usual without hesitation.

Despite years of hardship that accompanied drastic economic change during the 1980s, Tanzania has retained an infrastructure of self-determining and public-spirited political and administrative leadership. I think it was this, along with Philippe's courage and determination, that brought about such a dramatic reversal for those who felt most threatened by his revelations.

Right in the midst of this battle, however, the Krynens suffered a great loss. On 27 March, Joseph, their adopted child, died of pneumocystic pneumonia. He was six years old and had lived for five years after his original Aids diagnosis. A card carrying a wonderful picture of him, with his arms round Evelyne's neck, stated: 'He was unique, marvellous, unforgettable. He is resting now in our country, France, and we come back to his place, Tanzania, where he entrusted us with so many little ones who resemble him.'

Was it Aids? It would be called so almost anywhere else in the world. Two other children being cared for in a 'transit home' attached to the project had also died of immune system failure. I spoke to Philippe on 29 April – the day after he had been served the prohibited immigrant notice. He sounded deeply distressed, and was reappraising his position. He would not let go of his demand for a rethink of what was going on, however.

> We still don't believe HIV is the cause. Joseph was the hope we could do something with kids with Aids. Now my position will be different when it comes to speak about the possibility for children to survive, once they have Aids. It doesn't change my view about the relationship between HIV and Aids. It changes my view about the fact that once you have Aids, what we did is not effective. My fight is to find out the cause.
>
> My position is that HIV is a marker for immune suppression. It is not the cause of it. Not all HIV-positive people react the same way. Some may have immune suppression for a while, and without any treatment, recover. Others, with a background of malnutrition and very low vital strength, and on top of that a toxic exposure, fall over the point of no return with immune suppression.

The truth is always good to be said. I don't think it was a mistake. I deny 'Aids orphans', because the definition has to be rethought. Aids should be renamed. As long as you don't rename it, rethink what it is, you will never find a cure. It is misleading the people, misguiding the government. As long as we have stocks of 'Aids tests', as long as we have to make trials with a vaccine for HIV, we need Aids in Africa. Aids has become a political and commercial issue.

A few days later, I received the following letter from Philippe:

I never knew how long Joseph would survive, but I always believed his life, day after day, was a gift of Providence.

The gift had an end.

I don't know its meaning. I don't know why it ended. I don't know why life and suffering are entwined together.

I am left with a certainty in my bleeding sorrow: the only two forces of the universe are death and love. The death of Joseph hurts at the level we loved him: immensely. And the tears of today are nothing but the overflow of a tiny cup, a too tiny cup of six years, that Joseph filled up with immense love.

In a postscript, he wrote that what they learnt from Joseph during his five extra years, 'and from the many others who survived, is what makes me tell you today that Aids is not HIV'.

It is now September 1995. Philippe Krynen is still in Kagera, although Partage Tanzania has had to separate from the parent organisation in France and he is now running it as an independent organisation. That change has meant the loss of about a third of the sponsoring families, but there are still 4,000 children being helped, with a service stretched rather thinner than before. Research work continues, in particular into a possible link between multiple vaccination and subsequent immune depression.

Evelyne has returned to France. 'When Joseph died, she resented this and could not gather enough strength to continue,' Philippe says. He is attempting to avoid further controversy that would embarrass the authorities, but is continuing to emphasise in his organisation's internal publications the need to focus their work on primary health care 'and not speak about Aids as long as we don't know what it is'.

'My position today is not much different from when we met,' he says. 'I admit immune depression is a problem in this region, in young children as well as adults, but it is not a major problem as far as numbers are concerned. The cause of it has still to be found. I don't call it Aids, because the definition of Aids is linked with HIV. I am not going to state that there is no immunodepression, but I still state that there is no Aids. I refuse to apply the terms "Aids orphans" or "Aids epidemic" to the mortality and morbidity of this region. Immunosuppression in this region has to be studied as an end in itself, not related to any virus.'

Krynen is still searching for a toxic agent as the critical factor in precipitating collapse of the immune system, against a backdrop of social and biological deprivation. It is possible, however, that one need look no further than severe malnutrition during foetal development to understand deaths such as Joseph's. In the *Lancet* in 1983, evidence was presented that nutritional deprivation very early in life, and even pre-conceptually, has a big and lasting detrimental effect on the body's subsequent resistance to infection. 'This has been observed in both man and animals,' said the author, Ranjit Kumar Chandra, of the department of paediatrics, Memorial University of Newfoundland, Canada, and the department of nutrition and food science, Massachusetts Institute of Technology. Babies born very small because of being premature, but whose size is appropriate for their period of gestation, develop normal immune defences within three to four months of birth; but small-for-gestation low-birthweight babies have depressed T-cell numbers and function that may persist for months or years.

Chandra's own work has shown that nutritional deprivation before conception and during gestation in mice and rats impairs T-cell-dependent immune responses of the first and second generation offspring.[5] The deficiencies seem to be mediated by damage to the lymphatic system: the thymus gland, which programmes T-lymphocytes, does not form properly, and areas in the spleen and the lymph nodes that depend on the thymus have depleted function. The *Lancet* paper documented numerous other immune system abnormalities, and their harmful consequences, observed in malnourished adults as well as children. The whole field of nutritional immunology, in which Chandra is a world leader, was activated as a result of observations that the thymus is involuted (shrunken and deformed) in people dying of starvation. The fact that people who die of Aids in Europe and America show similar degeneration of the thymus suggests that this may be a mechanism of immune deficiency common to people who develop Aids for a variety of different reasons. Health workers in underprivileged communities have noted 'the mutually aggravating interaction of malnutrition and infection'. Chandra remarked:

> This is particularly evident in young children in whom nutritional status is a critical determinant of both mortality and morbidity; for example, in children with wasting (defined as weight-for-height less than 80 per cent of standard) the incidence of diarrhoea in one study was more than twice that of non-wasted children. Malnutrition increased the duration of diarrhoea by 33 per cent in underweight Nigerian children (less than 70 per cent of standard weight-for-age), and by 37 per cent in stunted children (less than 90 per cent of standard height-for-age), and by 79 per cent in wasted children.

His paper, which was based on the Hoffman LaRoche award lecture of the Canadian Society for Nutritional Sciences, listed TB, diarrhoea, leprosy, herpes, *pneumocystis carinii* and Candida, among others, as infectious diseases demonstrated to be influenced by nutritional status. As far back as 1974, long before pneumocystic pneumonia became identified in our minds with Aids, research demonstrating that protein-calorie malnutrition is 'a host determinant for *pneumocystis carinii* infection' was published in the *American Journal of Diseases of Childhood.*[6]

There was nothing in the Medical Research Council study of 'HIV' deaths in Uganda villagers telling us of their current nutritional status, let alone of previous nutritional deprivation that might have caused irreversible immune deficiency and consequent vulnerability to the multitude of infections seen in the African context. Since a number of these infections cause cross-reactions with the 'HIV' test, we may have here a complete picture of how the whole sorry story of an African 'HIV/Aids' epidemic came about. Philippe Krynen is almost certainly right: 'Aids' in Africa, as a new, infectious, epidemic condition, is a myth. Warnings that 'Aids now kills more people in Africa than famine', that it 'could wipe out an entire generation in developing countries', and that 'high-risk carrier groups like overseas students' will accelerate its spread in other countries, such as were promulgated in Britain by the Aids educational charity ACET as recently as 1992,[7] are sheer fantasy.

Despite completely undocumented, unresearched claims of an Aids epidemic affecting well-off Africans, the huge weight of evidence points to the immune deficiency that is so often wrongly called 'HIV/Aids' in Africa as being primarily a disease of poverty. As Charles Geshekter, professor of African history at California State University, Chico, has put it, 'It is the political economy of underdevelopment, not sexual intercourse, that is killing Africans... African poverty, not some extraordinary sexual behaviour, is the best predictor of Aids-defining diseases.' In Africa, 'Aids' is a collection of illnesses, some well known, others perhaps yet to be identified as implicated in the syndrome, brought together under an artificial umbrella by their shared tendency to trigger a positive result in what has come to be known as the HIV test. The syndrome is nonetheless deserving of whatever help wealthy nations may find it in their hearts to offer; but to terrify half a continent with a fictional epidemic of a purportedly lethal, new, sexually transmitted microbe has been a disaster, far outweighing any benefit reaching African people from the millions of dollars entering the continent for 'HIV'-related research.*

In December 1993, *New African* magazine ran a cover story, 'Aids: The Epidemic That Never Was', based on the 'hullabaloo' in the medical world over the Krynens' astonishing confession. The article, by Anver Versi, said that the stigma of an Aids epidemic had caused enormous harm to African self-esteem and had battered already fragile economies. On the other hand, the article acknowledged that 'to assume prematurely that Aids does not exist in Africa could be the recipe for an unimaginable catastrophe'. The story brought protests from a number of Aids-related organisations in western countries, in the wake of which the magazine's correspondent in Ghana, Kwabena Sarpong Akosah, interviewed Professor P. A. K. Addy, editor-in-chief of the *African Journal on Sexually Transmitted Diseases*, about the Krynens' claims. Addy, head of clinical microbiology at the University of Science and Technology in Kumasi, Ghana, was first asked if he took their confession seriously:

* Out of more than $1 billion a year devoted by the US National Institutes of Health alone to Aids research, more than $10 million supports clinical studies in Africa.

ADDY: Why not, I am really impressed that the very people who first blew the alarm bells that Africans were dying of Aids in fantastic numbers now say they got it all wrong.

N.A.: Have you been to Uganda, Kenya and Tanzania where the medical world claims is the epicentre of Aids?

ADDY: I have been to Uganda. And I've worked as a WHO personnel at the East African Virus Research Institute. I've known for a long time that Aids is not a crisis in Africa as the world is being made to understand. But in Africa it is very difficult to stick your neck out and say certain things.

N.A.: Why?

ADDY: Some of us get funding for our research projects from some institutions in the West. So it is suicidal for us to stand up and challenge the advanced parts of the world on certain issues.

N.A: Don't you think the Krynens' confession is meant to divert attention from the efforts at fighting Aids in Africa?

ADDY: I won't rule that out. But let me say that the West came out with those frightening statistics on Aids in Africa because it was unaware of certain social and clinical conditions in Africa. The Western medical 'experts' came to Africa with their minds already made up. I call this textbook knowledge. In most of Africa, infectious diseases, particularly parasitic infections, are common. And there are other conditions that can easily compromise or affect one's immune system. Malaria, malnutrition, tuberculosis, leprosy are all conditions which suppress one's immune system. These clinical conditions are what is deceiving the Western experts.

In answer to other questions, Addy said: 'These Europeans and Americans came to Africa with prejudiced minds and so they are seeing what they always wanted to see... The diagnosis itself, merely being told you have Aids, is enough to kill, and is killing people. So we must find ways to address the false positives. The moment you tell somebody you are HIV-positive, the person loses his or her psychological capacity to fight diseases.'

The interview with the Krynens was 'pivotal' for most Aids specialists, according to an article by Colin Meek in the British Medical Association's *News Review of* February 1994. At first, he wrote, they took me for a maverick, mistaking smaller than expected HIV infection rates among heterosexuals as evidence that there was little threat to most people whose lifestyles did not put them at risk. But after 'The Plague That Never Was', they felt our articles were making such an impact that they could no longer go unchallenged. 'The massive spread of HIV in Africa among heterosexuals underpins what they see as the potential threat to all communities and their demands for public safe sex campaigns everywhere. For them, the *Sunday Times* campaign was no longer simply "irritating" or "unbalanced", it became a danger to public health.'

Was that really their concern? Not according to Yolande Agble, a nurse who wrote to the *British Medical Journal* about the controversy (her letter went unacknowledged). Nor did she think there was any genuine concern for Africa. There was a difference of opinion among researchers on all the issues the newspaper had raised, she said, and we were right in bringing this to the notice of the reading public. She wrote:

> Several... doctors working in Africa (which is more than could be said of the critics here, many of whom consider Africa to be one big village, and not a continent of thirty-six countries, with a population of 504.5 million), have echoed these same concerns. The fact that no attempt is made to differentiate between those countries in Africa where Aids may be a problem, and those where it is no more of a problem than in this country, raises doubts and concerns as to the real reason behind this dogmatic attitude. The whole continent is by no means engulfed by an Aids epidemic... Could it be altruism and concern for the people in Africa which is causing some doctors and researchers to behave in an almost hysterical manner (one talked of the paper killing people) on the subject of Aids in Africa? Or is it a desire for scapegoats and guinea pigs?

The Krynens had nothing to gain other than a clear conscience, and a lot to lose, from attempting to lift the 'HIV' curse put upon African people by western scientists, who had unwittingly acted as witch-doctors of the worst kind. My own experience in Africa did not show me anything that was inconsistent with the description and analysis offered by the Krynens, and there was much to support it. I salute them, and others like them in Africa and elsewhere, who have been prepared to risk everything for the sake of fighting a deadly deception*.

* ADDENDUM, November 2022: The charity survived and nearly 30 years on it continues the work of caring for needy orphans, though now with a focus on development through education. 'The Aids issue is totally buried in dusty files, at least for us here in Partage Tanzania,' Philippe says. 'The distributors of antiretroviral drugs are still doing their business in the country but the pandemic tale is dead. As for the Covid tale, it didn't last long. In 2020 a short epidemic of acute respiratory tract infection was taken care of by a cocktail of common antibiotics. The combination of very few tombs per community, and a patent lack of statistics, dismantled the scarecrow. Prevention (masks and soaps) was quickly abandoned and business as usual never interrupted... Tanzania today is seen as a peaceful African jewel.'

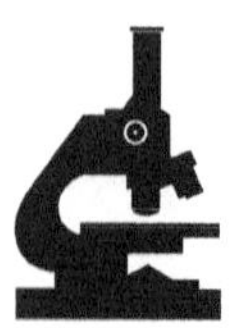

11: CONSTERNATION AT THE COURT OF HIV

The mental blocks afflicting the scientific community in its understanding of Aids have caused some uncharacteristically narrow-minded and sometimes repressive and decidedly unscientific behaviour by leading professional journals. They have behaved like noblemen at the court of HIV, anxious first to ignore, then ridicule, and finally to try to silence the small boy who kept insisting the emperor had no clothes. The strategy worked for several years and the difficult questions being asked by those such as Callen, Sonnabend, Lauritsen, Duesberg, Eleopulos, Farber, Root-Bernstein, Stewart and the Meditel team were never adequately explored, let alone answered.

The British-based journal *Nature* has been particularly aggressive towards dissident viewpoints. I have wondered sometimes if this is because John Maddox, its editor during most of the Aids years, knew in his heart that the HIV theory was deeply flawed. As previously described, he once appeared ready to recognise the implications of experiments showing that animals could readily be made 'HIV-positive' without the presence of 'HIV', but backed away from that line of thought after being strongly criticised for having expressed it in his pages.

Whatever the reason, when driven to respond to the debate, *Nature* regularly invoked the emotive argument that to question HIV was to imperil patients, ignoring the equally imperilling possibility that millions were being falsely terrorised by the HIV story, and inappropriately treated as a result of it.

In April 1988, for example, a news story mentioning Duesberg's 1987 critique stated that his ideas had been largely ignored by scientists, but had gained credibility 'mainly among patient populations with the greatest interest in learning that HIV infection does not lead inevitably to a fatal disease. But many researchers now feel that Duesberg's arguments must be confronted, as the consequences of acting on his advice may be fatal'. In June 1990, a commentary by Robin Weiss and Harold Jaffe declared that Duesberg was offering 'a perilous message'. Again in May 1993, in an editorial explaining why Duesberg was being refused a right of reply to a fresh attack on his views by *Nature,* Maddox stated: 'Duesberg has made his debating technique thoroughly intolerable by advertising his position to the Aids community, thus giving many infected people the belief that HIV infection is not in itself the calamity it is likely to prove.'

Duesberg had been trying to respond to a 'commentary' published in *Nature* on 11 March 1993 purporting to disprove his hypothesis of a causal link between drug use and Aids. A new analysis of data from a long-standing men's health study in San Francisco was said to show that heterosexual men had roughly equivalent drug use to homosexual and bisexual men, and yet HIV-positivity, and Aids, were almost exclusively concentrated in the latter group. The commentary, however, was not a scientific document. As its authors acknowledged, the analysis was conducted in order to test Duesberg's drug-Aids hypothesis; it bore the hallmarks of having been put together specifically to try to silence Duesberg, concluding with the remark that 'the energies of Duesberg and his followers could better be applied to unravelling the enigmatic mechanism of the HIV pathogenesis of Aids'. The authors did not quantify drug use beyond a broad self-assessment by the study participants, and the households sampled were not chosen completely at random, but came from neighbourhoods 'where the Aids epidemic had been most intense before 1984'. Moreover, there was a much higher level of general drug use (including heroin and cocaine) among HIV-positive men than their HIV-negative counterparts; almost 100 per cent of the men who died had used poppers; and a very high proportion of the latter were on AZT, a highly toxic drug which Duesberg insisted could cause 'Aids by prescription'.

These qualifications were not mentioned in a press release, headlined 'Drug use does not cause Aids', issued by *Nature* a week before publication. The release had its desired effect, however. Around the world, the study became quoted as evidence that the drug-Aids hypothesis had been knocked on the head. The *New York Times* ran a story headlined 'Debunking Doubts That HIV Causes Aids', and the *San Francisco Chronicle* declared 'Biologist's

Theory On Aids Attacked – Conventional View On HIV Supported'. The latter received, but did not use, a letter from Richard Strohman, professor emeritus, molecular and cell biology, University of California at Berkeley, pointing out that the article was not a scientific paper that had survived any vigorous review process. 'It was instead part of what is called "scientific correspondence" that gets by with often cursory review by journal editors,' Strohman wrote. 'Second, as a result of lack of thorough review there is no detail given on methods used to collect data. Third, without details on methods we cannot evaluate the data itself, never mind conclusions drawn from that data. Thus, all standards of real science are violated.' What remained was at best a mechanism for developing opinion or debate. 'In the mainstream of science or in a court of law it would be thrown out as hearsay evidence.'

As the behaviour of those who controlled the main channels of scientific communication became increasingly emotional, a few calmer voices from the higher echelons of science began to make themselves heard. One of these, who was later to become a kind of avenging angel on behalf of a sense of reason and even of common decency, was Dr Serge Lang, professor of mathematics at Yale University. In a complaint to the council of the National Academy of Sciences about 'science by press release', he said the press started calling Duesberg to get his comments on the forthcoming drugs article several days before it was made available to him by *Nature*. 'Thus does *Nature* and the authors of the article use the media to manipulate public opinion before their article has been submitted to the scientific scrutiny of other scientists, especially Duesberg who is principally concerned...I wish to warn you here against Maddox's unscientific, irresponsible, and manipulative journalism.'

Correspondence in *Nature* showed that other readers felt uncomfortable about the journal's treatment of Duesberg. D. J. Silvester, of Hammersmith Hospital, London, wrote that to reject an intended publication and then submit its author to the kind of criticism levelled at Duesberg 'smacks of the non-religious Inquisitions of the twentieth century' that had been referred to elsewhere in the magazine. Another, V. Koliadin, of Kharkov, Ukraine, wrote the following perceptive analysis of the situation, which was to become even more relevant in the light of subsequent events:[1]

You state that Peter Duesberg wrongly uses tendentious arguments to confuse understanding of Aids, that his debating technique is intolerable because he asks unanswerable rhetorical questions and that he should stop. The tone and logic of your leading article seem inappropriate to a scientific journal, and *Nature's* position on Duesberg's theory seems prejudiced.

The rhetorical questions Duesberg has posed are in fact statements – that the widely accepted hypothesis that HIV is the cause of Aids is not consistent with the facts. If, for instance, someone asks the question 'Why cannot the theory explain the facts A, B, C...?', that is not only a stimulant of further research, but a serious objection against the theory.

The reasoning behind Duesberg's theory occupies sixty pages of text and refers to more than 600 papers by other authors... The attempt to prove that the theory is wrong, based on references to a few studies by Duesberg's opponents, is not persuasive: there are no criteria to estimate these as more authentic than those to which Duesberg refers...

The real motives for the rejection of Duesberg's paper remain unclear. Neither the peculiarities of his rhetorical style nor 'nonauthenticity of information' can explain why the paper has been rejected. The real cause seems to be connected with the question (non-rhetorical and answerable) of whose interests may suffer if Duesberg's theory is true.

Duesberg's paper highlights a much more general problem: the effectiveness of the procedures used by scientific journals to select papers for publication. Even for ordinary works, the modern system seems ineffective. If a work expresses an unorthodox view, its chance of being published is quite small. As the history of science demonstrates, most landmark works have been at first regarded as wrong and intolerable. Open discussion of this problem in *Nature's* pages would be very useful.

Rather than listening to Koliadin, Maddox seems to have preferred the advice of two Italian Aids specialists, Luigi Chieco-Blanchi, of the Institute of Oncology, University of Padova, and Giovanni B. Rossi, a Rome virologist, who suggested Duesberg 'should be stopped'. For example, they wrote, 'should he somehow be prevented from appearing on television to misinform individuals who are at risk from the disease? One approach would be to refuse television confrontations with Duesberg, as Tony Fauci and one of us managed to do at the opening day of the VIIth International Conference on Aids in Florence. One can't spread misinformation without an audience'.

Duesberg has noted several examples of such censorship, when invitations to TV discussions have been cancelled at the last moment because of 'unforeseen circumstances'. Television news, with its enormous dependency on having the right camera shots, seems ill-suited to the exploration of ideas and has contributed minimally to the Aids debate. Television documentaries, which have extensive resources at their disposal relative to most newspaper inquiries, do often break new ground – the Meditel programmes on Aids for Channel 4's 'Dispatches' were classic examples – but because they may take months to prepare they cannot put across challenging ideas with the same consistency and flexibility as a newspaper.

Call for a Reappraisal

The steady stream of abuse against the *Sunday Times* that had appeared in *Nature* and elsewhere in British scientific and medical journals had so far failed to stem the tide of stories questioning the HIV theory. On 28 November 1993 – just before World Aids Day – the newspaper was at it again: a front-page news story reported Dr Kary Mullis, winner of the 1993 Nobel prize for chemistry for inventing the PCR genetic test used world-wide by Aids researchers, as saying it was not even probable, let alone scientifically proven, that HIV caused the disease. What had started out as a working hypothesis, based on the isolation of HIV from a French homosexual with swollen lymph glands, 'has now become a sort of religious position,' he declared. 'If there is evidence that HIV causes Aids, there should be scientific documents which either singly or collectively demonstrate that fact, at least with a high probability. There is no such document.' Mullis's own theory was that Aids arose through an enormous level of exposure to human viruses and bacteria. 'If you test Aids patients for just about any of those that are known, you find they have it – or have had it.' So it was not surprising that HIV was often seen.

The story added that Mullis was one of about 350 people, including many distinguished scientists, who had joined an international group that was pressing the scientific community to re-examine the orthodox view. This was the Group for the Reappraisal of the HIV/Aids Hypothesis, whose membership had grown more than seven-fold since we first reported its existence eighteen months previously.

Also on 28 November, a feature article, 'Aids: The Emperor's Clothes', summarised various 'dissident' viewpoints in the challenge to the conventional medical view and highlighted the simple, four-sentence letter the group had asked leading scientific and medical journals to publish. All of them – including *Nature* – had turned it down.

The following Sunday, among a selection of letters published on the issue, two in particular stood out as demonstrating the way thinking about Aids had diverged. The first, from John Godfrey, of Edinburgh, showed very clearly the practical inadequacies of what medical science had so far offered people with Aids:

> No, the messenger does not deserve to be shot! Neville Hodgkinson and the *Sunday Times* deserve great thanks from those of us categorised as having Aids who question the conventional view of its cause and effect and its treatment by orthodox medicine.
>
> After a brief bout of illness over two years ago I was told that I had Aids and that without treatment I might live less than a year. I was panicked into accepting treatment. My great fortune was to find myself on a drug trial that alternated medications. I quickly realised that various symptoms of being unwell which I was feeling could be directly attributed to a particular drug and disappeared when I wasn't taking it.
>
> After nine months of pharmaceutically induced sickness I decided to call it quits and find other ways of coping. Another great fortune was happening on Peter Duesberg's critique of the theory that HIV causes Aids. If it doesn't, then maybe there was another explanation for my brief bout of sickness – and other treatments. Fortunately, there has long been a small but growing body of dissident literature which details alternative therapies.
>
> Of course not all of it can be right. Several theories are conflicting. Lots of suggested treatments are half-baked. Many are impractical for those who want to go on maintaining their lifestyle and particularly their working

lives. What is important is that there are alternatives, and many people are managing to live healthy, enjoyable and productive lives by preferring some of these to conventional treatment.

The importance of Hodgkinson and your newspaper is that you continue to empower and encourage those who are determined not to accept conventional treatment with all its side-effects by putting the criticism from 'dissidents' in the public domain, whereas there has been deafening silence from the rest of the mainstream and scientific press. Also – I fervently hope – you are thereby giving more and more people who find themselves diagnosed HIV-positive or with Aids a cause for hope and a defence against the fatalism of the Aids orthodoxy.

The second letter, from Julian Meldrum, research and information officer with the National Aids Trust, expressed clearly why the Aids 'establishment' felt the newspaper was wrong to persist in airing dissident viewpoints. He wrote:

The reported comments of Dr Kary Mullis, while providing an insight into the thought processes of one scientist, do not amount to a useful contribution to our thinking about HIV and Aids. The best explanation of the known facts is that the world is experiencing a global series of epidemics of HIV infection, leaving a series of Aids epidemics in their wake. The pattern of transmission is similar to that of other known viruses, and is no more – or less – mysterious than for any other disease.

The best advice that can be given to an HIV-negative person wishing to avoid Aids is that if you can avoid becoming infected with HIV, then your chance of contracting an Aids-like illness is trivial. The main behaviour changes advocated to control HIV, such as the wider use of condoms and an end to needle-sharing by drug users, are both harmless and convey other benefits.

If the 'conventional' view is right, then the use of HIV tests by blood transfusion services, especially in countries where heterosexual transmission of HIV is commonplace, has already saved many thousands of lives. If the so-called Aids dissidents have any credible and testable alternative explanations of the facts about Aids, we should all support calls for the necessary research to be done. Until and unless such an alternative emerges, we have a right and a duty to ask them to stop confusing the public with unfounded speculation that is actually contradicted by many of the known facts.

If I had not known by this time the history of Procrustean distortion and suppression that had prevented the 'facts' about Aids from being known, Julian Meldrum's letter would have seemed reasonable. As indeed it did to James Fenton, a professor of poetry at Oxford University and *Independent* columnist, who quoted it approvingly the following morning in attacking 'the *Sunday Times* campaign on Aids', which he ascribed to 'a kind of *folie a deux* between the editor and his science correspondent, a shared hysteria in the face of unfolding events'.

Fenton's sniping did not bother me too much, but I did find it frustrating to see untruths repeated as fact again and again. Why were there not more scientists, acquainted with the facts, trying to stem the tide of nonsense? An answer came in this letter, addressed to me personally, from a London immunobiologist:

Another World Aids day has gone by and the question is how many more will pass before the biomedical world recovers some of its bygone sense. On Tuesday's BBC-2 Late Show, the science correspondent of the *Independent* was confident enough to claim there is no debate within the scientific community about the causative role of HIV in Aids. I am afraid that many scientists like myself have unconsciously supported such claims by choosing to play the fully employed chicken instead of risking to be the jobless hero. Most of us remember quite well how the day after Ceausescu's death the previously silent Romanians proclaimed worldwide that the former Genius of the Carpathians had been nothing more than a sick fool all the time. So let's hope that in the near future we – biomedical scientists – will behave as newly freed Romanians, at least for one day.

I hope your newspaper will carry on with a lucid and open-minded approach towards this muddled issue.

The Empire Strikes Back

At this point, an extraordinary event occurred. In a two-page editorial, headlined 'New-style abuse of press freedom', *Nature* declared that 'A British newspaper, the *Sunday Times,* has so consistently misrepresented the role of HIV in the causation of Aids that *Nature* plans to monitor its future treatment of this issue, if only to save readers the trouble of buying it'. The editorial, which singled me out as the prime mover in what it claimed had now been dignified as a 'campaign', announced a drive to bring our 'perverse' line of reporting to an end. A boycott of sales of the newspaper would be ineffectual, the journal said, and picketing its offices impracticable. Instead, each week, brief reports on our articles would be published in *Nature* 'to let readers judge whether the newspaper's line on HIV and Aids shows signs of being modified'. Letters of protest rejected by the paper would also be considered for publication in *Nature.*

The magazine acknowledged that 'the causation of Aids has been a profound disappointment to the research community'. Nearly ten years had passed since HIV was recognised, and the evidence that it caused Aids was still epidemiological; 'the mechanism of the pathogenesis of the disease has not yet been uncovered'. However, 'the vast majority of the evidence is consistent with the view that HIV is a cause (and probably a sufficient cause) of Aids. How, in these circumstances, can the *Sunday Times* so consistently assert the opposite?'

The newspaper replied gamely. On 12 December it published a big resume of the argument, strikingly presented under a page-wide block with 'Aids' in red letters on a black background, and the sub-heading 'Why we won't be silenced'. In it, I wrote of the wave of attacks that had accompanied our attempts to widen discussion on the cause of Aids. The sensational possibility that the medical and scientific communities might have picked the wrong target in their 1984 call to arms against HIV had been largely ignored by the British media, and suppressed almost entirely in the United States.

> Not content with failing to report crucial developments in the science surrounding HIV and Aids, several broadsheet newspapers, normally supporters of balance and objectivity, have uncritically reflected views

> hostile towards this newspaper expressed by scientists who have built careers and reputations, and fortunes in some instances, from the HIV theory.
>
> The science establishment considers itself on high moral ground, defending a theory that has enormous public health implications against the 'irresponsible' questioning of a handful of journalists. Their concern is human and understandable, even if we might expect our leading scientists to retain more concern for the truth while pursuing public health objectives.
>
> But neither the quality press nor mainstream science would be so sure of themselves if one magazine had been doing its job properly. That magazine is *Nature,* the British weekly science journal of prestige. *Nature* is the bible of the church of science, and its editor, John Maddox, is the high priest. He has persistently refused to publish letters and articles from doctors and scientists who question the HIV theory of Aids, and its corollary that heterosexuals around the world are at risk from a new infectious agent. To him, the theory is fact...
>
> If science does one day prove that HIV causes Aids, the *Sunday Times* will of course report the fact. So far it has not...Yet on the basis of an unproven hypothesis, *Nature* has led a propaganda war which may have unnecessarily stigmatised millions of HIV-positive people by implanting the idea that they are harbouring a new and deadly virus which threatens everyone. Despite being supported by billions of dollars of research funds, the hypothesis has got nowhere in ten years. It is in those circumstances that Maddox seeks to silence the *Sunday Times.*

The newspaper reprinted the *Nature* editorial in full, under the heading 'The science establishment says: Don't read the Sunday Times'. It also published a respectful, and penetrating, profile of Maddox by senior reporter Greg Hadfield. It paid tribute to his achievements at *Nature,* but included a description of an attack he had mounted on the French biologist Jacques Benveniste over an experiment that appeared to demonstrate a scientific basis for homoeopathy. In 1988, after publishing the findings with an editorial saying they could not be true, Maddox had spent a week in Benveniste's laboratory with two other biological 'ghostbusters', including James Randi, a magician and 'seasoned debunker', as Hadfield put it, to try to prove his point.

I had been to see Benveniste shortly after their visit. Regardless of the rights or wrongs of the research findings, the Frenchman was devastated by what he had experienced as ill-mannered and insensitive behaviour, bordering at times on loutish, by the *Nature* team. Maddox sought to justify this exercise by telling Hadfield: 'A speculative suggestion that rings an intellectual bell is one thing, but the claim by Benveniste was an assault on reason.'

At least the row between the *Sunday Times* and *Nature* widened awareness that the HIV 'gospel' had been challenged. The story was reported around the world, including a straightforward description of it in the *New York Times*, although I remember a long conversation with their correspondent in London in which he repeatedly pressed me on our 'lack of balance' on the issue. I could not see his point of view on this, and he could not see mine when I pointed out that hardly a word of the 'revisionist' theory and information we had reported had been put before the *New York Times* readers.

Andrew Neil made a similar point in a letter responding to a *Guardian* article on the controversy. He welcomed a recognition by the reporter, Madeleine Bunting, that there was 'a debate worth having' about the causes and nature of Aids and that the *Sunday Times* had been a lone voice trying to promote that debate. 'Ms Bunting is wrong, however, to claim that it is the supposed lack of balance in the *Sunday Times's* coverage which has alienated the Aids establishment. It is that establishment and its media supporters who lack balance: those who promote the orthodox line rarely, if ever, acknowledge there might be another point of view, much less give it space. The idea that there is some doubt – and nothing proved – about the role of HIV in causing Aids has been suppressed in most of the media with all the rigour of a one-party state.'

I was grateful for a story issued by the Press Association news agency, 'Papers at War on Aids Theory', which gave me a chance to correct some of Maddox's misrepresentations, such as that we had mounted a campaign in support of the view that HIV was 'irrelevant' to Aids. 'That is untrue,' the PA's health correspondent, Amanda Brown, quoted me as saying. 'If there has been a broad theme running through many of our articles over the past two years it has been that scientists do not yet understand Aids. We have reported a range of views and arguments relevant to this theme of which the hypothesis that HIV is irrelevant is only one. Maddox also accuses us of encouraging teenagers not to bother with condoms. This is another falsehood.'

Eminent Toxicologist Backs Dissidents

The attack elicited considerable support for the *Sunday Times,* as well as some sharp criticism. Six letters published on 19 December, all clearly carrying their authors' conviction, illustrated the wide divergence of opinion.

Dr Dennis Parke, emeritus professor of biochemistry at the University of Surrey and one of Britain's most experienced toxicologists, supported the call for a wider discussion on the causes of Aids. He said his own knowledge of the disease began in the early 1970s, when a few patients presented with strange symptoms of immune deficiency at a London hospital where he had worked for eighteen years.

> All were homosexuals, using various recreational drugs, and active in anal intercourse with the use of nitrite vasodilators. It was this last aspect which led us to consider that the nitrites were a key factor in the pathogenesis of this condition. Our hypothesis, twenty years ago, was that the nitrites reacted with faecal amines to form mutagenic nitrosamines, which then resulted in mutations of faecal microorganisms and viruses and to DNA damage in leucocytes. More recently it has been shown that nitrite also led to the formation of nitrosoglutathione, thus depleting the body's natural defence (glutathione) against toxic chemicals and drugs, and against the toxicity of the ubiquitous oxygen radicals.
>
> My own lifetime's experience of medical science has led me to believe that most disease states are multifactorial in their pathogenesis. Cancer is now known to be associated with genetic factors, with viruses, carcinogenic chemicals, oxygen radicals and dietary deficiencies (choline deficiency is hepatocarcinogenic in rats). Thus HIV infection, and the mutagenic effects of drugs and chemicals, coupled with the complex biological and biochemical interactions inherent in anal intercourse, might all be involved in the pathogenesis of Aids. The current drug treatment, AZT, I believe, is also a known mutagen.
>
> As the founding editor of the scientific journal *Xenobiotica,* I have published several controversial papers rejected by other journals for their heretical views. I considered this to be my duty as the editor of a scientific journal and as a practising medical scientist. Science is the quest for truth,

> and should be beyond the reach of censorship from vested interests. I hope Hodgkinson's courage in widening the debate may eventually elucidate the true pathogenesis of this dreaded disease.

Parke had been an adviser on drug safety and chemical toxicity to the British and American governments for nearly twenty years, had helped draft medicines control legislation, and had had more than 450 papers published in scientific journals. I rang this authoritative and experienced scientist to write a news story about his disclosures. He told me that the Aids cases he had seen could date from as far back as 1968 or 1969; but after HIV was taken up as the cause, 'nobody wanted to know' about other theories, and he had decided not to pursue the matter. An informal approach to the US National Cancer Institute brought a dismissive response, in spite of his having a lengthy association with the institute. 'There is a lot of bigotry in science and medicine,' he said. 'If you don't follow the consensus they don't want to know.'

Another letter that gave no comfort to our critics was from Anthony Tucker, science editor emeritus of the *Guardian*. He wrote: '*Nature* may be seen as the most important and distinguished general science journal in the world, but healthy science depends on hypothesis and challenge. For its editor to attempt to control views published in newspapers or anywhere else is bizarre, arrogant, dangerous and potentially corrupting.' Tucker added that during a public scientific meeting at the Royal Society in London on 3 December – when Maddox was assembling his attack on me and the *Sunday Times* – he and *Nature* were accused of blocking papers essential to analysis and reconstruction of the patterns and content of radioactive fallout from the Chernobyl accident. The charge was that he failed to publish between sixty and 100 papers on fallout that had been formally accepted and in some cases had reached the stage of proof correction.

> The ethics of scientific publishing are well understood. If a paper is accepted by a journal it cannot be submitted elsewhere unless it is specifically released. Thus formal acceptance followed by failure to publish is an effective form of censorship ... Maddox, in addition to his self-elected role as newspaper censor, is thus cast as a leading player in a sinister game of nuclear obfuscation.

John Moore, of the Aaron Diamond Aids Research Center in New York, who had roundly condemned me for writing the original April 1992 article on problems with the HIV theory and abused me subsequently in *Nature,* now wrote to say it was not the role of a newspaper to complain about the rejection by a scientific journal of nonsensical articles. 'For all practical purposes, there is no controversy on the cause of Aids; the case for HIV was settled beyond reasonable doubt years ago and this continued debate is sterile. Intellectual masturbation by the likes of Duesberg is all very well, but working scientists and physicians simply don't have the luxury of unfettered time to waste on him any more... For the *Sunday Times* to play Goebbels to Duesberg's Hitler is quite unnecessary.' Another correspondent, Karl Sabbagh, saw the newspaper's Aids coverage as 'more a result of efforts to revive a flagging reputation for investigative journalism than of any real concern for the facts of the story, or indeed, for people infected with the HIV virus... Self-righteousness ran rampant as Hodgkinson presented the issue solely as if the *Sunday Times* was exercising some public service or other in devoting thousands of words to the dissident views'.

Meditel's Michael Verney-Elliott suggested that Maddox might benefit from having two brief quotations pinned to his office wall in large letters. One was from John Stuart Mill: 'We can never be sure that the opinion we are stifling is a false opinion; and even if we were sure, stifling it would be an evil still.' The other was from the geneticist C. H. Waddington: 'The most formidable barrier to the advancement of science is the conventional wisdom of the prevailing group.' Finally, Richard Milton, author of a scientific challenge to evolution theory[2] that had also aroused Maddox's ire, wrote urging members of the scientific community to 'unhesitatingly close ranks and put their weight behind' the attempts to give a public platform to the voices of scientific dissent in the HIV/Aids controversy. At stake, he said, was the right of all scientists to report their findings, regardless of their political implications. He added: 'It would be hard to credit that the editor of the world's leading science magazine is publicly advocating a policy of scientific censorship over this issue, were it not for the fact that Maddox has openly pursued this policy for many years... under the cloak of appearing to represent the rational faction.'

Unpublished Gems

Scores more thoughtful and informative letters arrived on the issue. It saddened me that most were not published, but with such limited space in a Sunday newspaper, covering a multitude of new issues every week, and with 4 million readers to please, there was a strict limit. In that sense, I could agree with one scientist who wrote that there *was* a case for questioning HIV, but a newspaper was not the right place to do it (nor would it have been doing it in the same way, if the science journals had done their job properly).

Unlike previous correspondence, which had tended to come roughly as two letters against to each one in favour, the proportion was now reversed in the wake of Maddox's outburst. The overwhelming impression I obtained from them was of the contrast between the way the public generally thinks of science, as an objective search for truth, and the passionate reality of a struggle between a multitude of viewpoints and interests, with facts and reason playing decidedly secondary roles. There is probably nothing new in that; what seemed to be so wrong was that this reality was not acknowledged and allowed for by HIV's protagonists, who tended to portray themselves as the only reasonable party and therefore the only one entitled to have their case put before the public.

Several of the letters were from scientists who had their own personal and professional reasons for feeling aggrieved with *Nature*. One such was Professor R. A. Lyttleton, of the Institute of Astronomy at Cambridge University, a Fellow of the Royal Society (FRS), who wrote that 'Your criticism of the scientifically challenged editor of *Nature* is more than timely. His cavalier attitude on the subject of Aids is not limited to medical matters but extends to other fields of science, including astronomy and geophysics – in which I may be thought to have some experience, if the Halley lectures are any indication'. He felt ill-treated by the journal because of its rejection of a recent challenge he and Sir Hermann Bondi had submitted 'properly rubbishing the fashionable fairy tale of plate tectonics'. On the Aids row, he wrote that Maddox had 'succeeded in making journalists seem like paragons of scholarship... The advice of Sir Peter Medawar FRS to young scientists should be added to that of Mill and Waddington (quoted by Verney-Elliott) that the intensity of conviction that a hypothesis is true has no bearing on whether the hypothesis is true or not.' To leave any stone unturned in the search for real succour for thousands, perhaps millions, of souls afflicted by Aids was criminal.

Another scientist who felt ill-treated by *Nature* was Jeremy Dunning-Davies, senior lecturer in applied mathematics at Hull University. 'This is by no means the first time in recent years that *Nature* has pursued one view to the complete exclusion of alternatives,' he wrote. Together with some other scientific journals, the magazine had refused to report a controversy surrounding a theory associated with Stephen Hawking on the thermodynamics of black holes. 'Although the theory has been shown to violate the celebrated Second Law of Thermodynamics, *Nature's* belief in what it regards as conventional wisdom seems unshakeable.' Dunning-Davies said he and an Italian professor, Bernard Lavenda, had written three times to *Nature* pointing out errors in an editorial, but had received no acknowledgement. He added: 'Scientific controversy should be open and should be settled openly by scientists; disagreements should not be hidden away at the whim of an editor.'

A letter from an Englishman living and working at a hospital in Zambia reminded me of how the non-specificity of the HIV test lay at the root of misunderstandings on the part of many who had no particular axe to grind. He acknowledged that we had given good coverage to some of the responses to the articles on Aids in Africa, but complained that whereas 'your story was repeated in countless other publications', the denials had not appeared. 'My wife is daily battling with the mounting number of HIV-positive TB patients,' he wrote. 'Could you please consider commissioning an article to correct some of the harm done?' It is now clear that the real harm lay in the imposition on a continent of a diagnostic test purporting to be specific for 'HIV' while actually detecting antibodies associated with chronic and active TB infection (among others).

A letter from London dated 13 December said: 'What world do you at the *Sunday Times* live in? Your Aids coverage suggests it is a fantasy world created by wilfully ill-informed and dangerously short-sighted people, who are prepared to substitute wish-fulfilment for a sane and realistic analysis of the facts. I suggest you read the latest issue of *Nature* and seriously re-examine your policy, or perhaps appoint a new science editor. Until then I will cancel my order for the *Sunday Times* and take the *Observer* instead.' The loss of this 'reader' did not seem too serious, since he was apparently unaware that we had not only read the latest issue of *Nature* but reproduced its editorial in our own pages the day before he issued his threat.

Graham Ross, a Liverpool solicitor acting for patients alleging damage by AZT, wrote: 'Whether HIV is the sole cause or, as some mainstream observers are now conceding, merely a co-factor, or even a totally non-causative element in Aids, the fact remains that many asymptomatic HIV+ patients throughout the world are being prescribed the highly toxic drug AZT, the only justification for which being that HIV causes Aids. What is not in dispute is that AZT causes severe damage. For this reason alone an open mind is urgently required whatever the consequences for professional reputations.'

A comment made to me at about this time by Chuck Ortleb, the battling editor of the New York *Native,* seemed relevant to some of these letters, and indeed to *Nature's* outburst. He told me that he had detected 'intense anxiety among the leaders of the Aids establishment at present'. They were losing credibility on several fronts – AZT, HIV, predictions of spread, Africa. 'They feel they are losing control of the debate and they are trying to manage communication about the disease rather than the disease itself,' he said. 'HIV calmed everyone down; no one wants to go back to the panic of not knowing what was going on.'

Perhaps this also helped to explain a question put to me by Chris Dunkley, television critic of the *Financial Times,* who wrote on 12 December that he was sitting at his desk cheering – 'hardly a habit on wet Sunday mornings' – having just read 'every word' of our response to the *Nature* editorial.

> What IS it in the Aids saga which makes people (even those who would normally see themselves as liberal intellectuals) turn into totalitarians? Could it be the Nazi connection? "Nazis persecuted homosexuals as well as Jews, consequently anybody who says anything which might reflect a poor light on homosexuals runs the risk of being compared to a Nazi"? It must presumably be something at this emotional level because they seem to have lost all sense of balance and reason.

He enclosed a copy of his column from the previous week, 'as encouragement and proof that there are outcrops of non-Aids-industry thought elsewhere, however tiny'. Headed 'When political correctness is all', and triggered by a crop of television programmes marking World Aids Day, it contained an analysis of why 'television does not dare to get to the nitty gritty of the Aids phenomenon: sexual practices which are not usually mentioned in polite society'. He went on:

> Among the scores, probably hundreds, of Aids programmes so far screened I have never yet seen one which had the courage to say that (leaving aside infected blood banks and needle sharing) the disease appears to spread where you find (a) a group of abnormally promiscuous people, (b) where anal intercourse is commonplace or even the dominant practice, the lining of the rectum being more prone to rupture than the lining of the vagina, allowing the spread of the infection into the bloodstream, and (c) where either drug abuse or old venereal diseases weaken resistance to Aids or even provide a vector for the new disease. Where these three factors coincide, whether among heterosexuals or homosexuals, Aids will spread quickly unless preventive measures are taken...
>
> The preceding paragraph is not a moral judgement, nor a condemnation of any group. It is a statement of the facts as perceived after reading everything about Aids that it was possible to lay hands on and which was comprehensible to the layman. But if you expressed it on one of television's Aids programmes there would be an outcry, not from the audience, but from the 'agenda setters'. These people – producers, editors, heads of television departments – believe that it is wrong to tell the public the truth about Aids because, in their view, the public is already appallingly careless about 'safe sex' and dreadfully homophobic. Tell viewers the truth and the heterosexual majority will take this as a signal to forget all thought of danger to themselves, abandon 'safe sex', and increase the persecution of homosexuals. In television today it is more important to be seen to be politically correct than to be seen to be truthful.

Dunkley acknowledged that there had always been one exception to the rule: 'From the beginning Joan Shenton, a lone independent producer, working with her own company, Meditel, has stuck insistently to the old idea of journalism, reporting whatever she finds.' In a passage relevant to my own experience, he went on:

> As with any subject where there is one overwhelming school of thought and a number of fringe dissenters you run the risk of becoming identified wholly and only with the dissenters. Because they are the underdogs and receive so little attention elsewhere you tend to concentrate on them in an instinctive attempt to right the balance, whereupon the dominant group anathematises you and drives you more into exclusive concentration on the fringe.

Dunkley added that Shenton's latest film, *Diary of an Aids Dissident*, screened by Sky News, which showed how the Aids establishment were now so nervous that they were trying to suppress dissident publications (documents prepared by dissidents Robert Laarhoven from Holland and Peter Rath from Germany were confiscated by the organisers of the 1993 International Aids Conference in Berlin), 'suggests that we may be near to a breakthrough of the truth in the larger public domain'. Unfortunately, much misinformation still remained to be put before the public by those determined to keep the HIV hypothesis alive.

Five-year Half-life in Medical Ideas

Medical support for the dissident case was rare, but included a letter from a Sudanese doctor working in Manchester, Bushra Habbani, who questioned how a blood-borne disease could be endemic in central Africa and yet (according to orthodoxy) not spread by the most notorious blood carrier, the mosquito; a letter to *Nature* from Dr K. Ghattas, of London's Harley Street, who declared that 'many people are worried, asking for the case to be properly studied' and that 'If HIV does turn out to be the sole cause of Aids, it will be a sort of miracle. Historically bad science reveals little but harm'; and the following pithy comment from Dr Robert Lefever, a London physician:

As John Maddox, the editor of *Nature,* should know, the half-life of any new clinical recommendation is about five years. Each hospital registrar comes in time to prove that his chief was misguided. Such is the course of medical progress.

In twenty-five years of general medical practice, on the recommendations of my scientific elders and betters I have had to tell my patients that high dose oestrogen contraceptive pills are dangerous after all, that a high fibre and low fat diet is now considered as important as a low refined carbohydrate diet in diabetes, that inhaled steroids should be the first rather than the last resort in the treatment of asthma and that benzodiazepines are now recognised to be addictive. The recommendations on treatment for raised serum cholesterol have swung from one pole to the other with the predictability of a pendulum.

I do not expect my superiors to be right first time on every issue but I do expect them to look at their own track record before they get into a blather when their most recent fervent belief is challenged. Neville Hodgkinson may well be right and the Aids establishment wrong and that could prove to be good news for both clinical and scientific reasons.

A number of correspondents recognised that the issue went much further than controversy over the cause of Aids, or even over the attempts to silence 'dissident' views. It penetrated to the core of how science functions in today's society.

Professor C. I. J. M. Stuart, an emeritus professor still active in scientific research, wrote from County Kildare, Ireland, to say that at issue in the disagreement between Maddox and Hodgkinson was 'the integrity of the manner in which the scientific community reports its findings to the world'. It was greatly significant that the public press should challenge a major scientific journal over the logic of its scientific reporting, if the challenge were done responsibly and capably, which seemed to be the case in this instance. 'However, it is an undertaking likely to hit upon deeply laid prejudices within the scientific community and the general public alike.'

Contrary to widely held belief, the advance of natural science is not driven solely by considerations of logic. Because science is a human activity, we

> ought not to be surprised to find its advance sometimes marred by human frailties. Science is also a social activity; the individual's work is presented to the international scientific community with an implicit invitation for that community not only to judge its merit and relative significance, but also to participate in the work of correcting it or further developing it. But because it is a social activity, we ought not to be surprised to find in it the emergence of social ploy and prejudice interacting with individual self-interest.
>
> In reality, such social factors play an important role in determining what does, and what does not, become part of the established scientific outlook. It is a complex issue making deep connections with the role quite rightly played by scientific conservatism. That form of conservatism acts to protect against ideas that are ill-founded or otherwise lacking discernible merit. But, then, discernibility is itself shaped by the climate of social opinion. In short, the scientific community has its own popular causes – which often harden into dogmas – and it can often ignore ideas that seem to run counter to those dogmas.

The process of peer review – pre-publication vetting by acknowledged experts – was itself part of the sociology of science, Stuart added, and a major criticism was that the contemporary outlook tended to favour technically competent work that was in line with the views of 'the scientific establishment' while tending to ignore work that ran counter to the establishment. 'The British journal *Nature* and the American journal *Science* share a prominent role in determining the character of that establishment.'

> It is important to recognise that in its sociologic aspect, modern science strongly reflects the values esteemed by modern society as a whole. Ours is the Age of Management in which the values of the administrator are highly esteemed. Those values have become part of the cultural climate of the modern universities and, thereby, that of modern science. Today, the scientist has to deal with a great deal more than doing good scientific work; there is great pressure to work at becoming prominent in the intensely competitive world of achieving grant support and publication in journals deemed prestigious. Administrators determine the scientist's merit by

annually counting the number of pages published and the size of the grants obtained for research support. Absorbing the values imposed upon them, the scientists have in turn adopted this arithmetical evaluation of their own merit and that of their colleagues - who have now all too often become viewed as competitors.

The perspective I have drawn is not a happy one, but I know it to be shared by many of my colleagues in a wide range of scientific fields. I have no expertise at all in the field of Aids research. My work has been in the area of theoretical biology and, for the past twenty-odd years, in the foundations of physics. But over a period of more than thirty years I have observed profound changes in the character of scientific life and in the practice of scientific publication.

The more the public became aware of the sociology of modern science, Stuart concluded, 'the more likely it is that public pressure will urge that science return to the life of the mind instead of the life of the marketplace'. In those terms, he thought the newspaper had initiated a significant act of public service.

An even more revolutionary outcome of the controversy was contemplated by David Quinn, another correspondent from Ireland:

The scientific establishment... bears an uncanny resemblance to Medieval Christiandom. It is as totalist and unified in its world view as was the Medieval Church. While heretical movements exist, as they did in the Middle Ages, they are kept at the outer margins of the scientific world via various time-honoured devices for maintaining doctrinal control such as censure, ridicule, and *de facto* excommunication. Organs such as *Nature* act as a sort of Holy Inquisition.

But the early symptoms of a schism are beginning to develop. The authority of the Catholic Church was challenged over an issue which is to us relatively unimportant, i.e. the doctrine of justification. Yet once that authority was successfully challenged on one issue, it did not take too long for the great unified world view of the Middle Ages to unravel. One can envisage the current scientific 'Magisterium' being successfully challenged over an issue such as Aids, and then, with its credibility damaged, finding itself challenged over a host of other issues. One can then imagine a whole new paradigm, a sort of scientific equivalent of Protestantism developing in competition to the established 'Church'. For example, at present an excessively materialist cosmology dominates scientific thinking. It is not at all beyond the bounds of possibility that a less rigidly materialist cosmology will gain some currency in the years to come.

Perhaps the *Sunday Times,* in challenging the received wisdom on the issue of Aids, will help to spark off a scientific Reformation.

'Aids Plagued by Journalists'

It was greatly frustrating that much of this stimulating correspondence languished unused – all the more so since *Nature* was at this time carrying out its threat to publish letters rejected by the newspaper. Most of these were of course hostile to us; the journal did not see the numerous unused letters that favoured our position. Apart from the ever-present constraint of space, the reason for not continuing with the correspondence was that contrary to Maddox's claim, we had not taken up a genuinely campaigning stance on the issue. In this we were unlike both Meditel, which really had entered into a campaigning alliance with Duesberg and other members of the 'reappraisal' group of scientists, and *Nature,* which had taken upon itself the task of resisting the HIV critique.

When a campaign is pursued, articles whose news value is not necessarily great are nevertheless given space so that the issue is not allowed to die and the objective of the campaign can be followed through to the point of fulfilment. That was not the case with the HIV/Aids controversy at the *Sunday Times.* As long as fresh stories, of high news value in their own right, continued to be generated, the newspaper was happy to use them. When I reported new developments, that was news; and when others attacked us, that was also sometimes news, if their stature was great enough. But a campaign needs a clear objective, and the newspaper had not taken a position on the debate beyond that of insisting that the HIV hypothesis was in serious trouble and that a reappraisal was needed.

In January 1994, after *Nature* picked up on a report in the *Independent* about Father D'Agostino's statement of faith in HIV, I wrote to the journal correcting several errors (*Nature* had even distorted the *Independent* account, quoting D'Agostino as accusing me of 'terrible' journalism when the word he had been reported as using was 'irresponsible'). Maddox refused to publish that letter. He did, however, accept the following:[3]

> Because of your interest in our reports on HIV and Aids, I should like to make it clear that, contrary to some reports, the *Sunday Times* has never presumed to pass judgement on whether or not HIV causes Aids. We do however believe that a strong scientific challenge has been mounted to the consensus view that HIV is the cause of Aids, and consider the issue so important as to merit wide discussion and examination. We will continue to report views and findings relevant to this debate.
>
> Many such developments occurred over the past twelve months, and as we have been almost alone among the media in challenging the orthodox view that accepts HIV as the cause of Aids, we have often found ourselves left with a clear field in writing about them. This has given the impression that we are running a campaign on the issue, but the view here is that all our articles have been of legitimate news interest, given our fundamental position that there are real uncertainties over Aids causation.
>
> I should like to add that my own doubts about HIV's role have grown stronger over the twenty months since we first set out the 'dissident' views, not least because of the unreasoning way mainstream science has reacted to the challenge, at first dismissive and then, when the 'problem' refused to go away, openly censorious.

This letter was run beneath another, four times as long, in which Cambridge University's Dr Abraham Karpas attacked Simon Jenkins, a senior writer with the daily *Times* newspaper, over what had really been a quite moderate and eminently reasonable article on the controversy. 'It is about time that *The Times* and *Sunday Times* realised that, through badly informed and irresponsible journalism, they could mislead millions of their readers about HIV infection and Aids,' Karpas wrote. *Nature's* headline to the page was 'Aids plagued by journalists'.

In the wake of this correspondence, a letter arrived at the *Sunday Tunes* from Dr Christophe Benoist, director of research with the French National Centre of Scientific Research (CNRS) in Strasbourg, who said he was appalled by our ludicrous attitude over 'the Duesberg affair'. He suggested I shift my doubts to less dangerous matters, such as 'Benveniste's endless dilution story', flying saucers, or talking dogs.

A professor of biology from Brandeis University, Massachusetts, wrote:

> 'Mainstream science' includes experts in virology and immunology, 99 per cent of whom are convinced that HIV causes Aids. If your opposition to this view causes some people to reduce their precautions, you will have murdered them in the same way that the officials of tobacco companies murder people by misleading them about the dangers of cigarettes.

In reply, I wrote of 'the unnecessary damage being done to young people and their relationships – and to whole communities in Africa – if the HIV scare should turn out to have been ill-founded'.

A British doctor wrote to ask: 'Do you accept that if your "challenge to the orthodox view" is wrong and if as seems certain you encourage people to neglect precautions against contracting Aids, then you will be as surely responsible for some deaths from Aids as if you had gone out into the street and selected people for execution, even though you would never know who and how many?'

Yes, I answered, there was that risk, 'though from the start our articles have accepted that the "safer sex" message is common sense. However, since we believe the challenge to be well-founded, I have also to ask myself the consequences of failing to report it for the reason you suggest. One consequence would be that millions of HIV-positive people would continue to be inappropriately treated, and to suffer an unnecessary feeling of having been sentenced to death. In Africa, many give up and die on the basis of an HIV diagnosis; families throw HIV babies and mothers out, and hospitals refuse to treat them'.

I had to try to remember that what the paper wanted from me was to report what was going on, and not get distracted by the hurt and angry feelings of the doctors and scientists whose authority was being challenged so strongly. Besieged with so many letters, I was not always successful in this.

An Embarrassing Silence

The biggest challenge, however, came from within. Despite the editor's unflinching support, some colleagues felt profoundly uneasy about the HIV critique, in the face of so much professional and media criticism. They found it impossible to believe the entire world could have been so misled. There was also concern that I might be boxing myself into a corner on the issue, becoming too involved in the fight. This had some truth in it. I became angry one day when in the midst of fielding all the flak from *Nature* and elsewhere, I was pressed by a senior executive in charge of news to give more time to general science stories.

During the first few months of 1994, despite the boldly defiant initial reaction to *Nature's* attack, the *Sunday Times* went embarrassingly silent. A handful of news reports appeared, covering newly highlighted evidence on the damaging effects of the nitrite inhalants (bravely taken up by the Royal Pharmaceutical Society, but ignored by the Health Department and the rest of the press); and developments in the AZT controversy.

The first substantial article was a feature published on 3 April, headlined 'Conspiracy of Silence', about the growth – and continued ostracising – of the reappraisal group. In two years, a large and growing network of 'dissidents' had become established world-wide, and the article summarised the range of positions they had taken up. More than 450 had now put their names to the reappraisal letter, including more than seventy PhDs, scores of medical doctors and numerous other health workers and scientists, along with Aids patients, activists and others who had been working for years with those most affected by the epidemic. Most of the names were American-based, but overall the list spanned twenty-three countries. It was the tip of an iceberg of dissent: the group's newsletter had a mailing list of more than 2,000.

The article emphasised that although signatories of the letter were united in wanting a change of direction, they differed in the extent to which they rejected the HIV theory. Some, like Dr Charles Thomas, a molecular biologist and former Harvard professor of biochemistry who helped found the group, said it was complete nonsense. 'The HIV-causes-Aids dogma represents the grandest and perhaps the most morally destructive fraud that has ever been perpetrated on the young men and women of the western world,' he told me (a comment which led his wife, on seeing it in the paper, to joke something to the effect that one day he would say what he really meant). Thomas has given immensely of his time and energies seeking a new look at Aids, as has Phil Johnson, senior professor of law at the University of California at Berkeley, who told me: 'One does not need to be a scientific specialist to recognise a botched research job and a scientific establishment that is distorting the facts to promote an ideology and maximise its funding. That establishment continues to doctor statistics and misrepresent the situation to keep the public convinced that a major viral pandemic is under way when the facts are otherwise.'

Others, like Dr Lawrence Bradford, a biology professor in Atchison, Kansas, and Dr Roger Cunningham, a microbiologist and director of the centre for immunology at the State University of New York at Buffalo, thought the virus could be one factor among many, but maintained an unbiased assessment was urgently needed. Dr Alfred Hassig, former professor of immunology at the University of Berne and director of a Swiss blood transfusion laboratory, said multiple stresses on the immune system provoked an acute reaction, allowing latent microbes, including HIV, to proliferate. He believed dietary measures could reverse this process, and urged that 'the sentences of death now accompanying the medical diagnosis of Aids should be abolished'. Hassig has also worked long and hard to try to crack the consensus on HIV.

Most of the signatories, such as Dr Henk Loman, professor of biophysical chemistry at the Free University in Amsterdam, deplored the neglect of non-HIV lines of research. 'There are many people with Aids but without HIV, and a great many people with HIV but without Aids,' he said. 'These two facts mean that HIV = Aids is much too simple. Plausible, alternative, testable causes of impairment of the immune system which may ultimately lead to Aids should become part of regular Aids research.'

An Italian signatory, Dr Fabio Franchi, a specialist in preventive medicine and infectious diseases in Trieste, declared: 'I am not agnostic; I am well convinced, above all by the arguments of Professor Peter Duesberg.' (The previous November, Italy's *Corriere Della Sera* ran a challenging exposition of the controversy, producing a furious reply from the country's leading Aids researcher to which Duesberg was asked to respond.) Equally sure of

HIV's innocence was Dr Bernard Forscher, formerly managing editor of the *Proceedings of the National Academy of Sciences.* 'The HIV hypothesis ranks with the "bad air" theory for malaria and the "bacterial infection" theory for beriberi and pellagra [caused by nutritional deficiencies],' he said. 'It is a hoax that became a scam.'

The fact that the HIV theory was now being questioned by a large and growing group of scientists encouraged further media coverage internationally. An excellent account of the controversy appeared in *Die Woche,* a German highbrow weekly, on 21 April (sent to me with a note of encouragement from Peter Schmidt, a Berlin Aids 'dissident'). Germany has been relatively well served with information about the challenge from Duesberg, in particular, with articles that included a cover story in the magazine *Raum & Zeit* as far back as June 1992. In Sweden, journalist Ola Deråker, another tireless dissident, faxed scores of copies of 'Conspiracy of Silence' to members of all seven of the country's political parties.

The science editor at the *Australian* decided to run the article along with a fuller statement from Professor Hiram Caton, head of the school of applied ethics at Griffith University in Brisbane, Australia, and a fellow of the Australian Institute of Biology, whom I had also quoted. Caton had concluded as far back as 1988 'that Aids was not a disease entity, that the CDC definition of Aids was diagnostic codswallop, and that there was no compelling evidence that HIV causes immunosuppression'. He believed the orthodox view would collapse, 'because it flunks the practical tests... The hype will exhaust its credibility'.

Caton's intervention had many consequences, as he recounted in the January 1995 *Reappraising Aids* newsletter. 'The Aids mandarins sent faxes flying denouncing the *Australian* for printing such "loony fringe" opinion. I did four radio news interviews and one talk-back. Producers from three television networks rang to sound me out about a documentary on the challenge to Aids science. However, the mandarins, when contacted, threw such a tantrum that all three producers backed away.' Not intimidated, however, was the editor of the University of New South Wales Press, who commissioned and later in 1994 published a book from Caton on the controversy, *The Aids Mirage.* He summarised its themes as follows:

> The gay men who presented with wrecked immune systems in 1981 were pursuing a 'live fast, die young' lifestyle, as they well knew. Common health sense would have put them, and others living as they did, on a rigid diet and fitness regimen to detoxify their bodies and rebuild the immune system. Instead, doctors invented a causality in which lifestyle is neutral to disease causality and to therapeutics. Why? Because conventional medicine defines sickness as conditions that respond to pharmaceutical and surgical procedures in the medical armamentarium. Patients are sidelined as spectators in the healing process managed by doctors. They are told that they can do nothing to escape the iron grip of scientifically confirmed disease agents. This thinking leads to a therapy consisting of highly toxic drugs that attack the very immune cells whose rehabilitation is wanted...
>
> The few studies of long-term survivors of HIV infection indicate that they either abandoned or never commenced AZT therapy. The survivors also commenced diet and fitness regimes. This means that they maintain health by rejecting standard therapy, and by becoming doctor-free agents of their own health. There is a need to assemble as many such cases as possible, and to support client groups who will carry the message into the corridors of medical self-esteem.

On 1 May I wrote a rejoinder to assurances by health ministers that homosexual men using nitrites to boost their sex lives did not face any increased risk of developing Aids, apart from being more exposed to HIV through having more partners. Their advisers had cited the San Francisco study, which *Nature* highlighted with a press release declaring that 'Drug use does not cause Aids' and claiming that the findings 'seriously undermine' Duesberg's arguments. The officials could not have known that a re-analysis of the data by Duesberg and others had reached conclusions that directly contradicted those in the original article, since the journal refused to publish it. A second study quoted by ministers to justify their inaction on poppers had appeared in the *Lancet* as a 'short report'. It too was aimed at torpedoing Duesberg's claims, which it described as 'a hindrance to public health initiatives'. But as Duesberg pointed out in a letter accepted by the *Lancet*, 88 per cent of the HIV-positive men in this survey, which was among homosexual men in Vancouver, had used nitrites, and up to 100 per cent had used drugs of some sort. Drug use was also widespread in men who did not get Aids, but that might just mean other factors, such as genetic susceptibility, were involved, as with smoking and cancer.

My growing sense of frustration betrayed itself in this article, called 'Poppers and Propaganda', in which I also referred to the *Lancet's* purported 'squelching' of the questions on Aids in Africa with a study in which only five cases were diagnosed. 'A kind of collective insanity over HIV and Aids has gripped leaders of the scientific and medical professions,' I wrote. 'They have stopped behaving as scientists, and instead are working as propagandists, trying desperately to keep alive a failed theory... when will this madness end?'

Later that month Gallo himself gave comfort to Duesberg, when both took part in a scientific meeting on the toxicity of nitrite inhalants as a possible cause of some 'Aids-defining' diseases, particularly Kaposi's sarcoma. Much that implicates poppers in KS was heard at the National Institute on Drug Abuse (NIDA) meeting,* though as John Lauritsen wrote in his account of it for the *Native,* KS remains a puzzle in Aids, and no hypothesis so far put forward seems fully adequate to explain it. HIV 'obviously' played a role in the disease, Gallo said – 'I think the epidemiology is not debatable' – but he acknowledged that poppers could be a primary cause in KS, and urged that studies proposed by Duesberg for testing the role of nitrite inhalants in Aids should be supported (NIDA had turned down, and deemed unworthy of further review, a detailed proposal for these experiments, despite high-level endorsements for the funding application). Lauritsen concluded that despite the uncertainties, the drugs theory Duesberg had espoused 'is very much alive, more than a decade after its precipitous rejection by the CDC'. So too, from Gallo's comments, is the multiple risk factor hypothesis pursued by Sonnabend before the editorial coup that ousted him from *Aids Research* all those years ago.

In an additional report on the NIDA meeting, published in *Bio/Technology,* Lauritsen cited data from the Multicenter Aids Cohort Study showing that HIV-negatives had, on average, twenty-five months of nitrite use, HIV-positives had sixty months of nitrite use, and Aids patients had over sixty-five months of nitrite use.

* See Chapter 4

Rage and Distortion

Not a word of this meeting surfaced in any other mainstream journals. Instead, counter-information had started to flow thick and fast – from the science and medical journals, from the parliamentary group on Aids, from other specialist writers and broadcasters – in a concerted campaign to rehabilitate the HIV hypothesis after the setbacks it had suffered, a campaign that continued right through the following year. As Serge Lang wrote, in a letter expressing sympathy for Duesberg's position, 'It's like the video games – one can't shoot fast enough.'

An insight into the states of mind involved came when *Nature*, in rejecting a paper on 'Why There is Still an HIV Controversy', jointly authored by Charles Thomas, Kary Mullis, Bryan Ellison and Phil Johnson, enclosed reactions from two Aids researchers to whom the journal sent the manuscript for comments. One was courteous enough, and quite open about 'the huge amount of poor research in the Aids field', adding: 'If the HIV research community is against the non-HIV hypothesis it is far from united and certainly has no unified field theory of Aids pathogenesis. The cacophony of ideas being kicked around is proof of the discord.' Nonetheless, 'we all accept that the HIV theory has the upper hand. If others care to believe that the majority of Aids researchers are mistaken then it is up to them to show where the community has gone wrong'.

This was hard to do, however, when their work was being repeatedly refused publication, especially on such 'scientific' grounds as the following (sampled from the second reviewer's comments):

> Let us accept their premise [that HIV is not the cause of Aids] at face value: the inescapable conclusions are as follows. Either the thousands of scientists world-wide are members of an enormous conspiracy designed to suck research dollars into our laboratories, or we have deluded ourselves into believing that what we are doing is scientifically justified. A stark choice: we are either utterly evil, or we are morons... The *Sunday Times* has acted as Duesberg's mouthpiece for years, with serious effects in Britain and Africa... What would another article achieve? It would delude a few more members of the public into believing there was a controversy when

> there isn't one, the scientific issues being long since resolved ... If Aids testing in Africa is not what it should be, that's a shame but not a critical point ... If a fuss was made of a few cases of ICL (Aids without HIV) at a charged press conference, what of it? ... If people have been 'very slow to answer his (Duesberg's) science', it is because most of us have better things to do. Like working on an Aids cure or vaccine for instance... You people should spend time talking to HIV-infected people, living with and dying of Aids, as we do here in our city... Our friends in the HIV-infected population are sophisticated and intelligent; but they represent others with less access to knowledge and more susceptibility to the poison you purvey. Come and talk to these people, who know what HIV has done and is doing to their friends. For it is they that you damage with your luxurious intellectual masturbation, not Aids researchers: we merely find you boring.

This, from a magazine that purported to be the world's leading science journal, to a group that included the current Nobel prize-winner for chemistry. How could *Nature* bring itself to send such anonymous abuse to a group of scientists working, unpaid, to end what they believed to be a terrible mistake with horrible consequences for patients? *Nature* even tried to make a virtue of its behaviour, arguing in a rejection letter that whereas the referees showed a 'sense of commitment' in trying to understand Aids and help those with the disease, 'your article seems to imply that the most important priority is to establish that some Aids researchers are unprincipled in adhering to the idea that HIV causes the disease'. It was plain from the article, which was packed with factual evidence countering the HIV theory as well as with proposals for settling the controversy, that in no way was that the priority. Certainly, some polemics came into it, but in view of the way the reappraisal group had been treated that was hardly surprising. The rejection letter, from executive editor Dr Maxine Clarke, also stated condescendingly: 'I think that these comments speak for themselves, and I hope you find them helpful in thinking about how you intend to proceed with your campaign.'

The science establishment's anxiously censorious stance came to the fore again over plans for a one-day symposium in San Francisco at which speakers were to dispute the link between HIV and Aids. The symposium was organised by Professor Charles Geshekter, chair of the section for the history and philosophy of science of the American Association for the Advancement of Science, Pacific Division, as part of the division's 75th annual meeting in June 1994.

The line-up, which included Duesberg, Mullis and several other HIV sceptics, had been put together over previous months in consultation with division chiefs. But beginning in mid-May, 'an extraordinary chain of events unfolded that was unprecedented in my twenty-six years as a university faculty member and conference organiser,' Geshekter wrote later in a complaint to the division's council. Criticisms were lodged with the AAAS both in San Francisco and Washington complaining about 'imbalance' among the speakers. 'The critics were primarily journalists, Aids activists, and the very Aids researchers whose ideas and theories would be thoroughly scrutinised at the session.'

In the 26 May issue of *Nature,* AAAS executive officer Richard Nicholson indicated that the session might be called off. 'All options are still open, including cancellation,' he said. *Nature* also quoted Bernie Fields, professor of microbiology at Harvard Medical School, as saying the fact that such a meeting should take place under AAAS sponsorship 'makes it sound like a real issue when it's not; I think it's a disgrace'. David Baltimore, of Rockefeller University, New York, said he could not understand why the association had allowed itself to sponsor a meeting that did not represent scientific opinion. 'This is a group of people who have denied the scientific facts,' he said. 'There is no question at all that HIV is the cause of Aids. Anyone who gets up publicly and says the opposite is encouraging people to risk their lives.' (To which Mullis subsequently responded:[4] 'So what? I'm not a lifeguard, I'm a scientist. And I get up and say exactly what I think. I'm not going to change the facts around because I believe in something and feel like manipulating somebody's behaviour by stretching what I really know ... If you can't figure out why you believe something, then you'd better make it clear that you're speaking as a religious person, not as a scientist.')

In fact, 'despite all the backroom manoeuvring to sabotage it', as Geshekter was later to describe it, the symposium went ahead successfully. But changes in the programme were imposed on him, without consultation, by divisional organisers. These included the addition to the programme of seven pro-HIV speakers. 'Eager to placate the media and acquiesce to outside critics,' Geshekter wrote, they 'operated in a capricious, non-consultative, arbitrary, and anti-democratic manner. Their authoritarian and deceptive practices violated the principles of open scientific discourse which we assure our members and the public are scrupulously upheld by the AAAS.'

In his opening address as chairman, Geshekter told the symposium:

> HIV and Aids are now part of our daily vocabulary. They figure prominently whenever Americans are urged to practise 'safe sex'. Many of us have worn red ribbons, participated in quilt dedications, and watched films such as *And the Band Played On* and *Philadelphia.*
>
> Major debates have erupted among scientists trying to understand Aids. Some biologists question whether HIV does anything to cells. Virologists insist that other critical factors must be present to bring about full-blown Aids. Biochemists wonder whether HIV is really so mysterious? Does it actually remain latent, hiding in cells, only to mutate wildly, killing cells by strange mechanisms? Researchers from around the world have shown how unreliable the primary HIV tests can be. Finally, cell biologists are unable to detect significant amounts of HIV in the semen of HIV-positive men.
>
> Actuaries who assess risk factors for life insurance companies scrutinise the distribution of Aids cases and conclude that *most* people are not at risk. African physicians and public health officials dispute the alleged extent of Aids in Africa because its definition and symptoms often make it indistinguishable from tuberculosis, malaria, or malnutrition, tragically common conditions in modern Africa.

The aim of the symposium, he said, was to provide a *public* forum for viewpoints about Aids 'which have been excluded from previous AAAS meetings and, until recently, ignored by much of the media... Our objective was to assemble a diverse group of scientists united in one goal: to help save lives by arriving at the truth of the matter'. Geshekter, who is professor of history at California State University, Chico, added:

> 'HIV and Aids' is a deadly serious and controversial topic. Aids has claimed many lives, threatened others, and terrified communities. Aids activist

> Ian Young noted that the tragedy of Aids has produced many dubious assertions and not enough free inquiry. Treating hypotheses as dogma serves neither science nor the public good.

Nature, despite having published a critical and subversive report *before* this historic event, did not carry one word about the symposium proceedings themselves. Perhaps that was because, as Lauritsen later reported, 'the Aids-sceptics achieved a critical mass, and spoke with confidence and authority. Those who attempted to defend the official dogmas were confused and defensive; they failed to rebut or even acknowledge the points made by the sceptics'. It was not just long-established dissidents like Lauritsen who saw the proceedings in that light, either, as a column by Susan Gerhard in the *San Francisco Bay Guardian* made clear:

> Kary Mullis, the man with what *Spin* described as a 'party boy surfer demeanour', stepped out of those pages and on to the stage with the same casual, contrarian, inquiring mind he'd demonstrated courtesy of Celia Farber's article [an interview with Mullis in the July 1994 issue]. His question – the one that keeps him in the pages of *Spin* as opposed to the pages of the establishment science journal *Nature* – is whether there really is a connection between HIV and Aids. Here, he and Dr Peter Duesberg continued to grind the axe: The problem with the $2 billion-a-year HIV research industry, they argued, is that it looks more like a religion than science.
>
> While it may be OK for me and most of my friends to *believe* in science – we have to, as we're not equipped with our own labs and sets of petri dishes – we expect more than blind devotion from the men and women of Reason. It was truly frightening to watch how, with a few pointed questions, they made that religion – my religion for many of the last ten years – look as arcane as the Vatican's.
>
> Duesberg asked how, if HIV replicates in twenty-four hours, the disease can take up to ten years to incubate, and why he could find 4,500 HIV-free Aids cases in the medical literature. Mullis simply asked anyone in the room for a reason why HIV moved from being the 'probable' cause of Aids

to the definite cause of Aids without any experiments that actually verify that relationship.

As panellists from the other side of the HIV/Aids debate attempted to answer HIV's critics with lengthy descriptions of HIV's mechanism of action in the body, recaps of studies that drew the association between HIV and Aids, and descriptions of the history of the disease as it's already been told, I flashed back to the early 80s and the murky warnings about a disease both we and they didn't really understand. As scientists at the conference defensively droned on about the trees, I realised that their understanding of the forest was pretty dim.

In mid-1994, Andrew Neil left the *Sunday Times*. Although his successor, John Witherow, made a loyal response to some new attacks in the *Independent* while he was still acting editor, the challenge to HIV was not a fight of his own choosing and it was quickly made plain to me that I would no longer be able to spend so much time on the issue. In July 1994 I stepped back from the fray, quitting the paper that had given me such extraordinary support against so much top-level criticism for so long. At a retreat centre near Oxford, I soon re-established peace of mind (which had tended to be obscured by the relentless nature of the controversy), and began to take stock of what had happened.

It was not before time. The attacks had become increasingly personal, and my credibility as science correspondent difficult to maintain. A reminder of this came the following October, when I was invited to address a group studying the practice and philosophy of science at University College, London University (UCL). The invitation came from Dr Luca Turin, of the department of anatomy and developmental biology, whom I had met in the United States and who was well aware of the genuineness of the uncertainties over Aids causation. One of the flyers he had put up advertising the meeting came back to him with a note scribbled on it from Lewis Wolpert, professor of biology as applied to medicine at UCL, a radio pundit on science and author of books aimed at increasing public understanding of the subject (the last of which[5] concluded that 'once one rejects understanding and chooses dogma and ignorance, not only science but democracy itself is threatened'). Wolpert wrote:

Dear Luca,

If you are not careful you might end up asking a real scientist to talk. I find your choice of topics and speakers bizarre. Why not get Uri Geller?

- Lewis

P.S. But that is just what I expect from Philosophy of Science.

The Ones Who Refused to Fit

As I contemplated the intense experience of the previous two and a half years amid the tranquil beauty of the Oxfordshire countryside where much of the writing of this book has been done, I marvelled at the resilience of those journalists and other commentators who had understood at a much earlier point that the HIV paradigm was seriously flawed, who had withstood similar attacks, and who were still fighting for a return to sanity.

Celia Farber is the prime example. She has been covering the HIV debate in detail since 1987, when she first interviewed Duesberg for *Spin* magazine. Since that time, she has written countless articles on the subject, including investigative reports and interviews with leading figures in the debate. From 1986 to 1991 she was the editor and primary writer of *Spin's* monthly Aids column 'Words from the front'. Subsequently, she has been an associate editor of the newsletter *Rethinking Aids,* later renamed *Reappraising Aids,* and a member of its editorial board. She has argued for a reopening of the question of what causes Aids on numerous radio and TV shows. Her articles have twice been the focus and reading material for college courses on critical science reporting. 'If you call up scientists asking simple, intelligent questions about the cause of Aids you get a kind of irrational fury,' she says. 'It is like holding a cross to a vampire. If you give any credence to these ideas you lose your contacts in the medical establishment and for a full-time medical reporter this is a problem. Investigative journalism and science haven't met before... What we are up against is a multi-billion-dollar infrastructure.' Bob Guccione Jr, editor and publisher of *Spin,* concurs: 'A terrible tragedy is being perpetrated because our government and health agencies, the pharmaceutical industry and the research industry are unwilling to allow any debate to get in the way of their fantastic profit-making.'

John Lauritsen, in a magnificent report on the AAAS symposium in the *Native,* headlined 'Truth Is Bustin' Out All Over', quoted Farber on the pressures a journalist can face in bucking the establishment:

> The big journalists are the least likely to rock the boat, and in fact I was educated on this by none other than Robert Gallo, who called me in 1988, after he'd read something I'd written. And he said that he just wanted to have a heart-to-heart talk. He said, 'You seem like a nice girl – and you seem to have your head on straight – and I want to advise you that this is no way to make a career for yourself.' He said, 'Don't you want to be like Barbara Walters? How do you think Barbara Walters got to be where she is? It certainly wasn't by attacking and criticising and following lunatics around.' [laughter from audience]

North America has also been particularly well served by the work of Colman Jones, an award-winning Toronto-based writer and broadcaster. He has made many diligently researched, questioning contributions to the Aids debate, disseminated mainly through the Canadian Broadcasting Corporation's *Ideas* radio programme and through *Now* magazine. In particular, he has pursued a case for investigating the role in Aids of *Treponema pallidum,* the organism which causes syphilis. Repeated reinfection with this agent does not always produce the classical symptoms, and some scientists believe syphilis may have gone untreated in thousands of gay men during the 1970s, with long-term consequences contributing, perhaps centrally, to the immune system breakdown seen in Aids. A similar mechanism may be at work in some African communities. Katie Leishman, of the *Atlantic Monthly,* has also made superhuman efforts to persuade the Aids community to look at the easily testable syphilis theory.

One of Jones's most recent contributions has been to investigate the case of Kimberley Bergalis, a young college student whose case terrified the US when government health officials reported that she had contracted HIV from her dentist – the only dentist-to-patient transmission ever reported. He documented how genetic data generated by the US Centers for Disease Control, allegedly linking six cases of HIV transmission to the dentist, David

Acer, had been called into question by leading researchers, and how internal CDC papers, obtained under the Freedom of Information Act, pointed to gaping holes in the version of events made public by the agency. The records appeared to confirm what many observers had suspected all along: that Bergalis and other patients said to have been infected by Acer had other risks for becoming HIV-positive. 'This is no idle matter,' Jones wrote in an article on the affair for *Spin*. 'The implications of the Acer case have been far-reaching, ranging from calls for mandatory HIV tests of health-care workers to changes in infection-control machinery in dentistry. If Acer did actually transmit a deadly virus to his patients, there is indeed cause for concern. But an equally disturbing scenario seems to be emerging; one that suggests David Acer was condemned on the basis of fragmentary, circumstantial evidence, perhaps driven more by hysteria than science.'

Other investigators have reached similar conclusions. Stephen Barr reported in an eight-page article in *Lear's* magazine in April 1994 that documentation on the case 'demonstrates that David Acer was convicted largely by hysteria, and that the public has been misled'. In a TV documentary by CBS's *60 Minutes,* broadcast on 19 June, presenter Mike Wallace said there was 'compelling evidence that was either never discovered or completely ignored by the CDC; compelling evidence that casts doubt on the stories told by Dr Acer's patients, and also calls into question the reliability of the scientific techniques used by [the CDC] to accuse the dentist'. The CDC's Dr Harold Jaffe, who had headed the investigation that purported to implicate Acer as the source of infection in his patients, was asked by Wallace how many other HIV-infected professional health-care providers had passed the virus on to their patients. The answer was: 'In no other case do we have evidence of transmission from the provider to their patients.'

Charm, humour, intelligence and solidarity seem to have been the secrets of the Meditel team's ability to maintain their courage in the face of many obstacles. Ever since Michael Verney-Elliott first took the story of defective Aids science to Meditel's London offices in 1986, he has been a backbone for the team's research efforts, loyally aided by biochemist Hector Gildemeister. Joan Shenton, as team director and front woman, has taken some tremendous knocks but stays free of hostility. I saw her in action once with the parliamentary advisory group, socking out her points with great force but without rancour. 'We have certainly experienced the censorship,' she says. 'We have been dragged through the Broadcasting Complaints Commission accused of being unfair in our treatment of the subject of Aids, we have been denied a basic right of reply in the letters pages of national newspapers, and we have been publicly denounced as murderers.' Jad Adams, whose book *Aids: The HIV Myth*[6] arose out of the work for the first Meditel documentary on the subject, says he had never before experienced so much resistance and hostility from his own colleagues or from the establishment. 'There is even resistance,' he says, 'to the reporting of the fact that there ARE dissidents.'

For a while, the *Sunday Times* found the authority and strength to break that resistance. As a result, the fact that there was a challenge to HIV became much more widely known around the world. In the end, however, acceptance of the inadequacies of the HIV paradigm by those most affected by Aids, both patients and researchers, may be more likely to come through quiet dissemination and assimilation of information than through newspaper headlines.

A hopeful sign for the future of the debate in Europe is that several health activist groups have taken up responsibility for that task, both within and outside the gay community.

Continuum, the group founded in the UK by Jody Wells in late 1992, continues to go from strength to strength, despite Wells's death from pneumonia in August 1995 (eight years after his Aids diagnosis – when he was told he had a year to live if he was lucky – and two weeks after he had written off his car in an accident). The *Continuum* magazine,[7] under editors Huw Christie and Molly Ratcliffe, publishes a serious-minded mixture of personal experience and scientific findings directed towards 'changing the way we think about Aids'.

The longest-established British group is Positively Healthy,[8] founded in 1987 by Cass Mann 'to counter the death wish philosophy and anti-science agenda encoded by most of the other "Aids" organisations in the UK'. By the mid-1990s, PH was focusing its campaigning efforts against the use of nitrite inhalants, still at that time an enormous business in the UK. Mann says none of the group's hundreds of members is taking AZT, 'and the vast majority are completely well and living full, normal and healthy lives. The few that get ill are treated only for the presenting illness, and the consideration of being treated for HIV is not part of our scientific model, as HIV's pathogenicity has never been proved'. Wayne Moore, Positively Healthy's co-chair, says that in eight years since he was diagnosed HIV-positive, he has never been asked by his doctors about any aspect of his lifestyle including diet and nutrition, smoking, alcohol intake or recreational drug use. This lack of interest, he says, is 'wholly due to the belief that HIV is the sole, sufficient and necessary cause of Aids'.

Deconstructing Aids

An authoritative newcomer to the debate in the UK is the HEAL Trust (London),[9] an alliance of scientists, researchers, health-care professionals and people with an HIV or Aids diagnosis. Directed by Gareth James, a registered homoeopath, it has produced a well-referenced critique of the orthodox Aids paradigm, entitled *Deconstructing Aids*. The London trust is modelled on the HEAL (Health Education Aids Liaison)[10] organisation founded in New York City in 1992 by Michael Ellner, a medical hypnotherapist who has worked with thousands of people with Aids-related conditions and fears, and who speaks of 'the constant terror, and the programming to get sick and die', induced by the HIV=Aids=Death equation. Another founder member, Frank Bouianouckas, professor of mathematics at City University, New York, organised the first conference to question HIV as the cause of Aids as far back as 1988, after seeing many of his friends die from drug toxicity.

In Holland, Robert Laarhoven, of the Dutch Foundation for Alternative Aids Research, has for years been collating and distributing photocopied packs of articles relevant to the HIV and AZT critique. At the Berlin conference in 1993, his press pass was confiscated and he was threatened with deportation from Germany for 'criminal trespass' – placing copies of *Rethinking Aids* on an unauthorised table. Many other groups had put literature on tables in the same area, but the conference officials did not intervene with them. On Berlin's Open Channel TV, however, nine hours of Aids-critique programmes were aired, produced by Peter Schmidt and Kawi Schneider.

In the US, the newsletter *Reappraising Aids* continues to serve magnificently. Tom Bethell, the *American Spectator's* Washington correspondent and a media fellow at the Hoover Institution, has lent additional journalistic weight to the editorial board, as well as contributing some fine articles on the controversy since hearing a Duesberg lecture in 1992.

The newsletter seeks to expose 'the facts behind the hype', as Dr Mark Craddock put it in a recent article entitled 'HIV: Science by Press Conference'. He analysed in detail the latest example of this hype, a 12 January 1995 event in which David Ho and George Shaw were presenting the results of studies purporting to show (after ten years of contrary findings) that HIV was an incredibly active virus, producing billions of offspring every two days, but which were simultaneously dealt with by billions of T4 cells. This battle was postulated to go on for the many years during which an HIV-positive person stays well, but ultimately to lead to immune system failure and death. (Nearly two years earlier, Ho had pleased a rally of 700 HIV researchers in Albuquerque, New Mexico, by announcing plans to make a button reading 'It's the virus, stupid', a phrase taken up by *Science* in headlining its report of the meeting.)

Craddock, of the school of mathematics and statistics, University of Sydney, Australia, wrote:

> As a mathematician, I was intrigued by the claim of John Maddox, editor of *Nature,* that the new results provide a new mathematical understanding of the immune system. Unfortunately, my confidence in this claim was badly shaken when it turned out that on the very first page of the Shaw paper (Wei *et al.,* p. 117, *Nature,* 12 January 1995) they make an appalling mathematical error. And in the same paragraph make an assumption which turns out, by their own admission, to have no basis in observation, and which they give no justification for...As bad as these mistakes are, they are only the beginning.

After demonstrating his case mathematically, Craddock pointed out that the whole basis for the measurements given in this and another similar paper was an unvalidated technique, called quantitative competitive polymerase chain reaction (QC-PCR). Because tiny variations in sample size were magnified exponentially, 'there is simply no way of knowing whether a given estimate is correct or 100,000 times too high!' He also pointed to several other illogicalities in the methods used and assumptions drawn, concluding that

> ... HIV 'science' has declined so far that these elementary questions are addressed neither by the research groups themselves, nor the referees at *Nature* whose job it is to critique the papers before publication. Is nobody at *Nature* bothered by the fact that neither paper contains any hard data which can be independently analysed? ... Nobody in the HIV research community is at all bothered by this. They seem to have learned like the mad hatter to believe six impossible things before breakfast and so one more makes no difference. One gets a remarkable sense of being disassociated from the real world when entering the realm of Aids research.

Finally Craddock, whose research includes the mathematical behaviour of infectious diseases, demonstrated that according to the disease model and calculations as set out in *Nature,* Aids should develop in days or weeks after infection, not years. 'There is no possible way it can take ten years. This emerges from Ho *et al.'s* own model. They seem blissfully unaware of the prediction that their own results give. They probably have not bothered to look at tedious questions like "do our results correspond with what we observe in patients?".' He concluded:

> Science is about making observations and trying to fit them into a theoretical framework. Having the theoretical framework allows us to make predictions about phenomena that we can then test. HIV 'science' long ago set off on a different path. It seems as if nobody bothers to check the details in this field. Nobody is asking the fundamental questions, and nobody wants to. People who ask simple, straightforward questions are labelled as loonies who are dangerous to public health... My question is this. Just what exactly will it take to get the people doing HIV research to turn away from high tech, unproven methods, arcane speculations about

> molecular interactions and so on and ask themselves 'Do any of us have the faintest idea what we are doing?'

Another powerful challenging force in the US is Serge Lang. Through what he calls his 'cc list', he has relentlessly pursued *Science,* in particular, with allegations of giving improper information to its readers on various counts, including inadequate and tendentious reporting on the Gallo case and the HIV/Aids controversy. He circulates his comments, and relevant documents, to key players in the controversy, including Broder, Gallo and the council of the National Academy of Sciences, of which he is a long-standing member.

In the autumn of 1994, *Yale Scientific* published a long article by him, 'HIV and Aids: Questions of Scientific and Journalistic Responsibility', in which he wrote of how 'some purported scientific results concerning 'HIV' and "Aids" have been handled by press releases, by disinformation, by low quality studies, and by some suppression of information, manipulating the media and people at large. I am not here concerned with intent, but with scientific standards, especially the ability to tell the difference between a fact, an opinion, a hypothesis, and a hole in the ground'. He added: 'For a decade, billions of dollars have been spent investigating HIV as a cause of diseases lumped together under the name "Aids", without success. At the same time, proposals for funding research on other possible causes have been rejected... The mainstream and official scientific press have promoted the official view about Aids, mostly uncritically. When the official scientific press does not report correctly, or obstructs views dissenting from those of the scientific establishment, it loses credibility and leaves no alternative but to find information elsewhere.'

Tens of thousands of scientists have now been struggling for more than ten years to understand HIV and its role in Aids, and to find a treatment for the condition and a vaccine to protect against it. The fact that these efforts have so far proved fruitless does not mean HIV is not the cause of Aids, nor that those who have worked hard within the HIV paradigm are to blame for its unproductiveness. However, since HIV has become the most heavily investigated virus in history, it does strongly suggest a reappraisal is needed. The stubborn refusal to hold other possibilities in mind, both now and in the earliest days of Aids research, and the hysterical response to criticism, has been the real failure on the part of the institution of science as it is currently organised.

The public have repeatedly been told, on the basis of the 'lethal virus' theory, that all sexually active people could be at risk as the virus follows its predicted spread away from the original groups afflicted by Aids. The fact that those predictions have not been confirmed by experience does not mean HIV is not the cause of Aids, or that the spread will not one day occur. However, after a decade of HIV-monitoring and at least fifteen years of Aids, it does make it extremely unlikely that HIV is a new pathogen spreading through a defenceless population.

Leaders of the scientific and medical professions have behaved repressively towards those such as Sonnabend, Duesberg and Stewart who have sought to keep non-HIV (and non-AZT) options open. The fact that they have done so does not mean the mainstream was wrong about HIV, but their defensiveness does suggest that unscientific factors have been prominent in the maintenance of the HIV theory. It has been particularly scandalous that, with so much circumstantial evidence implicating chronic drug abuse with so many Aids cases, the theory that drugs can cause Aids through cumulative toxicity should have been so neglected for so long.

In the same way, Duesberg's persistence in pointing out the anomalies, and dangers for patients, in conventional thinking on Aids does not mean he is right in every aspect of the critique he has mounted. In particular, his argument that whereas the epidemic of chronic drug use is new, homosexuality is not, and that therefore the 'safe sex' campaigns have been to no avail, does not carry conviction. Gay liberation brought an explosive increase in anal intercourse, in settings that could in themselves be expected to foster disease, along with drugs that facilitated that explosion. As Brandy Alexander said, 'The sex got to be unstoppable.' It *was* a new phenomenon. Furthermore, there is much evidence that Aids risks are far higher in men who habitually play the role of passive, receptive partner in anal sex than in predominantly insertive partners. Duesberg's claim that this reflects greater use of nitrites among the former, because of the drug's muscle relaxant properties, is similarly unpersuasive: nitrites are also widely used to promote and prolong erections. Thirdly, although the limited way in which Aids has spread supports Duesberg's case against the cause being a new infectious disease, there has been persistent evidence of a transmissible component, through which close contacts of high-risk individuals have themselves become at risk.

Finally, despite the problems with circular reasoning over HIV's purported role in Aids, and the confounding effects on the immune system of a doom-laden diagnosis and the potentially lethal treatments that have accompanied it, there has seemed from the earliest days to be more significance to the presence of 'HIV' antibodies in the circulation than Duesberg's argument – that these antibodies simply indicate a successful response to a harmless passenger virus – would allow. A new way of looking at what that significance might be is the subject of the final chapters in this book.

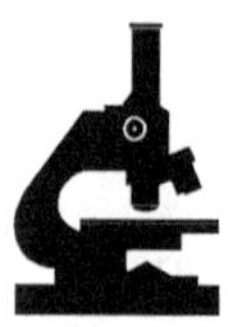

12: THE VIRUS THAT NEVER WAS

The historian and television producer Jad Adams has written[1] of how, at the beginning of the Aids epidemic, scientists working in the field of retroviruses, principally Gallo and Montagnier, were led by their preconceived notions and experience into developing faith in a particular organism as the cause of Aids. 'They were not the only ones who came with an already full agenda,' he says. Duesberg, a father of retrovirology and now arch-critic of HIV, had previously followed a similar pattern, performing pioneering work in the field of cancer-causing genes and then questioning their role in cancer. Adams, too, had been involved in analysing basic science and then questioning the public policy based on it. 'When Aids arrived, each of us played the roles we had been preparing for ourselves.'

In Perth, on the south-western tip of Australia, 2,000 miles from any city of comparable size, a small group of scientists have been preparing themselves for what may prove to be the most remarkable role of all in the Aids saga. They are developing a challenge that goes beyond the question of HIV's role in Aids, beyond issues of co-factors, or the triggering of harmful auto-immune processes or other mechanisms of disease that have been attributed to the virus. They question the very existence of the entity that has come to be known as 'HIV'.

Their standpoint is so radical that most of their published work to date has only hinted at the potential bombshell that underlies it. With so many billions of dollars having been spent on 'HIV'-predicated research and treatment, they are aware of the credibility gap that has to be crossed before the scientific community will be able to consider their arguments. Paradoxically, however, their point of view gives more credit to the conventional explanation of Aids, and is in some ways closer to the conventional picture, than Peter Duesberg's fiercely argued position. In fact, it is likely to put to the test an implied claim by Duesberg and his supporters that they hold the high ground of scientific open-mindedness, because it may challenge some of the basic assumptions in the field of retrovirology that Duesberg pioneered.

The story centres around Eleni Papadopulos-Eleopulos, a tiny lady of Greek origin, who joined her family in emigrating to Australia in the late 1960s after training in nuclear physics at the University of Bucharest, Romania. She was employed by the department of medical physics at the Royal Perth Hospital to research and establish improved radiation treatments for cancer patients. The work led her into a deep examination of some fundamentals of biology, in particular into studying how the body's cells maintain healthy function, and the mechanisms involved when their activity and growth become disordered. After reading much of the classical literature on cell function as well as more recent data and ideas, she developed a theory in which actin and myosin, two major proteins whose interaction was well known as causing muscle contraction, were also seen as a key factor in regulating the activity of cells, including mitosis, the process by which cells divide and reproduce.

Her theory, published as a sixteen-page paper in the high-prestige *Journal of Theoretical Biology* in 1982, proposes that cellular processes have a cyclic nature controlled by a periodic exchange of electrical charge between actin and myosin. This exchange is governed by a well-established oxidative mechanism called redox (short for reduction/oxidation). It is mediated mainly by sulphur-containing compounds that are adept at either giving up or receiving electrons (oxidation causes an atom to lose electrons, while its counterpart reaction, known as reduction, causes an atom to gain electrons). In the cell, oxidation causes activation and expenditure of energy, while reduction brings about a relaxed state in which the cell is able to absorb and store energy. Redox also contributes to the regulation of genetic activity – DNA synthesis and transcription – within the cell.

The paper concluded that the actin-myosin system, and its redox state, appeared to be the unifying factor in muscle function, impulse transmission, metabolism, cellular membrane activity, cell division, 'and indeed the basis for biological function'. Each tissue had its own characteristic cycle, with feedback mechanisms to keep its activity within healthy limits. Changes in the factors regulating these cycles, beyond the point where homoeostatic safety mechanisms were breached, could lead to a variety of disorders, including cancer, which was postulated to involve an excess of oxidising agents. Further scientific papers on the role of the redox state in the contraction and relaxation of muscles[2] and blood vessels[3] were published subsequently by Eleopulos and fellow researchers.

When Aids appeared in 1981, 'it wasn't too big a jump to see that oxidative mechanisms had the power to explain much about Aids and perhaps even 'HIV' itself,' says Val Turner, an emergency physician at the Royal Perth Hospital who has worked closely with Eleopulos in recent years. The oxidative theory of Aids offered a way of tying in the seemingly disparate observations about patients, and laboratory observations as well. It argued that both Aids, and the various biochemical phenomena that had given rise to the HIV theory, were caused by the many oxidative agents to which Aids risk groups were exposed.

However, whereas the HIV theory offered hope that drugs or vaccines might repair, protect or cure patients, the oxidative stress theory put the blame on toxins – anally deposited sperm, injected and ingested drugs, nitrite inhalants and Factor 8 preparations. These are all powerful oxidants, and for gay men and drug users theoretically avoidable, although because of the lifestyle changes demanded if these risks were to be removed the 'germ' theory proved more attractive to many, in the short term at least.

During the 1980s, Eleopulos wrote six papers from the perspective of this oxidative theory of Aids, in addition to drawing evidence from retrovirology, immunology and epidemiology that challenged the 'HIV' hypothesis. Only one was published, and even then only after protracted arguments in which she had to counter criticism from referees. Entitled 'Reappraisal of Aids – is the Oxidation Induced by the Risk Factors the Primary Cause?', it was mostly written in 1985 and twice rejected by *Nature* during 1986. It finally saw the light of day in 1988 in the journal *Medical Hypotheses,* which, although a serious scientific publication, does not carry the same weight as the mainstream journals. In it, Eleopulos argued that there was no compelling reason for preferring the viral hypothesis to one based on the activity of oxidising agents – and in fact the latter was to be preferred, since it led to possible methods of prevention and treatment using already available therapeutic substances.

For example, the epidemiological finding that Aids in homosexual men was directly related to the number of homosexual partners, and to frequency of receptive anal intercourse, had been interpreted back in 1984 as evidence for the disease being caused by a sexually transmitted virus, which happened to be transmitted more easily through the lining of the rectum. However, the finding could be equally well or even better accounted for if sperm itself was considered a causative factor. Several studies had shown that homosexual men who took an exclusively 'active' (sperm-donating) role in sex did not develop Aids, whereas immune suppression was common in promiscuous anal sperm recipients. Anal intercourse could also explain why the female partners of some men with Aids also developed immune suppression, but the disease did not seem to spread any further: the reason was that women could receive sperm, but not donate it. (Sperm presented a risk in anal intercourse but not, normally, in vaginal intercourse because whereas the vagina was thickly lined, semen in the rectum was separated from blood vessels and the lymph system by only a single, easily penetrated layer of cells.) These patterns of spread were different from those present in all sexually transmitted infectious diseases, where both partners were equally susceptible.

The paper cited several studies involving carefully designed animal experiments which 'leave no doubt that sperm is a strong immunosuppressive agent'. Sperm was one of the best-known agents for promoting mitosis (cell division) and like all other mitogens was an oxidising agent; its ability to take electrons from the surface of the egg was a prerequisite of fertilisation.

Furthermore, many of the agents used for treating the infectious illnesses that were much more common among homosexuals than heterosexuals – gonorrhoea, syphilis, hepatitis B, herpes, amebiasis, bowel infections – were oxidising, mitogenic and immunosuppressive. On top of that, viruses themselves caused oxidation of their host's tissues, and an accompanying immune suppression, in the course of their growth process. Two viruses in particular, cytomegalovirus (CMV) and Epstein-Barr virus (EBV), were universally active in Aids patients, and both produced clinical and immunological abnormalities similar to those seen in Aids: fever, rash, swollen lymph glands and extra vulnerability to other infections. Both in humans and animals, these viruses produced T-cell abnormalities as seen in Aids; and both could be isolated from many tissue sites in almost all Aids patients – unlike 'HIV', which had never been isolated in fresh (as opposed to cultured, highly stimulated) Aids tissues.

The diseases fitting the Aids definition appeared in homosexuals before 1981, but it was from that time that their symptoms started to be reported in the medical literature under the inclusive term of Aids. The increasing incidence, and the clustering of cases around New York and California, had been interpreted by 'HIV' theorists as evidence for a microbial cause. But promiscuity had increased greatly during the 1970s, and so had exposure to recreational drugs, especially nitrites, whose use became widespread around 1975. The nitrites – oxidising agents which played a significant role in many biological functions, and which were known to be immunosuppressive, mitogenic and carcinogenic – were first manufactured in California and then transported to New York, the two areas with the highest incidence of Aids.

Thus as far back as 1986, Eleopulos had been offering a multifactorial theory of Aids causation in which the various contributory factors were unified by their shared ability to put the body's tissues under a chronic oxidative assault. She had described mechanisms through which this process could become progressively destructive. She had also provided a solution to a puzzle that was already troubling some researchers at that time, the failure of predictions that Aids, like other sexually transmitted diseases, would spread by any type of sexual intercourse and that more and more cases would appear among heterosexuals. 'So far this has not happened,' she wrote. Unlike many viral diseases, Aids could not be spread even by prolonged, close exposure to Aids patients. According to US acting assistant secretary for health James O. Mason, quoted in *Science* in 1985, 'this is a very difficult disease to catch'.

The answer to the puzzle was that although anal intercourse could contribute to the oxidative stress in various ways, Aids was not a sexually transmitted disease.

How 'HIV' Came into Being

Eleopulos went further. She described a variety of mechanisms, associated with oxidative stress, whereby proteins attributed to 'HIV' – whose antibodies were detected by the HIV test – could be expressed by cells without any need for a virus to be present.

For a start, viruses shared proteins with normal host cell components, a phenomenon known as molecular mimicry. The most prominent and persistently detected antigen in the HIV tests was a protein of molecular weight 41 (p41), which is the molecular weight of actin. Since actin is found in all cells, including bacteria, and since there are studies demonstrating that actin plays a key role in activity at the surface of a stimulated cell, there was a strong possibility that what had been taken to be a signal of the presence of HIV might actually be a signal of cell tissues undergoing oxidative stress.

Eleopulos also pointed to studies showing that when normal cells are stimulated into dividing, substances associated with supposed cancer-causing viruses (oncoviruses) are expressed by the cells, without the synthesis of the virus as such in the form of virus particles. Antibodies to such substances are commonly found in the blood of healthy people, and a variety of factors that can cause their expression have been identified, including age. One group of researchers, discussing their work on these antibodies, concluded: 'The results are consistent with the idea that the antibodies in question are elicited as a result of exposure to many natural substances possessing widely cross-reacting antigens and are not a result of widespread infection of man with replication-competent oncoviruses.'

Was the same true of the antibodies attributed to 'HIV'? Neither of the two blood tests routinely used for detection of Aids risk, Elisa and western blot, detected the virus itself, and both gave persistent false positive results, even when simply tested against each other. It was significant that the false positives increased with the 'stickiness' (viscosity) of the serum samples tested, and the stickiness increased with oxidation. Most importantly, the probability of having a positive Elisa increased with age, poverty, and the general level of immune complexes circulating in the blood, and especially with malaria and other parasitic diseases.

According to Eleopulos, the only sensible conclusion from this and other evidence of the non-specificity of the tests was that 'seropositivity does not mean virus positivity'. In other words, the 'HIV' test had not been shown to signify the presence of a virus. This astonishing but logical conclusion was buried in the text of the *Medical Hypotheses* paper and a further five years were to pass before it would be drawn to the attention of the scientific community in the *Bio/Technology* paper described in Chapter 9.

Having shown that the antibody test could readily give positive results without the presence of virus, Eleopulos went on to demonstrate that there was little, if any, of the virus readily detectable in Aids patients. She recalled that the initial reaction to the retrovirus hypothesis was sceptical *(Nature* turned down the Montagnier team's paper that was later held to have been the first to demonstrate the presence of HIV). However, after the publication in *Science* on 4 May 1984 of Gallo's batch of four papers staking out his own claim to have discovered the virus responsible for Aids (a claim subsequently discredited on several counts), the theory became almost universally accepted. In those papers, experimental evidence for the detection and isolation of HTLV-3, later to be known as HIV, was documented. But in another *Science* paper the following December, the American group reported failing to find HIV in fresh peripheral lymphocytes, lymph nodes, Kaposi's sarcoma tissue, bone marrow and spleen from patients with Aids and Aids related complex (ARC). They concluded:

> Thus the lymph node enlargement commonly found in ARC and Aids patients cannot be due directly to the proliferation of HTLV-3 infected cells... Whether the lymphocyte proliferation in lymph nodes occurs in response to infection with HTLV-3 or another agent, or both, is not known. Similarly, the absence of detectable HTLV-3 sequences in Kaposi's sarcoma tissue of Aids patients suggests that this tumour is not directly induced by infection of each tumour cell with HTLV-3. Furthermore the observation that HTLV-3 sequences are found rarely, if at all, in peripheral blood mononuclear cells, bone marrow and spleen provides the first direct evidence that these tissues are not heavily or widely infected with HTLV-3 in either Aids or ARC.

For similar reasons the French group had also admitted, in a 1986 article in *Nature,* that it was unlikely that Aids was the result of a direct progressive destruction of T4 cells by the virus. 'Thus,' Eleopulos stated, 'the originators of the viral theory of Aids agree that there is no direct evidence to support their theory.'

If that were the case, however, what had led Gallo and his collaborators to conclude that HIV *was* the cause of Aids? They had based their opinion on laboratory findings that had been interpreted as meaning that despite the admitted difficulty of detecting the virus in fresh tissues, it *could* be isolated from most HIV-positive people 'after some unusual and drastic manipulation of the lymphocytes obtained from the patients', as Eleopulos put it. All the experiments for detecting, characterising and isolating HIV, and for its continuous production, were done on these 'drastically manipulated' laboratory cultures. Furthermore, the cultures were not just prepared with T-cells from Aids patients, but were co-cultures with highly selected, usually cancerous (in order to get continuous production) T-cell lines.

Unlike other viruses, HIV had never been isolated as an independent, stable particle. In the vast majority of cases where 'isolation' was claimed, the basis of the claim was the detection of the enzyme reverse transcriptase (RT). This had been thought to be associated exclusively with retrovirus activity, but there was evidence (amply confirmed since) that all cells were capable of expressing it. Apart from RT, the cultures also had present in them almost every other enzyme implicated in DNA synthesis.

Some purported 'isolations' had included seeing virus-like particles budding from cell walls, but if any of them were HIV, they had never proved stable enough to be separated from the rest of the culture and thereby characterised with certainty. Such particles were not only hard to detect, but at least in some cases had been demonstrated to be normal organelles – discrete, membrane-bounded parts of the cell – and not viruses.

There were also studies showing that actin-myosin interaction, induced by oxidising agents, could trigger cells into producing particles. Most importantly, researchers had shown as far back as 1971 that normal, virus-free cells could be induced to produce particles 'which resemble RNA tumour viruses in every physical and chemical respect'. What had come to be called 'retroviruses' could arise spontaneously in virus-free cell cultures, and their rate of appearance could be increased a million-fold by the use of radiation, chemical mitogens, or infection of the culture with other viruses.

What did all this mean? It meant that the heroic measures Gallo's team had described to get 'HIV' to appear and grow, which included pooling T-cell samples from several Aids patients, manipulating the culture conditions with mitogenic stimulants, and the selection of special cell lines to which to add the rest of the cocktail, might simply have triggered natural cell mechanisms, including activation and replication of genetic sequences naturally present in the cells, whose results were mistakenly interpreted as indicating the presence of 'HIV' and which had nothing to do with a new, infectious agent.

This possibility was greatly strengthened by further findings. One was the fact that co-cultures of blood samples from Aids patients that were *not* stimulated did not show evidence of infection. Another was the fact that co-cultures of apparently uninfected cells had been persuaded to express 'HIV' when stimulated. And in a study co-authored by Gallo, it had been shown that when T4 cells from healthy people were exposed to supposedly infected cells and then 'immunologically activated' (stimulated), they would produce 'HIV' and die; but when the same infected cells were not stimulated, they did not express the 'virus'.

Since this was the case, even assuming that HIV existed and could be transmitted from a sick person to a healthy one, the healthy person would never become ill unless exposed to high concentrations of stimulatory agents. 'In other words, [HIV] by itself cannot produce ill-effects, while the mitogenic agents would produce the immunological and clinical abnormalities associated with Aids irrespective of [HIV] infection.'

Some years later, Montagnier made known that he had also reached the conclusion that 'HIV' on its own was harmless, and that it needed some other factors before it could contribute to Aids. In fact, in a 1991 paper in the journal *Virology,* he and his colleagues showed that activation, in the absence of 'HIV', can induce the same cell-killing effects. In other words, HIV is neither necessary nor sufficient to induce the cell-killing effects in 'HIV-infected' cultures.

Most leading Aids researchers, including Gallo, have now come around to a similar position. They still hold fast to the idea that 'HIV' *must* play a central role, but to this day, no one knows how, as an August 1995 report in *Science,* 'Researchers Air Alternative Views on How HIV Kills Cells', confirmed. The mystery is compounded by the fact that the virus is supposed to be producing the range of twenty-nine indicator diseases that qualify a person for an Aids diagnosis, which include cancers as well as opportunistic infections. As *Science's* Jon Cohen put it, 'the meeting focused on what has been one of the most puzzling and controversial scientific questions raised by HIV: How does it destroy the immune system and cause Aids?'. According to Phil

Johnson, of the Reappraisal Group, 'Official explanations of how an ordinary retrovirus can kill cells it never infects have grown ever more complicated as the prospect of a cure or vaccine has grown ever more distant'.

By contrast, as Eleopulos argued, an assault on the body by oxidative, mitogenic agents like sperm and nitrites could account for general viral activation, Aids-related malignancies such as KS and lymphoma, *and* loss of immune cell activity, since lymphocytes are highly sensitive to oxidative stress.

Haemophiliac patients could also be expected to show immunological activation, since all clotting factors were oxidising agents, the strongest being Factor 8. The latter had been found to be immunosuppressive both in laboratory studies and in patients. But the proportion of HIV-positive haemophiliacs developing Aids was smaller than among HIV-positive gay men, presumably because they were not facing the same multiple immunological assaults. Similarly, transfusion patients other than haemophiliacs faced well-documented immunological risks; but what was now reported as 'Aids' in haemophiliacs and transfusion recipients was only manifested as opportunistic infection (they do not suffer from KS or other Aids-related malignancies). Cases appearing before 1981 would not have been identified as Aids.

Finally, Eleopulos presented evidence that opiates, like nitrites, were oxidising agents, and that immune system abnormalities and clinical symptoms similar to those seen in Aids had been reported in drug abusers for many years prior to Aids.*

At every step in her paper, Eleopulos gave references to the scientific documents that supported her assertions and it is a real tragedy that her conclusions went unheeded. She had recognised, independently, that the virus – should it exist – was inactive to the point of oblivion, even in patients with Aids. She pointed to the dangers of using the non-specific 'HIV' test in Africa, dangers which have only recently been driven home by others, and the paucity of Aids cases in that continent despite high levels of 'HIV'-positivity.

* As documented in detail by Gordon Stewart in Chapter 5.

Anti-oxidant Therapies Proposed

Eleopulos also raised the possibility that prevention, and even cure, of Aids might be achieved with appropriate anti-oxidant agents – a strategy that has gained an increasing level of both scientific and patient support in the 1990s.

Health activist organisations such as HEAL, Continuum and Positively Healthy have insisted for years that improvement in the quality of diet plays a central role in long-term survival of HIV-positive and Aids patients, and much of the focus of that improvement has been with respect to fresh fruit and vegetables, which contain many anti-oxidant substances, and anti-oxidant supplements such as vitamins C and E, beta-carotene and selenium.

On the scientific side, a November 1993 conference at the US National Institutes of Health heard a description of 'factors supporting the existence of oxidative stress in HIV/Aids', looked at how oxidative stress 'contributes to promotion of viral replication and immune cell death', and discussed proposals for therapies and clinical trials based on plant products with anti-oxidant properties. Chairing one of the sessions was Dr Leonard Herzenberg, of Stanford University School of Medicine, who the following May reported in the *Proceedings of the National Academy of Sciences* studies implicating a drop in the body's concentration of glutathione, one of the main mechanisms for protecting against oxidative harm, as playing a critical role in the decay of the immune system seen in Aids. Glutathione is ordinarily abundant inside all body cells, where it plays a role in synthesising new genetic material as well as disposing of unwanted oxygen molecules ('free radicals') generated during cell activity.

To see how its loss affects T-cell performance, Herzenberg and other Stanford researchers isolated T-cells from healthy people and lowered their stores of glutathione chemically. They found that with about a 25 per cent reduction, the cells failed to respond to signals that would normally stimulate them into multiplying to mount an anti-microbial attack. At the same time, the manipulated T-cells became inappropriately sensitive to other signals, including tumour necrosis factor, a chemical normally associated with inflammatory reactions and which imposes a further oxidative burden on the cells. Eventually, this vicious cycle results in the confused and damaged cells committing suicide in a process known as apoptosis or programmed cell death. Montagnier was the first to draw the attention of the world Aids community to the role of apoptosis in Aids, now often cited by mainstream researchers as central to the loss of T-cells.

Thus, the picture really begins to come together. Observers such as Lauritsen had noted the particularly prominent role of nitrite inhalants in the lives of most gay men with Aids. Scientists like Dr Dennis Parke* had concluded that the nitrites were a key factor in the pathogenesis of Aids, noting that the chemicals led to the formation of nitrosoglutathione, which robbed the body of its natural defence (glutathione) against toxic chemicals and drugs, and against the toxicity of oxygen radicals. Montagnier's group had identified T-cell 'suicide' (apoptosis) as a key factor in Aids. Gallo had puzzled over his lab's data pointing to the presence of immune stimulation, triggered by inflammatory cytokines (of which tumour necrosis factor is one), in T-cells thought to have been crippled by HIV, adding: 'But we have learned – this should be of interest to everybody that isn't completely married to HIV – that the inflammatory cytokines are reportedly increased in gay men even without HIV infection...I wish I knew what else was increasing them before a gay man was ever infected with HIV. Maybe it's nitric oxide [from poppers], maybe it's a sexually transmitted virus, maybe it's all of them, maybe it has to do with rimming (oral-anal sex) because it's immune stimulation with non-specific infections...'

Now researchers such as the Stanford team were showing precisely how loss of glutathione causes T-cells to self-destruct. Furthermore, although grossly neglected by mainstream research, and subject to much ill-informed criticism by HIV (and AZT) zealots, considerable evidence has already been collected that some plant-based medicines, with proven antioxidant action, can bring dramatic improvement even in patients already gravely ill with Aids.** Finally, gay health activists had long insisted that when HIV-positive

* See Chapter 11

** Dr Howard Greenspan, of the US company Advanced Biological Systems, which markets two such products from a Swiss-based research research physician, Dr Jozsef Roka, has been battling for several years to draw this research to the attention of Aids organisations. When I met him in London in 1993 he told some horrific stories of the rudeness and prejudice he had encountered from AZT-promoting, Wellcome-funded organisations both in the US and Britain.

and even Aids patients cut out drugs and improved their diet, as well as implementing safer sex practices, they frequently stayed or became well.

The one remaining problem, that may now be all that stands in the way of an understanding of Aids, and rational preventive and therapeutic measures, is the continued belief in 'HIV'.

Challenge to HIV Isolation Claims

In 1989, Eleopulos further developed her questioning of the virus's very existence, although still not making that challenge explicit, in a long, brilliantly argued letter to the *Lancet*. Despite complimenting her on her 'interesting' and 'detailed and well-referenced' letter, however, the journal decided not to find room for it.

To understand the full power of her critique in this and subsequent papers, we need to look in some detail at the conventions that have arisen surrounding virus isolation. In the 1950s, in fresh, uncultured tumour tissue and in cell cultures derived from it, particles later attributed to retroviruses were readily detectable with the electron microscope. In the 1960s, the technique of spinning biological material in a density-graded centrifuge (the further the materials travel down the test-tube, the greater the density) was introduced, and found capable of separating and isolating such sub-cellular particles, including viruses. However, because some cell constituents were found to separate out at the same density as viruses, when viruses were isolated from cell cultures the best results were obtained with a preparation containing a lot of virus, and few cellular contaminants The method used involves first separating out the liquid part of the cell culture (called the supernatant), then putting that through the centrifuge.

When these conditions were met, one could obtain – at a density of 1.16 grams per millilitre, using sucrose as the separation medium in the centrifuge – a relatively pure concentration of retroviral particles. Even so, the presence of other cell constituents, including fragments from disrupted cells, could not be avoided. So to prove that the material which banded at the relevant density really did contain little else but the particles, and that these were indeed retroviruses, every such preparation underwent three more steps. These were:

1. Examination with the electron microscope to see how many particles were present and ensure that they all looked roughly the same.
2. Biochemical analysis to look for reverse transcriptase, and viral and cellular RNA and proteins, so as to be able to characterise the particles and any contaminants.
3. Biological tests, to ensure that the isolated material was genuinely infectious.

Since 'HIV' has proved impossible to obtain directly from fresh patient tissue, the isolation techniques used have been particularly fraught with confounding factors. The Aids patient's cells have to be co-cultured with other cells, usually from a highly abnormal leukaemic T-cell line. Even that was not enough: the work that led to the Gallo team's original claims of having isolated HIV involved pooling fluids from the T-cell cultures of no fewer than ten individual Aids patients with the leukaemic cells (this was not stated in the original paper, but came to light during subsequent investigations). Furthermore, Gallo and in fact all other HIV researchers have used stimulatory, mitogenic agents to drive the culture into expressing its 'HIV'.

After a few weeks, the resulting fluid, with intact cell material strained off, is separated out according to density by centrifugation, and the material that bands at 1.16 gm/ml is considered to be retroviral. In HIV work, detection out of that material of either reverse transcriptase (RT) activity, and/or proteins which produce an antigen-antibody reaction with sera from the patient, is considered equivalent to virus isolation.

Eleopulos argued that to infer the presence of a virus on the basis of such findings is faulty reasoning. Even to claim detection of proteins associated with HIV would be wrong if there were some non-HIV explanation for the presence of the reactive proteins (antigens) and RT – as is indeed the case. RT can be found in all cells, although its appearance and level of activity depend on the culture conditions which, in turn, depend on the type of cell used and its physiological state. It was those parameters which determined the detection of RT, not the presence of HIV. Similarly, the protein antigens attributed to HIV, although not usually detected in healthy tissue, *are* present in non-HIV-infected cells from people with other disease conditions, and can be induced in normal, non-HIV-infected cells by mitogenic stimulation (i.e. they are non-specific, as we saw in the discussion on the 'HIV' test in Chapter 9).

What, then, about the diagrams and photographs of 'HIV' particles, complete with mine-like receptor knobs, and an apparently well-documented, specific complement of genes? Once again, not all is as it has seemed. The diagrams are based to some extent on unproven assumptions. (The group that first put forward the model including surface knobs subsequently said these were only found in immature particles still budding from the cell wall, which were 'very rarely observed', and were seen only on 'metabolically impaired cells'. Furthermore, the mature particles hardly react at all with antibodies from patients with Aids.)

Most of the electron microscope photographs have only shown particles still in culture, not in the centrifuged material. Before the Aids era, many retrovirologists showed that finding a particle with features similar to retroviruses does not prove that they are retroviruses, nor that they are infectious. Particles of this kind have been reported in milk, in cultures of embryonic tissues, in sperm, and in most human placentas, as well as in cell line cultures used for 'HIV isolation' which have not been exposed to Aids patient material. Since neither Gallo's team, nor anybody else before or since, has published electron micrographs clearly demonstrating isolated HIV particles in the material derived from Aids cultures which bands at 1.16 gm/ml, 'it is impossible to know which, if any, of the particles band at that density'. Another problem is that although particles detected in stimulated Aids co-cultures are considered to be HIV, there are different views as to which subgroup and family of retrovirus they belong. Montagnier's group initially reported HIV as a Type C oncovirus, then a Type D oncovirus, and subsequently as belonging to the lentivirus family.

Particles can be seen in the lymph nodes of Aids patients, and researchers refer to these as HIV. But in the one carefully conducted electron microscope study[4] of this phenomenon, comparing samples from 'HIV-positive' patients with those from a control group of patients who also had swollen lymph nodes, particles attributed to HIV were found in 90 per cent of the patients and 87 per cent of the controls, leading the authors to conclude that 'such particles do not, by themselves, indicate infection with HIV'.

Even more importantly, it turns out that the DNA of normal, noninfected human tissue contains numerous genetic sequences that have been attributed to 'retroviruses', including several that are homologous (almost the same) as sequences attributed to HIV.

In other words, Eleopulos reasoned, the 'HIV' found in the mitogenically stimulated laboratory cultures may be no more than a package synthesised as a result of activation and recombination of some of these many, naturally present gene sequences. 'HIV may not exist in all Aids patients, if in any,' she wrote. That this might be the case was supported by the studies showing that mitogenic stimulation of cell cultures leads to the expression of 'retroviruses' (given the right conditions for the cell type and its physiological status) even though there is none initially present. It was also supported by evidence that no two identical 'HIVs' have been isolated, not even from the same individual.

It was this latter phenomenon that proved disastrous for Gallo's claims to have been the first to find the 'Aids virus'. The 'HIVs' identified by Montagnier and himself, although not absolutely identical, were eventually agreed to be so close as to have convinced the scientific community that they came from the same patient, a Frenchman. (That was not the case to begin with, however; Gallo's first paper sequencing 'the Aids virus, HTLV-3', published in *Nature* on 24 January 1985, gave the virus 9,749 nucleotides – the 'letters' of the genetic alphabet – whereas the Institut Pasteur group, led by British expatriate Simon Wain-Hobson, gave it 9,193 nucleotides in a paper published in *Cell* a few days previously.)

Exceptional Research Climate

Gallo's rush to stay ahead of the French created an exceptional research climate of which the full story has still not been told, despite the prodigious efforts of John Crewdson in the *Chicago Tribune*. The crazy events of the time included publication in *Science* of electron micrographs that purported to show Gallo's virus, but which subsequently turned out to be of particles cultured in Gallo's lab with the French patient's cells, sent to him by Montagnier for research purposes.

It was a strange twist of fate that Gallo's unseemly behaviour in the affair helped to convince the scientific community that his arch-rivals, the French team, really had cultured a genuine Aids virus, a claim that Gallo originally challenged. 'Bob never believed the French,' a scientist with close ties to both camps told Crewdson. 'He never thought LAV [the French group's original name for their 'Aids virus'] was real; he thought everything they wrote was wrong.'

'No one has ever been able to work with their particles,' Gallo wrote to the editor of the *Lancet* a few weeks before his 1984 *Science* papers were published. 'Because of the lack of permanent production and characterisation it is hard to say they are really "isolated" in the sense that virologists use this term.' Originally, when the French researchers published their first paper in *Science*, Gallo and others questioned whether the electron microscope pictures of particles accompanying the article were of a human retrovirus. In a letter to *Nature* in 1986 explaining how his own laboratory had come to have similar pictures, he wrote that 'Naturally, we wanted to check the material received from Dr Montagnier by electron microscopy to check this contention'. According to Eleopulos, he was right to doubt the French claims of isolation.

Gallo also originally dismissed as 'ridiculous' the French team's claims that they had identified a retrovirus specific to Aids on the grounds that their culture reacted with antibodies in blood samples from Aids patients. 'That's bad virology,' Gallo had said. 'Patient sera, especially in Aids patients, has antibodies to a lot of different things.' Once again he was right, as amply demonstrated by Eleopulos years later in her *Bio/Technology* dissection of the non-specificity of all 'HIV' tests. Although the French checked for cross-reactions with serum from patients known to be infected with other common viruses, patients with Aids have antibodies to numerous 'self' proteins as well as to an enormous range of microbes.

Amazingly, Gallo had been right all along! His mistake, however, was to enter what he later called the 'passionate' stage when his own candidate as the 'Aids virus', HTLV-1, proved a non-starter with the scientific community. It was just as unproven as the French candidate, but carried the additional burden of having previously been linked with the uncontrolled white blood cell growth of leukaemia, rather than the loss of cells seen in Aids. At this point, with the National Cancer Institute suddenly coming under acute pressure from the Reagan administration (previously neglectful of what had been seen as an exclusively gay problem) to do something about Aids, he seems to have allowed his competitiveness to overcome his judgement, leaping on to the bandwagon of the French 'Aids virus' – but naming it as 'HTLV-3' – once it appeared to have started to roll.

Whatever it was that the French had come up with, and which Gallo was now working with, Gallo's own attempts to identify it as a specific retrovirus were equally inadequate. As Montagnier had done, he also looked for reactivity with serum from Aids patients, and in addition, with antibody-containing serum obtained by injecting a laboratory rabbit with 'HTLV-3'. But 'HTLV-3' meant an unidentified isolate from the stimulated, leukaemic cell culture, whose contents could still be expected to include human cell proteins liable to trigger 'anti-self' antibodies or antibodies resulting from cellular activity independent of the presence of an infectious virus. As Val Turner has commented, 'How was it possible to ensure the specificity of rabbit antisera to a virus before the virus has been isolated?'

We saw above that the protein antigens attributed to HIV, although not usually detected in healthy tissue, can be induced in normal, non-HIV-infected cells by mitogenic stimulation; and also that the cell line cultures used for 'HIV isolation' can produce particles even when they have not been 'infected' with Aids patient material. If this evidence of 'virus' infection is in reality a consequence of naturally present, endogenous (originating from within) cell processes, why have the same phenomena not been reported more often in 'control' cultures, that is, in cultures not treated with sera from Aids patients?

One reason, Eleopulos has proposed, could be that the culture conditions have been optimised according to what best stimulates the Aids patient tissues into expressing 'HIV'. The physiological state of the T-cells and other tissue taken from healthy controls is different, and could be expected to require different culture conditions for the 'HIV' genes to be activated.

Another reason could be that the tissues from patients with Aids or from people in groups at risk of Aids are already mitogenically stimulated by their exposure to sperm, nitrites, opiates, Factor 8, and so on. Many of these patients also receive chemotherapy and/or radiation treatment, which have been shown to cause DNA damage that activates gene expression and facilitates 'retrovirus' detection, including 'HIV'. Val Turner argues that the most appropriate controls would be sick rather than healthy people, 'with lots of antibodies, low T4 cells, low redox, exposure to drugs and other agents, but not with Aids. That is, the circumstances must exist that might predispose to the development of "retroviral" phenomena'.

Finally, controls are not always used, and when they are the tests are not done 'blind', so the experimenters may be biased in what they see and how they interpret it by their expectations. Failure to detect reverse transcriptase in the controls is especially suspicious, given that with the right conditions, all cells can express RT activity. Normal human placenta, which has been extensively used in Aids research, contains particles attributed to retroviruses, and yet claims of 'virus isolation' are abundant in samples from Aids patients but never reported in non-Aids samples.

In 1991, the Institut Pasteur published in their journal *Research in Immunology* a paper jointly authored by Eleopulos, Turner and Papadimitriou, who as well as being professor of pathology at the University of Western Australia is an internationally renowned expert on electron microscopy. Entitled 'Oxidative Stress, HIV and Aids', the paper did not overtly challenge HIV's existence. It did point out, however, that HIV had only been 'isolated' from laboratory cultures, not from fresh tissues, and that this could not be done unless the cultures were subjected to oxidative stress.

A more explicit statement of the Eleopulos team's concerns about the claims made for HIV isolation had to wait until 1993, when the journal *Emergency Medicine* published an article entitled 'Has Gallo Proven the Role of HIV in Aids?', again with Turner and Papadimitriou as co-authors. This invited paper, which arose out of an address to the Australasian College for Emergency Medicine, Sydney, in November 1992, reached similar conclusions to the *Lancet* letter, but demonstrated them in the context of Gallo's original claims. The paper concluded: 'The data and arguments that have been presented by Gallo and his colleagues do not constitute proof of HIV isolation or an unambiguous role for HIV in the pathogenesis of Aids.' It added that although some researchers use methods of 'viral isolation' essentially the same as that described by Gallo's group, most use even *less* rigorous methods.

The *Bio/Technology* paper, which also appeared in 1993, further documented the scientific case against the existence of HIV, although the arguments were presented in the context of the critique of the 'HIV' test. It provided references to the work showing that normal, uninfected cells contain genetic sequences closely related to, or identical with, those of retroviruses. Depending on conditions, this 'provirus', as it has come to be called, remains unexpressed, partially expressed or fully expressed. Sometimes particles are produced without any genetic material at their core; sometimes the core genetic material has one or more genes missing. This means that finding antigens linked to such a provirus, and the associated antibodies, does not prove the presence of infectious virus. Furthermore, animal data show that new genetic packages arise, to which two or more 'proviruses' may contribute.

The genetic data on 'HIV' present many such problems, Eleopulos says. The data differ in different types of cell within a single individual. Studies have also shown that the type of 'HIV' isolated depends on the culture conditions used, as well as the type of cells. Howard Temin, the Nobel Laureate and discoverer of reverse transcriptase, stated in a 1993 book:[5] 'The data indicate that in any one Aids patient, at any one time, there are many different virus genomes' (more than 100 million genetically distinct variants, according to data published in 1995).[6] In one case where two sequential isolates were made from the same person sixteen months apart, none of the provirus in the first isolate was found in the second, leading one HIV researcher to conclude: 'The data imply that there is no such thing as an [Aids virus] isolate.'[7]

These findings also indicate that maps of 'HIV' genes, built up painstakingly by sequencing material derived from Aids patient cultures, are to some extent artificial, constructed according to precedents set by previous workers rather than according to biological fact. Indeed, Gallo's team had originally challenged the French interpretation of their sequence data. Crewdson, in his account of that event in his 1989 investigation, put one aspect of the problem very neatly: 'Constructing a gene map from a DNA sequence can be compared to translating poetry from a foreign language. The poet's thrust may be obvious, but the elegance of the finished translation will turn on words that can be interpreted in more than one way. For a multitude of reasons, it is possible for two scientists to look at the same DNA sequence and disagree about where a gene begins and ends, or even whether it exists at all.'

In the case of 'HIV', it seems that even the poet's thrust is far from obvious. According to a report in *Nature,* more than 99.9 per cent of 'HIV genomes' may be defective: that is, if one obtains 1,000 'HIV genomes' and subjects them to detailed analysis, only one would have the full complement of genes. Yet it appears to be only by convention that that one is considered to be the complete version, as opposed to containing extra sequences compared with others. Such enormous variation suggests that one is not looking at a particular species of 'virus' at all, but rather that one is seeing natural variance of genetic expression, within and between individuals, by the genetic machinery of stimulated cells.

To improve detection, the polymerase chain reaction (PCR) method was introduced by HIV researchers. It lies behind many recent claims of increased levels of detection. It cannot be regarded as signifying the presence of the whole 'HIV genome', since with PCR relatively small regions of genetic material can be identified, one gene at best. Besides, even if one did identify all the sequences attributed to 'HIV', that still would not mean virus was present. The cells may have the information needed to synthesise 'virus' particles, but foremost researchers are agreed that that does not happen unless some special circumstances are fulfilled.

Evidence has mounted that the positive PCR signals may be due to events triggered within the cell's own genes by the stimulatory, oxidative burden to which the Aids risk groups and cultures are exposed. For example, some studies have shown that a positive PCR reverts to negative when exposure to risk factors is discontinued.[8] Another has shown that cells from HIV-positive patients in which no HIV DNA can be detected, even by PCR, become positive for HIV RNA when they are co-cultivated with normal, stimulated T-cells.[9] This is powerful confirmation of the idea that 'HIV' is a consequence of a pathogenic process, not a cause – possibly even a reflection of an attempt by the over-stressed cell to protect the body against the stimulatory assault.

This requirement for cell activation before 'HIV'-type genetic sequences can normally be detected explains why early HIV researchers failed to detect such sequences in 'uninfected' cells, leading them to conclude that 'this virus is exogenous to man'.[10] In fact, more refined studies have shown that the human genome itself – the totality of genes in the cell – contains sequences similar to (and according to Eleopulos's way of thinking, contributing to the make-up of) those seen in 'HIV'. In one study,[11] researchers demonstrated the presence of 'a complex family of HIV-1 related sequences' in human, chimpanzee and Rhesus monkey DNA from normal, uninfected individuals.

In another, PCR testing of human genome DNA with probes specific to the reverse transcriptase sequences of HTLV-1, HTLV-2 and HIV proved positive, even under stringent conditions requiring a near-perfect match.[12]

Genes That Jump Generations

These and other similar findings raise the intriguing and challenging question: do *any* human retroviruses exist in the sense of genuinely infectious, pathogenic agents that invade us from outside? Is retro*virology* a misnomer for a natural mechanism of gene activation and replication, akin to the 'jumping genes' phenomenon that so surprised geneticists when Barbara McClintock first proposed it in 1947 that it took until 1983 for her discoveries to be recognised with the Nobel prize?

We saw in Chapter 6 that within the human genome, about 10 per cent comprises transposons, genes that can move both from one part of a chromosome to another, and from one chromosome to another. We also saw that some move around the cell in the form of an RNA intermediate, and use reverse transcriptase to integrate themselves as DNA at their new site. So-called retroviruses differ from transposons in that they have a protein coat facilitating their ability to leave the cell and travel elsewhere. It seems likely, however, that at least some of the phenomena attributed to and described as 'HIV', especially when the PCR detection method is used, are no more than signals of transposon activity, and not even evidence of the presence of a retrovirus as conventionally described. This would explain the high levels of 'virus isolation' claimed with PCR compared with traditional techniques that focus on extracellular phenomena.

Names are important. As long as mobile genetic elements are referred to as 'viral', the impression we have of them – scientists as well as the public – is of an unwanted invader. In some organisms, when these elements are seen to transpose through an RNA intermediate, they have been termed 'retrotransposons', which is appropriate. In mammals and birds, however, they are commonly referred to as 'endogenous retroviral elements'. This conveys a more sinister role for them, but there is no logic to the distinction. Exceptionally, as in all biological mechanisms, a natural process can produce a harmful result, such as when a 'jumping gene' switches on a genetic mechanism that ought to stay silent, or switches off a protective mechanism. But in general the mechanism appears to be benign.

There seems to be something about the present model of human biological functioning that makes it difficult for the scientific community to accept either that there is such dynamism present within the cell, or that it could have a benign purpose. Barbara McClintock waited decades before recognition of her 'jumping genes' concept. Similarly, Dr Ted Steele, an Australian immunologist, has experienced harsh treatment – especially from *Nature* – in trying to win consideration of a theory that he first put forward nearly twenty years ago, that useful changes to the body's immune system may be passed on to succeeding generations by genetic inheritance.

When the immune system responds to an invading microbe, a large number of genes are brought into action to synthesise an appropriate antibody. DNA rearrangements take place inside the lymphocytes, and the resulting sequences code production of a strip of RNA which provides the pattern from which the cell can make the antibody proteins. Steele first postulated in a book published in 1979 that genetic arrangements that had been successfully 'tested' in the body cells in this way were carried to germ line (reproductive) tissue in the gonads (the testes and ovaries), and integrated there into related DNA sites by reverse transcriptase, so that they could be passed on to offspring. Germ cells are traditionally thought to be quite separate from body cells such as lymphocytes, but Steele and co-workers at the Australian National University have demonstrated body cell patterns in the germ line cells, and are developing ways of tracking genes in transit. There is already strong evidence that the mechanism of transport is 'retroviral' – that is, through particles that bud from the cell and carry the desired genetic package to the reproductive cells. The idea that a main role of these 'retrovirus' particles is to pass useful genes to offspring is strengthened by the detection of such particles – and reverse transcriptase – in a variety of normal human reproductive tract tissues and secretions including placenta extracts, amniotic fluid, ovarian follicular fluid and semen.

It is interesting to speculate whether in a stressed immune system, the same mechanism comes into play in order to amplify a desired immune response within the individual, by transferring useful genetic packages from cell to cell. A central part of the response that became misinterpreted as 'HIV' may be played by the genes of the major histocompatibility complex (MHC), whose protein products are important to the control machinery that limits the immune system's destructive potential. If there is an auto-immune component to Aids, it probably lies in such territory: lymphocytes chronically exposed to semen and blood may start self-destroying, a reaction then brought under some control by the gene products attributed to 'HIV'.

Ted Steele confirms that 'when cells that make antibodies are put under stress, they certainly make large quantities of endogenous retroviruses'. (To avoid the confusing 'deadly virus' connotations, some other term for these endogenous agents is needed – 'extracellular jumping genes', perhaps, or 'enveloped transposons'.)

Eleopulos believes 'HIV' cultures are simply systems that propagate certain endogenous genetic sequences which come from cells subject to oxidative stress. It was one of these endogenously produced genetic packages that Montagnier's group originally succeeded in producing, and which Gallo's team propagated by transferring into a leukaemic cell line. That did not mean it was a virus, nor an infectious agent of any sort, nor even that the patient from whom it came was 'infected'. However, because the antibody test constructed on the basis of it often detected proteins produced by similarly stressed cells in people with Aids and at risk of Aids, and because genetic testing often picked up the presence of stretches of similar genetic material inside activated T-cells, perhaps part of a family of related genes, the virological community mistakenly developed the concept that a new, lethal virus was at large, which the world came to know of as the Human Immunodeficiency Virus.

Papadimitriou, Eleopulos's distinguished pathologist collaborator, summarises his view as follows: 'They have not proven that they have actually detected a unique, exogenous retrovirus. The critical data to support that idea have not been presented. You have to be absolutely certain that what you have detected is unique and exogenous, and a single molecular species. They haven't got conclusively to that first step. Just to see particles in the tissues, and fail to look for evidence that it is an infective virus, is wrong. Are these particles that cause disease? The proper controls have never been done. There is no evidence, ten years on, that the particles are a new infectious virus.'

Challenge to Data on Infectiousness

Peter Duesberg, despite being convinced of the harmlessness of HIV, has regarded it as a genuine infectious virus. When I asked him if there was any laboratory or other scientific evidence of its infectiousness, he called Jay Levy, one of the first virologists to claim independent isolation of 'the Aids-associated retrovirus' (ARV), as he had originally called his version of 'HIV'. Levy referred to a paper published in *Science* by himself and others in 1986 in which they described 'transfection' of a cell line with a laboratory-constructed molecular clone of ARV/HIV. They saw reverse transcriptase (RT) activity in the cell line, leading them to conclude that it was producing virus. Then, when this 'virus' from the cell line was passed to mitogen-stimulated, normal human cells obtained from healthy volunteers, viral antigens were detected. They also found that an infected cell line contained all the protein antigens associated with ARV, and showed cytopathic (cell-damaging) effects 'typical of Aids retroviruses'. They concluded: 'This clone gives rise to replicating infectious virus that has the biologic characteristics of ARV...These results indicate that ARV is the sole cause for these known properties of the Aids retrovirus.'

The Australian group challenge these conclusions. First, they question the idea that the molecular clone Levy had constructed had any relationship with a genuine virus. His team had taken a stretch of RNA, about the size postulated for a retrovirus, from the culture medium of an 'ARV-infected' cell line, but presented no evidence that it belonged to a retrovirus-like particle, with proteins and nucleic acids. Nor was there any evidence that the cells which were 'transfected' with the cloned material produced virus particles.

Given the stimulated culture conditions used, it would have been surprising not to see RT activity, irrespective of 'ARV', because RT was not specific to retroviruses. And the appearance of the protein antigens proved nothing, since they were also non-specific (for the many reasons described in Chapter 9), and neither Levy nor any other HIV researchers presented unambiguous evidence that the proteins were indeed coded by the stretch of RNA he used to construct his clone.

Even if Levy – and Montagnier, and Gallo – did have a genuine particle-like gene package capable of leaving one cell and entering others (an 'endogenous retrovirus', or enveloped transposon), that would still not make it an infectious, disease-inducing virus. The fact that Levy reported cytopathic effects was readily explained by the manipulation of the cells. As far back as January 1985, Montagnier cautioned that the 'Aids virus' did not produce such effects on its own, and that they could only be observed in activated, stimulated T-cells; and years later he showed that activation, in the absence of 'HIV', can induce the same effects.

The essence of the problem in Levy's procedure was the lack of acknowledgement that all cells contain 'retroviral' genomes, which under the right conditions may be expressed, producing RT and other proteins, without any need for an infectious or even 'transfected' agent. It could have been the act of transfection, and the cell-stimulating conditions of the experiment, that led to the appearance of 'retroviral' phenomena. To check that possibility, Eleopulos said, it was essential to have a 'control' culture, in which exactly the same procedure was followed but using a clone with different (non-'ARV/HIV') genes. According to the Eleopulos group, it is the lack of such control procedures that has bedevilled HIV research throughout the Aids years.

Eleopulos says that 'to me, the presently available evidence does not prove even that it is an endogenous retrovirus, because what we see, the phenomena collectively known as HIV, are non-specific. RT is non-specific; virus-like particles are non-specific; the antigen-antibody reactions are non-specific; PCR is non-specific. You can't even say you have a retrovirus there.' According to Val Turner, 'HIV is a metaphor for a lot of quasi-related phenomena. No one has ever proved its existence as a virus. We don't believe it exists.'

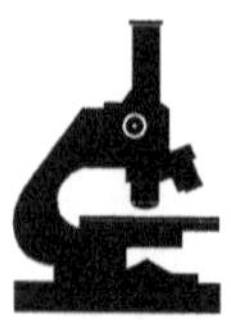

13: A BETTER FIT

The Australian group's theory that 'HIV' is a term for a collection of biological phenomena associated with an over-stressed immune system resolves many of the puzzles and paradoxes described in this book with which the orthodox theory has struggled.

Firstly, there is the lack of epidemiological evidence, fifteen years into the Aids epidemic, of the syndrome being caused by an infectious, bi-directionally sexually transmitted microbe. The 'lethal virus' dogma stated that HIV/Aids, as with other sexually transmitted diseases, could be transmitted both ways, from the active to the passive partner and vice versa. This led to the central prediction that the syndrome, although initially restricted to certain risk groups, would spread rapidly through the general population. Eleopulos emphasises, however, that around the world, several large, well-designed studies both in homosexuals and heterosexuals have shown without exception that the only sexual act directly related to the development of 'HIV'-positivity and Aids is *passive* anal intercourse.

Duesberg's theory that Aids is caused by long-term drug consumption may account for many cases of Aids, but does not have an adequate explanation for this observation. Eleopulos's oxidative stress theory, however, both accommodates and explains the data. Aids can be sexually acquired by a homosexual man who is a frequent passive recipient of sperm. The risk could come from the challenge to the immune system presented by the seminal fluid and sperm itself, synergistically increased by repeated exposure to sperm heavily infected with known microbes such as cytomegalovirus, which became hugely prevalent in promiscuous gay men during the 1970s 'gay lib' sexual revolution. But the theory predicts that sex in itself will not put at risk a gay man who never has sex as a passive partner.

Similarly, sex could never be an Aids risk to an exclusively heterosexual man, because he will never be a passive recipient of sperm. The syndrome *could* be heterosexually acquired by a woman, through exposure to the toxic effect – in anal sex – from sperm, or because of exposure to ejaculate carrying an immunosuppressive infectious agent such as CMV, or both, acting synergistically. But it can only go one way in heterosexual sex – the disease cannot be sexually transmitted in the usual sense of the word.

Today, fifteen years after the appearance of Aids as a recognisable disease, its heterosexual transmission – the main prediction of the HIV theory – is still unfulfilled. Aids, as we have seen, remains almost exclusively confined to the original risk groups. The promised heterosexual spread has not occurred – even into female prostitutes, in the European and American context, other than those who are also heavy drug users. Aids doctors *do* see cases among the immediate, close contacts of risk-group victims, but Eleopulos's analysis accommodates these one-way cases more easily than Duesberg's, with its exclusive concentration on the immunosuppressive effects of drugs. Relative to the total, cases in which men are reported as having developed Aids through sex with infected women are rare, and offer poor statistical support for heterosexual transmission, given much evidence in previous data of covert drug abuse, homosexual/bisexual practices and misdiagnosis.

A second major difficulty for the HIV hypothesis resolved by the oxidative stress theory is the enormously long and variable latency period between 'infection' and disease. 'It's not that HIV "hides" in cells for a long time, then suddenly creates havoc when it starts to reproduce, as HIV theorists have told us,' says Dr Stefan Lanka, a young German molecular biologist who supports Eleopulos's analysis. 'Rather, what they are calling HIV is simply a part of the cell's own function, which becomes expressed under certain conditions.'

A long-awaited book by Duesberg, *Inventing the Aids Virus,*[1] effectively dismantles the 'slow virus' concept, arguing that no such entity has ever been shown to exist, although conventional viruses can be *slow acting* in a defective immune system, or break out periodically, like herpes viruses, when the immune system is depressed. Even among animals, chronic retrovirus infections are restricted to inbred strains that have lost natural immunity.

'In both examples, only the weakened immune system of the host allows the infection to smoulder or occasionally reappear from hibernation,' Duesberg writes. 'By contrast, a "slow" virus is an invention credited with the natural ability to cause disease only years after infection – termed the "latent" period – in previously healthy persons, regardless of the state of their immunity. Such a concept allows scientists to blame a long-neutralised virus for a disease that appears decades after infection. The slow virus – never proven to exist – is the original sin against the laws of virology. It would help destroy our standards for determining if a disease is truly an infection, or caused by a particular germ, for it would allow researchers to blame a disease on a germ even if it was undetectable or barely present in a victim.' That is exactly what has happened with HIV, in Duesberg's view. In most people with Aids, no virus particles can be found anywhere in the body. Yet in all classical viral diseases, free particles are clearly detectable. In hepatitis B, for example, about 10 million such particles are present in each few drops of blood. In diarrhoea caused by rotavirus infection, between one and 100 billion virus particles are present in each gram of faeces.

Thirdly, no photograph of an *isolated* 'HIV' particle has ever been published, even from cultured material. This is disputed by some, who point to (very rare) electron microscope pictures of centrifuged material which they claim includes HIV particles. The example usually cited is from an article published in *Virology* (vol. 189, pp. 695-714) in 1992. Eleopulos, however, says that not only do the pictures not show pure particles, but more importantly they were not of material which bands at 1.16 gm/ml, 'the absolutely minimum requirement that a retroviral particle must satisfy'.

What is unquestionable is that it is so difficult to isolate 'HIV' to the point that it is free of everything else, and characterise its proteins unambiguously, that it has never been possible to do this routinely and thereby use virus isolation as a means of validating the 'HIV' test. Dr Steven B. Harris, an American physician who has exposed some deficiencies in the arguments of 'HIV' dissidents, revealed lack of awareness of the significance of this problem in a recent rejoinder to Lanka.[2] He confessed that 'I know of no really good photos of HIV isolated directly from humans, but the virus is present in low concentrations outside cells in humans, and contamination is great. What is wrong with culturing it first?'. The problem with culturing it first, as Eleopulos has demonstrated, is that the oxidative, stimulatory culture procedures and abnormal cell lines used introduce so many other factors as to make it extremely uncertain what the end products mean, and whether or not they signify the presence of a unique infectious agent or endogenously produced cell proteins and genetic elements. Because of this uncertainty – and because, in fact, no pure virus has ever been obtained – it is not clear what proteins are used in the 'HIV' test. This is why it has been beset with so many difficulties, as we saw in chapters 9 and 10.

Here, also, is the explanation for the dramatic 1991 findings described in Maddox's 'Aids Research Turned Upside Down'* article, in which mice and monkeys injected with immune system cells from other animals became HIV-positive, despite no exposure to 'HIV'. The antibodies that had been assumed to signify the presence of a virus did not necessarily do any such thing. If Maddox's call for 'heart-searching throughout the world's programmes of Aids research' in response to these findings had been heeded, and if he had stuck with his own gut reaction that the findings were hugely significant, the pathology at the root of Aids science might have been brought to light much sooner.

Aids researchers were encouraged in their belief in a viral aetiology for Aids, and in HIV, when a genetic sequence was ascribed to it. But according to Lanka, who obtained his doctorate at the University of Constanz after isolating new plant viruses, what really happens is that at the end of the complicated, stimulatory, co-culturing procedures, large amounts of unrelated sequences of RNA are present, from which a stretch corresponding to the 'correct' length of 'HIV' – that is, similar to that of the genome of other purported 'retroviruses' – is selected.

Thereafter, most researchers have worked exclusively with cloned genetic sequences, studying the effects of these sequences in the minutest detail, on the assumption that the original characterisation had been performed correctly, and unaware that the 'virus' they were supposed to represent was a natural cell product – a 'transposon' or 'enveloped transposon'.

Because the isolation and identification procedures used are finding a variety of naturally present genetic sequences rather than the presence of a genuine virus, sequences detected vary widely from one preparation to the next, a feature of 'HIV' work which sequence analysts have misinterpreted as indicating a phenomenal capacity of 'HIV' to mutate. A computer-simulated phylogenetic 'tree' (an evolutionary history of this non-existent 'virus') was constructed, but in Lanka's view it merely established what its designer sought to prove.

* See Chapter 1

The Search for the Virus

Ever since Peter Duesberg managed to push his HIV critique into the awareness of scientific peers in the late 1980s, virus theory protagonists have displayed great discomfort. Robert Gallo has consistently refused to share a platform with Duesberg although he has recently seemed to want to find some reconciliation with his old and previously much respected friend. Others have repeatedly tried to make out that the debate is over – yet Duesberg's main point, that there was little or no active virus present, even in patients with Aids, has continued to haunt them.

In 1989 the *New England Journal of Medicine* carried an article by David Ho and others purporting to demonstrate new evidence for the active presence of HIV in the blood of infected people, such that 'residual' doubts about the virus hypothesis were resolved. An editorial by Mark Feinberg and David Baltimore hailed the work as ending 'lingering' doubts. But the doubts persisted in a major way.

In March 1992 *New Scientist* reported that little or no virus could be detected in the blood, but that evidence was now mounting from work by Tony Fauci's group that the virus was nevertheless busy invading and destroying key components of the immune system – the thymus gland, and immune cells passing through the lymph nodes, where millions of virus particles lay hidden. According to Fauci, these results meant we should no longer talk about Aids, the final stage of immune deficiency, but instead talk in terms of 'HIV disease'. Nevertheless, the following July *New Scientist* headed a review of competing theories with the headline that 'Despite nearly a decade of intensive research, no one knows how HIV causes Aids'.

In July 1993 *Nature* gave us more details of work by Fauci's group and others. It turned out that what they were doing was using PCR to detect genetic sequences, attributed to 'HIV', in their DNA rather than RNA form – sequences which, as demonstrated by Eleopulos, have never been shown to be related to a specific retrovirus, let alone capable of destroying the immune system. Yet on the basis of these observations, leading Aids researchers Howard Temin and Dani Bolognesi claimed in a commentary: 'These results demonstrate that the extent of HIV-1 infection is very significant even during the early stages after infection, leaving little doubt that the virus itself is sufficient to bring about the disease.' Maddox, in an editorial headed 'Where the Aids virus hides away', commented that 'Duesberg... should now admit the likelihood that he is mistaken.' The *British Medical Journal,* in a news report on the research, stated that it 'puts paid to any notion that HIV does not infect enough cells to cause disease, as suggested by Peter Duesberg'.

Four months later, *Nature* published a letter pointing out that the 'HIV' was latent and non-culturable, and that 'instead of showing us "where all the cytopathic HIV has been hiding", recent results only strengthen the conclusion that most of the progression to Aids occurs in the presence of a very low level, albeit chronically active, HIV-1 infection'. There was no press release to proclaim this interpretation, nor Fauci *et al.'s* reply, which presented a far more uncertain picture than the original *Nature* coverage. They emphasised that they had made no claim to have identified precise mechanisms whereby T4 cells were killed. What they were able to say, however, was that with so many lymphocytes [presumed] infected, 'the ongoing activation of replication in even a small fraction of infected cells *could* gradually eliminate a substantial segment of the population, either as a direct consequence of viral replication or by indirect mechanisms... In addition, the persistence of a replicating virus *could* trigger a complex series of immunopathogenic events even involving uninfected cells, which *could* account for the progressive deterioration of the immune system...We do *feel*...that the virus has a central role in the pathogenesis of HIV disease either directly or indirectly by triggering a series of immunopathogenic events which contribute to the progressive immunosuppression' (my italics). Such caution was entirely justified, and perhaps in a way spoke of how Aids science had advanced in the ten years since Gallo described HIV infection as equivalent to being run over by a truck. But it was also a reflection of the great predicament the HIV theory had created for the world's leading researchers that they were now reduced to a *feeling* that 'HIV' had a central role in 'HIV disease'.

The leaders of opinion were still resisting the idea that there might be something fundamentally wrong in their assumptions, however, and in January 1995 *Nature* dedicated eleven complete pages to what may come to be seen as the ultimate expression of the pathological science that has grown up around the beleaguered HIV theory. On the basis of T4 cell counts, along with non-standardised, non-specific PCR counts of purportedly 'viral' genetic material, and with the use of drugs that block DNA synthesis, groups led by George Shaw, of the University of Alabama at Birmingham, and David ('It's the virus, stupid') Ho, of the Aaron Diamond Centre in New York City, came up with a new picture of how 'HIV'-positive people (and Aids patients) can stay well for years (up to twenty-five years, according to the latest estimates for haemophiliacs) despite being infected with a lethal virus (that is nevertheless impossible to isolate directly). According to their new picture, right from the start the virus and the immune system fight a pitched battle with each other. The virus produces between 100 million and 1 billion copies of itself each *day*, which infect and kill a billion immune cells. But the immune system fights back, pouring in a billion new T-cells. Aids only develops when the virus starts to get the upper hand.

I have already described Mark Craddock's devastating critique of these speculations. On 18 May, *Nature* published six pages of letters of response, almost all of them critical. They included a letter from Duesberg and Harvey Bialy, pointing out that the senior author of one of the papers had previously claimed that the PCR method used 'overestimates by at least 60,000 times the real titre of infectious HIV'. Other correspondents pointed out that T-cells were not necessarily being killed and regenerated as the researchers had assumed, but that they could for example be trapped and liberated from lymph tissue according to immune system needs and conditions.

But whereas *Nature* alerted the world's press to the original papers, leading to numerous news stories and follow-up features (boosted by an editorial in which Maddox declared that 'the new developments are (or should be) an embarrassment for Duesberg' because they 'resolve the paradox'), the subsequent rebuttals received no publicity.

Ho's group concluded their paper with the claim that on the basis of their results, 'Treatment strategies, if they are to have a dramatic clinical impact, must... be initiated as early in the infection course as possible', a call to pharmaceutical arms taken up in the *British Medical Journal* and no doubt elsewhere in the medical literature. Thus, a climate of acceptance was created for a return to the strategy of attacking a non-existent virus with chemotherapy as soon as a person tests 'HIV'-positive, a strategy previously discredited by the Concorde trial.

Sure enough, not long after the *Nature* papers appeared, new studies were released claiming to indicate that giving 'HIV'-positive patients a combination of AZT and other similar drugs offered the best way forward. One of these, the 3,000-patient 'Delta' trial, conducted by investigators in continental Europe, Australia and the UK, received a fanfare of publicity when it reported that while 17 per cent of patients taking only AZT died over a two-year period, 10 per cent of those on AZT+ddI (dideoxyintosine, a reverse transcriptase inhibitor) and 12 per cent of those on AZT+ddC (dideoxy-cytosine, also an RT inhibitor) died, representing a 38 per cent 'drop' in mortality. All of these figures, however, were for patients brought into the trial as AZT 'virgins'; the death rates were far higher, and the apparent benefits of combination treatment disappeared, in patients who had taken AZT previously. This strongly suggests that there will be an accelerating death rate in patients kept on the combination therapies. But since the Delta trial has been halted prematurely, once again the truth will be obscured, just as it was by numerous prematurely terminated, wish-fulfilling trials that previously held AZT on its own to be the 'gold standard' of treatment.

Furthermore, there was no drug-free control group to show what happens to patients who go without any of these 'therapies'. Since there has never been a substantial trial showing long-term benefit from AZT, and since several studies, including Concorde, have shown an increased death rate in AZT-treated patients, Delta cannot be said to have proved any benefit to patients. In addition, a parallel study in the US has reported contradictory findings: AZT+ddI did not improve survival, although AZT+ddC did. The latter, as with Delta, only 'worked' in patients who had not taken AZT before.

It is a sad reflection of the desperate state of Aids science that the Delta findings should be touted as an advance, not just by drug manufacturers but also by Britain's Medical Research Council, which took part in Delta and is now conducting a trial targeting 'HIV' with *four* anti-viral drugs.

Surge in Haemophiliac Deaths

The scale of the tragedy that may be unfolding before us was brought home by a recent report, published as a letter to *Nature,* on death rates among haemophiliacs in the UK.[3] The report showed dramatic increases in annual death rates among a group of 1,227 patients who gave a positive result after the 'HIV' test became available in 1984. There were 403 deaths in this group between 1985 and 1992, of which 235 were certified as being caused by 'Aids, HIV etc.' (although no evidence was presented in confirmation of these diagnoses). Because even the non-Aids deaths were also higher in this group than in the patients who tested negative, the study authors concluded that HIV was probably responsible for about 85 per cent of the deaths in the 'HIV'-positive patients.

Once again, *Nature* and the 'HIV' lobby took up these conclusions without question, as a stick with which to beat Duesberg, and as reason to propagate their view that 'HIV infection will eventually lead to Aids', as a *Nature* editorial proclaimed. 'Not for nothing is the knowledge often called a "death sentence",' the editorial said, concluding that the study 'will, for most people, be sufficient proof that the infection leads to Aids'. It added: 'Those who have made the running in the long controversy over HIV in Aids, Dr Peter Duesberg of Berkeley, California, in particular, have a heavy responsibility that can only be discharged by a public acknowledgement of error, honest or otherwise. And the sooner the better.'

The *Independent* quoted Paul Giangrande, a clinical scientist at the Oxford haemophilia centre where the MRC-supported study was based, as warning that 'HIV'-positive haemophiliacs who do not yet show symptoms of Aids are unlikely to remain healthy 'because the data showed no decrease in death rates over time'. The newspaper's science correspondent added that 'the research undermines one of the last remaining arguments of the Duesberg lobby', quoting one of the *Sunday Times* articles in which I reported the dramatic stabilisation in the immune systems of haemophiliacs switched to high-purity Factor 8 treatment. (As described in Chapter 8, the old product was made from concentrated extracts from the blood of thousands of people, and it had been estimated that a typical patient receiving forty to sixty treatments a year could be exposed to blood from up to 2 million donors annually.)[4]

It was wrong to think that the *Nature* report killed hopes that haemophiliacs switched to the new treatment would be spared Aids. As the authors of the report themselves pointed out, 'This study includes deaths only to 1992, and so does not permit examination of data following widespread use in the UK of high-purity factor concentrate'. The high-purity treatment was still considered experimental in 1992, and was only in use among a tiny minority of haemophiliacs in Britain. It came into more widespread use the following year, after the *Sunday Times* had drawn attention to studies in the US and Italy showing that the T-cell counts of some HIV-positive haemophiliacs did a U-turn, returning in some instances to healthy levels, after they were put on the new product. For the two groups studied, mean T-cell counts had levelled out for up to four years, whereas there was continued decline in those kept on the old product.

That discovery, rarely understood, acknowledged, reported or discussed by the Aids mainstream, is entirely consistent with Eleopulos's oxidative stress theory. Removal of the stress on the immune system of being injected regularly with other people's blood proteins also removed the stimulus for the T-cell abnormalities. Furthermore, Eleopulos's theory predicted that those haemophiliacs who tested 'HIV'-positive would be at increased risk of Aids compared with other haemophiliacs, as she saw their seropositivity as another indication of a cumulative stress on their immune system. The immune system stresses *preceded* their positivity.[5] That this could be the case was acknowledged as long ago as 1986 by Centers for Disease Control researchers, who concluded that 'Haemophiliacs with immune abnormalities may not necessarily be infected with [HIV], since factor concentrate itself may be immunosuppressive',[6] and by Montagnier in 1985 when he wrote: 'This [clinical Aids] syndrome occurs in a minority of infected persons, who generally have in common a past of antigenic stimulation and of immune depression before LAV [HIV] infection.'

The *Nature* study made no acknowledgement of this and other evidence* that 'HIV'-positive haemophiliacs had compromised immune systems before they became positive. It gave no details of the ages of the patients, or their cumulative dosages of Factor 8, as compared between the two groups, 'HIV'-positive and 'HIV'-negative. It is also reprehensible that in view of the revolution in Factor 8 treatment dating from 1993, the study included deaths only to 1992, despite publication only occurring nearly three years later.

Furthermore, the attribution of deaths to 'Aids, HIV etc.' has no meaning, unless HIV is to be held responsible not only for Aids but for all the other

* See Chapter 8

diseases from which these patients died. This is exactly what happens in practice, according to Frank Bouianouckas, of HEAL (New York), although there is no scientific basis for it. He says that once doctors know a patient has been designated HIV-positive, they have a strong tendency to ascribe almost any illness to HIV. 'An acquaintance recently told me that he had a breathing crisis. He went to a hospital but withheld the information that he is gay. They immediately determined that he had asthma. His own doctor was astonished, since he had been searching for an Aids condition for four months and asthma had not even been suspected.'

Why did the study draw such sweeping conclusions about HIV, when there were other, testable interpretations of the differences between the two groups? Why did they fail to discuss the impact of the introduction of high-purity Factor 8? Why did the researchers not wait to include data that would look at this impact? Why did the *Nature* editorial, and other commentators, not even acknowledge the potential of such a significant advance for transforming haemophiliacs' prospects?

Lethal Effects of 'HIV' Diagnosis

The answer to all these omissions and evasions may lie in a desperation to avoid facing what may have been the most important contribution to the increase in deaths in 'HIV'-positive patients: the lethal effects of an 'HIV' diagnosis. As many gay health activist groups have understood and observed, these effects are brought about by the combined burden on the body of AZT chemotherapy (directed against a non-existent pathogen) and the physiological consequences of psychological stress associated with being told you are going to die from what, in the late 1980s, was the world's most feared disease. Both of these toxic assaults were exclusively associated with 'HIV'-positivity. 'HIV'-negative haemophiliacs were spared both the chemotherapy, and the death sentence imposed by the orthodox model of 'HIV=Aids=Death'.

The rise in death rates began in 1986 among those with severe haemophilia, and in 1988 for those with moderate or mild haemophilia. In both groups the excess deaths increased progressively with time. These data correlate very well with the introduction of 'HIV' testing early in 1985 (by the end of that year, 78 per cent of potentially infected severe patients had been tested, and 52 per cent of moderate/mild patients) and the marketing of AZT, which was introduced for symptomatic Aids patients in 1987 and came into widespread use among HIV-positive haemophiliacs in 1989. The correlation is closer than for purported 'HIV' infection, which is said to have begun from 1979 onwards, according to information from stored blood samples. No information was given in the *Nature* report about AZT use, other than that 'it has been widespread for HIV-infected haemophiliacs since about 1989', but we know from the experience of people such as Sue Threakall, now suing Wellcome over the death of her haemophiliac husband, how it was pressed even on healthy 'HIV'-positive patients.

Information *was* given about AZT use in a study of US haemophiliacs published in the *Lancet*[7] in September 1994. The study, headed by Gallo's National Cancer Institute colleague James Goedert, made a complicated analysis of haemophilia clinic records covering 441 HIV-positive patients, over a four-year period dating from 1 January 1988. It purported to show 'no detectable clinical benefit' from high-purity Factor 8 in terms of the risk of Aids or death, but was meaningless from this point of view since it gave no details of how many patients had received the high-purity product and for how long (we were only told that 364 subjects were treated with a high-purity product at some point during the study period). However, the study did show that those taking AZT were four and a half times more likely to develop Aids, and nearly two and a half times more likely to die, than HIV-positive haemophiliacs who did not take the drug. The authors said this might be because it was given first to those at highest risk, but such a large disparity supports the more sinister interpretation that AZT was itself causing Aids in these patients.

Goedert *et al.* admitted that the high-purity Factor 8 might also have been given first to patients at highest risk, so that 'selection bias in the choice of concentrate purity cannot be excluded'. However, that reservation, in a study which in any case had so little data as to render it meaningless on the question of the life-saving, Aids-preventing value of high-purity treatment, disappeared in a subsequent *Lancet* letter from Goedert. He wrote (25 November 1995) that he and his co-authors had previously shown the use of the high-purity product 'had no effect on mortality among HIV-infected subjects'. That conclusion can be regarded as no more than wishful thinking. Yet because it fits the way the majority of Aids scientists wish to think, it is published without challenge in a respected journal and becomes the basis for a new and convenient myth to arise, defusing the dramatic implications of the finding that high-purity Factor 8 stabilises an immune system measure normally held to be vitally relevant to Aids.

It is a classic example of how Aids science has failed us. There is no plot to deceive, merely a particular group perspective which imposes itself on facts better interpreted, from the perspective of this book, in a quite different way. The fact that Goedert should be predisposed to attempting to dismiss data that does not fit the HIV theory is not surprising. As we saw in Chapter 3, he was one of the close Gallo associates appointed to the board of *Aids Research* in the 1985 coup that ousted Joe Sonnabend. Even by 1983, as Randy Shilts told us, Goedert's 'conversations with Jim Curran thoroughly committed him to the idea that a new infectious agent was causing the syndrome'.[8]

On top of bringing a strong risk of being put on AZT, an 'HIV' diagnosis has directly immunosuppressive effects in its own right, as the HEAL Trust (London), has documented in its *Deconstructing Aids* report. The diagnosis is associated with higher levels of psychological and social distress and leads to T-cell abnormalities and increases in latent viral activity. One study, from Cornell University, showed a suicide rate for people with 'HIV' or Aids sixty-six times higher than for the rest of the community. HEAL cited Luc Montagnier as recognising the role of psychological factors in suppressing immunity, and emphasising that 'If you suppress... psychological support by telling someone they are condemned to die, your words alone will have condemned them'. It also quoted Paul Lineback, counselling psychologist at Eastern Oregon State College, as commenting that 'Protecting and promoting the unproven hypothesis as fact is inducing unnecessary stress, probably emotional harm and maybe even psychological murder'. A Swiss immunologist, Professor Alfred Hassig,[9] who for many years was head of the Swiss Red Cross blood transfusion service, has also documented how stress hormones such as adrenalin, noradrenalin and cortisol can disrupt the oxidative and anti-oxidant balance in the body, depleting the effectiveness of immune system cells. 'The widespread view that HIV is a death sentence must be resolutely opposed,' he says.

'HIV-itis' Infects Asia

The epidemic of 'HIV-itis', as Zimbabwe's health minister called it, is a very real threat to health. Europe, the US and several African countries have now rumbled some of its worst manifestations, but the latest victims of the full-blown syndrome are Thailand and India. One million of Thailand's 60 million people are said to be infected, and the figure is similar for India, which has received a US$85 million World Bank loan for its Aids control programme. Despite shrinking levels of estimated 'HIV'- positivity in Europe and the US, these countries are said to have suffered an explosive spread of the virus. There is considerable evidence, especially from Thailand, that this explosion is entirely illusory.

In 1987, a careful 'HIV'-testing programme of Thai prostitutes attending VD clinics by a group of young US-trained biochemists, aware of some of the pitfalls of the test, revealed almost nothing. But incredibly, three to four years later, after a switch to cheaper test kits and introduction of widespread screening, hundreds of thousands were suddenly said to be seropositive. The main reason, according to *Bio/Technology's* Harvey Bialy, who knows both Thailand and the 'HIV-test' literature well, has nothing to do with a genuine viral infection. Rather, it is 'lousy screening tests and wild extrapolations', such that by 1993 half a million people were being said to have 'HIV', in a population one quarter that of the US.[10] By October 1995, some 3 million people were said to have been infected in Asia, most of them in Thailand and India, and the WHO says this will increase to 10 million by 2000.

Bialy's view is supported by Eleopulos *et al.*, who in a 1995 paper[11] show that different studies from Thailand use different criteria to define a positive test, including some that are far less stringent than required even by the variable and confused western standards. 'Thus, many HIV-positive Thais would not be HIV-positive in the West,' they state, concluding that 'unless and until the specificity of the HIV antibody tests in Thailand is determined it cannot be assumed that Thais are infected with HIV'.

In the region claimed to be worst affected, Chiang Mai province in the north, which borders the 'Golden Triangle', one of the world's major opium and heroin producing areas, 61 per cent of drug users were said to test positive in 1993. However, it has long been known that drug users often have high levels of immune complexes in their blood, and high rates of false positivity on a number of routine laboratory tests. A 1986 study[12] on stored blood samples from IV drug abusers dating back to 1971 found that many tested positive using the western blot kit, leading the authors to conclude that the addicts had either been 'HIV'-infected as early as 1971, or that 'the seropositivity detected in these specimens represents false positive or nonspecific reactions'. Furthermore, another study has shown that people who use cocaine non-intravenously are *more* likely to test positive with the western blot than those who inject.[13] Evidence available as far back as 1985 shows malaria is associated with false positive 'HIV' test results; and Thailand ranks fifth in the world in a WHO league table of countries worst affected by malaria. The problem is particularly acute in northern border areas, according to a 1993 report[14] on a study in three northern Thai villages. The author wrote: 'Data and observation indicate that land-poor families forced into sudden farming have greater contact with the primary vectors in Thailand ... In addition to agricultural activities on clearings near forested areas, clandestine forest activities and cross-border traffic contributes to the prevalence of malaria in the Thai border villages.' Like malaria, tuberculosis and to a lesser extent leprosy – both demonstrated to show 'significant cross-reactivity' with 'HIV' proteins – are also common in Thailand. Probably as a result of chronic infections, Thai people in general show signs of immune activation: Israeli immunologists have shown that Thai temporary labourers in Israel have greatly elevated (up to six times higher) levels of immune system activation markers compared with ordinary healthy Israelis.[15]

Faced with the fear created by what is almost certainly a totally unreal epidemic, Thailand is now 'aggressively looking for ways to thwart HIV', as a November 1995 report from that country by *Science's* Jon Cohen put it. 'Nowhere is this more pronounced than in the country's emerging role as the most important place in the world for testing Aids vaccines,' Cohen wrote. 'There's probably more going on here than anywhere,' said William Heyward, an epidemiologist with the US Centers for Disease Control, currently working for the WHO to help Thailand set up Aids vaccine trials. Cohen writes that while in 1994 the US National Institutes of Health scrapped plans to spend nearly $30 million on large-scale tests in the US of the two leading candidate vaccines after an expert panel concluded they showed too little promise, 'Thai researchers and officials feel that a different calculus applies here: in spite of an intensive education and public health campaign, infection rates are still high, and even a partially effective vaccine would be better than nothing.'

Thus, the tragedy marches on. A group of researchers at the Harvard Aids Institute, which has probably done more than any other organisation to fuel 'HIV-itis' world-wide with a series of hugely alarmist reports and statements, was recently defending a proposal to run a trial of AZT in 1,500 pregnant Thai women without studying a non-AZT group for purposes of comparison (some mothers and babies will simply receive the drug for shorter periods than others). 'We firmly believe that it would be unethical to incorporate a placebo arm in our study,' wrote[16] the researchers, who are collaborating with workers at Chiang Mai University. 'The Thai government has already provided AZT to Aids patients on a limited basis and recently stated its intent to continue to distribute AZT to HIV-infected pregnant women as needed to reduce the chance that they transmit the virus to their infants... While there is great uncertainty as to how AZT works and which treatment component is most important, all of the co-investigators agree that providing no treatment at all to HIV-infected pregnant women would subject their infants to a considerable risk.' In fact, there is no evidence that treating unborn babies with this highly toxic drug is of any benefit to them; the likelihood is that it can only do harm. But in the minds of the researchers, it seems unethical to withhold the drug.

This is understandable, because they equate 'HIV' antibodies with death. They have been taught to do so, through journals like *Nature* and *Science,* by an elite group of experts who seized command of Aids science during a public health emergency, and who have been unwilling to relinquish that command despite increasingly clear evidence that they were fighting the wrong enemy from the start. The AZT researchers do not know that the assumptions which lay behind the 'HIV=Aids=Death' equation were faulty, and that their basis for exposing unborn babies to a drug which by its very nature kills healthy body cells is a non-specific test for a non-existent virus. If they knew that, they would not wish to poison the babies in this way. The same is true of the entire HIV/Aids industry, and of its leading advocates. They would not assault the minds and lives of hundreds of thousands of people by telling them they are infected with a lethal virus if they did not believe that to be the case.

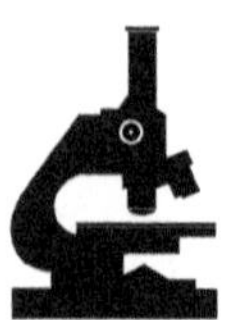

14: SHEDDING THE ILLUSIONS

'What they say is not unreasonable, but it all hinges on whether what they did at the beginning is true,' says Eleopulos's colleague Val Turner. The thrust of this book has been to present evidence, denied to the scientific and medical mainstream by the leading professional journals, that the original work claiming the isolation of an immune cell-destroying virus was inadequate, that the procedures which should have identified those inadequacies did not operate, and that a kind of censorship operated subsequently which grew more intense as the case for a reappraisal of the HIV theory grew stronger.

The theory came at a time of enormous growth in spending – much of it provided through central government agencies – on molecular biology, a field in which great technical advances are constantly taking place but which has so far yielded surprisingly few returns to humanity. According to some observers, there has even been a strong downside to some of this work, in which simple-minded interpretations of genetic findings can all too easily damage people's lives. The danger becomes particularly acute when those involved 'attribute excessive control and power to genes and DNA, rather than seeing them as part of the overall functioning of cells and organisms,' argues Ruth Hubbard, professor of biology emerita at Harvard University, in her cautionary book *Exploding the Gene Myth*.[1]

Richard Strohman, professor emeritus in molecular and cell biology at the University of California at Berkeley, goes further. He says the half-century-old pursuit of genetic explanations for illness has actually slowed the pace of progress towards genuine understanding, and within medical practice itself – essentially, causing doctors and scientists to miss more and more of the wood as they peer more closely at the trees and the leaves. Strohman began a 1993 paper[2] on the limits of the genetic paradigm – the major research paradigm governing modern biomedicine – with a 1970 quotation reminiscent of

Eleopulos's theories of cell homoeostasis and Aids causation:

> The reality [of disease] is the inability of one person's homoeostasis, conditioned by his genotype and a lifetime of special experiences, to maintain equilibrium; neither genes nor environment 'cause' disease, it is simply that the organism is unsuited for adaptive action in one, or several environments.[3]

In many ways, Strohman said, fundamental biology is currently rediscovering earlier insights about differences in complexity between living and non-living systems. It is trying to place individual genetic events in the larger context of the life of the cell and of the organism as a whole. For several decades, however, medical research and treatment has been governed by the essentially mechanistic genetic paradigm, which says:

DNA→RNA→Protein→Everything else, including disease.

By the late 1980s, the vast majority of the National Institutes of Health research budget was going to projects reflecting this dogma, with its implications that genes cause disease, ageing and death, and that genetic research will produce the means for eliminating disease and extending life significantly beyond current expectations. A split had developed between applied medical sciences and basic research biology that was potentially dangerous to the public health.

Strohman looked at how this split has affected approaches to several diseases, including Aids, on which he commented: 'It is impossible to dissect the HIV-Aids hypothesis here, but it is only prudent to raise the possibility that Aids may be another example of our biomedical paradigm's misplaced emphasis on genes as the cause of complex human disease. Only time will tell if the focus on genes – the genes of HIV – is misguided. It seems an obvious recommendation, however, that our research extend itself to environmental factors that might play an important, and perhaps a dominant, role in Aids.'

A new medical approach to diseases was needed, that would permit examination of the interaction between individuals and the environment. It would include molecular genetics as a crucial aspect, but recognise that genes are regulated by the responses of the cells in which they sit, which in turn are governed by the stress-related behaviours of the organism as a whole.

This new approach would model the possible ways in which cells can adapt to stressful environments, 'and identify conditions under which the entire cell or tissue moves from positive adaptation to negative or disease state'.

Disease, in this wider view, is seen as a result of an organism's frustrated attempts to adapt to hostile circumstances for which there is no adequate response. 'When the world presents information for which the genome and its interactive... network have no adequate informational response – for example, an overly oxidative environment – the result is maladaptation, regressive-state change in cell behaviour, and finally end-state disease.' Strohman regretted that at present there was no such science of the wider picture, nor even a theory about it.

The HIV story may eventually be seen as a classic example of the dangers of narrow-focus science. Maddox demonstrated an awareness of the problem in a 1988 *Nature* editorial, in which he wrote: 'Part of the trouble is that excitement of the chase [of molecular cause] leaves little time for reflection. And there are grants for producing data, but hardly any for standing back in contemplation.'

Perhaps when the illusions are shed and a clearer picture of Aids finally emerges, the enormity of what went wrong will be turned to good advantage by the world of science, as a catalyst for a radical rethink about its observational methods, assumptions, and institutional checks and balances. Perhaps, too, that may include reconsideration of the way society treats the human beings we call doctors and scientists. A training that focuses so much on specialised knowledge, to the detriment of wisdom (the wider picture), encourages a disregard for the wisdom of the body – the self-adjusting, self-healing capabilities of organisms given respite from the pressures that induce disorder.

A similar disregard – for the wisdom inherent in the Earth and its life systems – contributes to environmental disorder. This is probably now seen at its most acute within the former Soviet Union, where two other problems that featured in the mishandling of Aids also became acute: peer review systems that favoured conformity, and were therefore a fertile breeding ground for political correctness in science, and state domination of research funding.

Finally, the unrelentingly outward focus of science, by leaving subjective factors out of the picture, can compromise its objectivity, especially when it comes to tackling such an intensely emotional subject as Aids. The early investigators were understandably reluctant to get into the emotionally murky and politically dangerous waters of sex and drugs. As a result they were prevented from seeing what was actually staring them in the face. Subsequently, as more and more money, power and prestige rode on the HIV wagon, it became increasingly difficult for all involved to climb off, despite the Procrustean consequences.

The idea that science offers a purely objective description of reality, and the failure to take the feelings of scientists themselves into account, is a far deeper and more damaging illusion than HIV itself. Perhaps a day will come when Gallo, Montagnier and the other great players in the HIV story will be looked back upon, not without affection, as tragic heroes whose mistakes pointed the way to a scientific reformation; one in which it became acknowledged that the processes of rational observation and inquiry must be tempered by a less rigidly mechanistic outlook – a change that can only come when we reverse our tendency to treat scientists themselves as soulless machines. Regardless of what we ultimately come to understand about 'HIV', I feel sure that the benefits of such a reformation would extend beyond Aids patients, to the whole of medicine and indeed to all of human society.

The Way Forward

I have described the case for a different way of thinking about Aids with as much care and conviction as I could muster, in order to be true to the perspective I now hold on the issue, which affects the lives of millions. With more than 100,000 papers published on Aids from the perspective that accepts HIV as the cause, there is of course a mass of evidence arguing in a different direction. It is impossible for me to do justice to all this work. All I can do is ask the reader to see if a reasonable case has been made for a reappraisal of the assumptions that underpin the conventional approach.

Assuming for a moment that there is merit in the 'dissident' arguments explored in this book, what could persuade the scientific mainstream to re-examine the basic paradigm? Perhaps the process is already under way, and it is just a question of time while new thinking gradually filters through to wider awareness.

There are two predictions of Eleopulos's theory, however, which might be readily examined. One concerns the 'HIV'-positive haemophiliacs who have been switched to high-purity Factor 8. Although the precise reason for HIV-positivity in haemophiliacs is not known, if it was the impurities in their previous treatment that caused them to test positive originally, some or all could be expected to cease to test positive as their immune systems recover. After Montagnier had shown slides at the 1993 Berlin Aids conference of U-turns in haemophiliac patients' T-cell counts when they were switched to the new treatment, he told me that the patients still tested positive for antibodies to HIV; but it may have been too soon after the change for them to become seronegative.

A second way of testing the theory that what we call HIV is an endogenous phenomenon would be to stimulate normal, healthy cells in ways that parallel the conditions in which cells from Aids patients are persuaded to demonstrate 'viral' activity. This has already been done, and 'viral' phenomena sometimes demonstrated. Given the right conditions, it should be possible to show such phenomena routinely if Eleopulos is right. Stefan Lanka would particularly like to see Kary Mullis's PCR invention used to search for 'HIV' genetic sequences in such normal, appropriately stimulated, human cells. Such an experiment would be the equivalent of the 'control' studies which HIV researchers – steeped as they are in the conviction that the virus has been proved to exist – have almost always neglected to perform.

The Aids dissidents, despite – or maybe even because of – their marginalised status, seem to be growing in stature with the passing of the years. Joe Sonnabend has lost much of his rage and is working more closely with the mainstream, accepting that the roots of the disastrous developments he witnessed in the mid-1980s lay not in wickedness, but in political and social forces that were beyond the power of any individual to control. The tireless John Lauritsen continues to keep *Native* readers informed of developments with humour and optimism. His eight-page account[4] of the American Association for the Advancement of Science (Pacific Division) HIV symposium in June 1994 may have buried the HIV theory prematurely – concluding 'The HIV-Aids hypothesis is dead. Only in a genuine spirit of free inquiry can we discover exactly what "Aids" is and what its causes are' – but its description of a rout of HIV's defenders at that meeting marked a turning point in the debate. Philippe Krynen, having risked everything but his integrity to make such a valuable mark on the history of 'Aids' in Africa, is building bridges to the health officials he so took by surprise and taking care not to cause further upset that might jeopardise the future of his charity's work.

Kary Mullis's convictions on Aids have not been muddled or softened by his Nobel prize – in fact quite the reverse, as *Spin's* Celia Farber found on reaching him on the phone late one evening as he bade farewell to some dinner guests. He had recently been hired by ABC's *Nightline* programme as scientific consultant on a superb two-part series on the HIV debate, and continued to defend Duesberg passionately. 'I was trying to stress this point to the ABC people, that Peter has been abused seriously by the scientific establishment, to the point where he can't even do any research,' he told Farber, adding:

> Not only that, but his whole life is pretty much in disarray because of this, and it is only because he has refused to compromise his scientific moral standards. There ought to be some goddamn private foundation in the country, that would say, 'Well, we'll move in where the NIH dropped off. We'll take care of it. You just keep right on saying what you're saying, Peter. We think you're an asshole, we think you're wrong, but you're the only dissenter, and we need one, because it's science, it's not religion.'

He went on:

> I am waiting to be convinced that we're wrong. I know it ain't going to happen. But if it does, I'll tell you this much – I will be the first person to admit it. A lot of the people studying this disease are looking for the clever little pathways they can piece together, that will show how this works. Like, 'What if this molecule was produced by this one and then this one by this one, and then what if this one and that one induce this one' - that stuff becomes, after two molecules, conjecture of the *rankest* kind. People who sit there and talk about it don't realise that molecules themselves are somewhat hypothetical, and that their interactions are more so, and that the biological reactions are even more so. You don't need to look that far.

> You don't discover the cause of something like Aids by dealing with incredibly obscure things. You just look at what the hell is going on. Well, here's a bunch of people that are practising a new set of behavioural norms. Apparently it didn't work because a lot of them got sick. That's the conclusion. You don't necessarily know why it happened. But you start there.

Mullis was aware, Farber said, that his view of Aids – one that encompasses each person's history or 'lifestyle' – was rejected by virtually all Aids organisations, researchers, and activists, who considered it 'blaming the victim'. 'It's not blaming the victim,' he argued. 'It's not anybody's fault. They just did something that didn't *work*, that's all.'

Later in the interview, as Mullis pondered on the lives ruined by the HIV diagnosis and AZT (and other 'scary' medical practices seen 'through the glasses that you've developed through looking at this thing'), Farber realised that on the other end of the phone, this Nobel laureate, pioneer of the DNA revolution, had started to cry.

Mullis told her:

> God, I hate this kind of crap... Sometimes in the morning, when it's a good surf, I go out there, and I don't feel like it's a bad world. I think it's a good world, the sun is shining. I'm really optimistic in the mornings. But, you know, it's not because of you calling me. It's just thinking about this issue, it just drives me to – I'm making tears thinking about it. I don't see how to deal with it. I can't possibly write a book that will describe it to somebody. You can't do a damn 22.8-minute TV thing that is really going to have any effect except to get somebody to shoot through my window and hit me. I feel like I'm on a hostile planet.[5]

I have felt a bit like that, too, at times, when under attack on all sides, over a protracted period, for my reporting on the HIV/Aids debate. Even if it achieves nothing else, writing this book has helped me gain a sense of perspective. Not necessarily into the molecular mechanisms I have tried to explore, but at least into the fundamental goodness of those on all sides of the controversy who, despite their differences, and despite their failings, ultimately wish to do what is right by their fellow human beings.

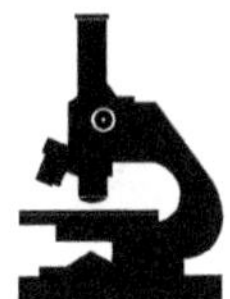

NOTES

Chapter 1: The Procrustean Bed

1. *Nature,* vol. 353, p. 297.
2. ibid., vol. 366, pp. 493-4.
3. ibid., vol. 373, p. 102.

Chapter 2: When Two Roads Diverged

1. Michael Callen, *Surviving Aids,* HarperCollins, New York, 1990.
2. From an untitled speech Michael Callen gave early in 1983.
3. Michael Callen, *Surviving Aids.*
4. Randy Shilts, *And the Band Played On,* St Martin's Press, New York, 1987; Penguin Books, 1988.
5. *Lancet,* 2 February 1980, p. 226.
6. C. Schmidt, 'The Group-Fantasy Origins of Aids', *Journal of Psychohistory,* vol. 12, 1984, pp. 37-78.

Chapter 3: An Editor is Silenced

1. Studies reported in the *Lancet* (vol. 2, 1982, p. 125) and the *New England Journal of Medicine* had shown antibodies to CMV in 94 per cent of male homosexuals, and fifteen out of fifteen autopsied Aids cases in one study had disseminated CMV infections.
2. Dominique Lapierre, *Beyond Love,* Century, 1991; originally published in French as *Plus grands que l'amour.*
3. ibid., pp. 48-9.
4. Randy Shilts, *And the Band Played On,* pp. 70-71.
5. ibid., p. 272.
6. J. Sonnabend, 'Aids: An Explanation for Its Occurrence among Homosexual Men' in *The Acquired Immune Deficiency Syndrome and Infections of*

Homosexual Men, ed. Pearl Ma and Donald Armstrong, Yorke Medical Books, 1983, revised 1989.

7. *Aids Forum*, vol. 2, no. 2, May 1989.
8. *The* New Scientist *Inside Science*, Penguin Books, 1992.
9. ibid.
10. S. Harris, 'The Aids Heresies: A Case Study in Skepticism Taken Too Far', *Skeptic*, vol. 3, no. 2, 1995.
11. *Lancet*, vol. 340, 17 October 1992, pp. 971-2.
12. *Science*, vol. 262, 12 November 1993.
13. *New Scientist*, 13 May 1995, pp. 36-40.

Chapter 4: Drugged

1. John Lauritsen, *The Aids War*, Asklepios, New York, 1993. Obtainable directly from the author at 26 St Mark's Place, New York City 10003, 820 (postpaid).
2. David Durack, *New England Journal of Medicine*, December 1981.
3. P. R. J. Gangadharam, V. K. Peruman *et al.*, 'Immunosuppressive Action of Isobutyl Nitrite' (presentation to the International Congress on Immunopharmacology, Florence, Italy, May 1985).
4. E. M. Hersh *et al.*, *Cancer Research*, March 1983, pp. 1365-71.
5. E. Lotzova *et al.*, *Cancer Immunology Immunotherapy*, vol. 17, 1984, pp. 130-34.
6. M. Marmor *et al.*, *Lancet*, 15 May 1982, pp. 1083-7.
7. U. Mathur-Wagh *et al.*, *Lancet*, 12 May 1984, pp. 1033-8.
8. J. R. Neefe *et al.*, *Federation Proceedings*, vol. 42, no. 4, 5 March 1983, p. 949.
9. G. Newell *et al.*, *Preventive Medicine*, January 1985, pp. 81—91.
10. J. Ortiz and V. Rivera, presentation to the American Public Health Association Convention, November 1985.
11. V. Quagliarello, *Yale Journal of Biology and Medicine*, 1982, pp. 443-52.
12. E. Sue Watson and J. Murphy, unpublished letter sent to the *Journal of the American Medical Association*, October 1982.
13. *Annals of Internal Medicine*, August 1983, pp. 145-51.
14. *Journal of Toxicology and Environmental Health*, 1985, pp. 835—47.
15. Randy Shilts, *And the Band Played On*, p. 87.
16. ibid., pp. 158-9.
17. 'The Poppers-KS Connection', *Native*, 13 June 1994.

18. E. Dax *et al., Immunopharmacology and Immunotoxicology,* 13, no. 4, 1991, pp. 577-87.
19. John Lauritsen, *The Aids War,* p. 179.
20. ibid., pp. 190-91.
21. ibid., pp. 192-3.
22. *The Columbia University College of Physicians and Surgeons Complete Home Medical Guide,* New York, 1985.
23. Robert Root-Bernstein, *Rethinking Aids,* The Free Press, New York, 1993, p. 128.
24. Jon Rappoport, *Aids Inc.: Scandal of the Century,* San Bruno, California,1988.

Chapter 5: A Conspiracy of Humbug

1. *Lancet,* 18 May 1968, pp. 1077-81.
2. ibid., 22 September 1984, pp. 682-5.
3. Robert Matthews, 'Storming the Barricades', *New Scientist,* 17 June 1995.
4. Phair *et al., Journal of Acquired Immune Deficiency Syndromes,* vol. 5, 1992, pp. 490-96.
5. *Lancet,* 14 February 1987, pp. 345-9.
6. N. Padian *et al., Journal of the American Medical Association,* vol. 266, 1991, pp. 1664-7.
7. *British Medical Journal,* vol. 304, 1992, p. 811.
8. Michael Fitzpatrick, *The Truth About the Aids Panic,* Junius, 1987.
9. *Journal of Public Policy,* vol. 13, no. 4, pp. 305-25.

Chapter 6: A Challenge from Within

1. John Rennie, 'DNA's New Twists', *Scientific American,* March 1993.
2. R. Schwartz, *New England Journal of Medicine,* 6 April 1995, pp. 941—4.
3. Bryan Ellison, *We Will Never Win the War on Aids,* Inside Story Communications, 190 El Cerrito Plaza, Ste 201, El Cerrito, CA 94530, USA.
4. A detailed discussion of Duesberg's criticisms of the claims for a direct relationship between HTLV-1 and T-cell leukaemia is contained in Jad Adams's book, *Aids: The HIV Myth,* Macmillan, 1989, pp. 41-9.
5. ibid., pp. 70-93.
6. ibid., pp. 89-90.
7. Bryan Ellison, *We Will Never Win the War on Aids,* p. 132.
8. ibid., pp. 245-7.

9. R. Pillai *et al., Archives of Toxicology,* vol. 65, 1991, pp. 609-17.
10. Martin Walker, *Dirty Medicine,* Slingshot Publications, BM Box 8314, London WC1N 3XX.
11. Bruce Nussbaum, *Good Intentions,* Atlantic Monthly Press, New York, 1990.
12. Peter Duesberg, 'Aids Acquired by Drug Consumption and Other Noncontagious Risk Factors', *Pharmacology and Therapeutics,* vol. 55, 1992, pp. 201-77.
13. *British Medical Journal,* vol. 301, pp. 1362—5.
14. Robert Gallo, *Virus Hunting: Aids, Cancer, and the Human Retrovirus,* HarperCollins, 1991.
15. ibid.

Chapter 7: Aids: Can We Be Positive?

1. Michael Fumento, *The Myth of Heterosexual Aids,* Basic Books, New York, 1990.
2. *Lancet,* vol. 338, pp. 1159-63.
3. ibid., 3 August 1985, pp. 233-6.
4. *British Medical Journal,* 25 November 1989, pp. 1312—15.
5. Victor Lorian, 'Aids, Anal Sex and Heterosexuals', *Lancet,* 14 May 1988, p. 1111.

Chapter 8: The Case Against HIV Grows Stronger

1. *Journal of Allergy and Clinical Immunology,* January 1989, pp. 165-70.
2. S. Seremetis *et al.,* abstract. The paper was subsequently published in the *Lancet,* vol. 342, pp. 700-703.
3. De Biasi *et al., Blood,* vol. 78, no. 8, 1991, pp. 1919-22.
4. *Blood,* vol. 73, 1989, pp. 2067-73.
5. *British Medical Journal,* vol. 309, 30 July 1994, pp. 309-13.
6. ibid.
7. J. M. Jason *et al., Journal of the American Medical Association,* vol. 255, 1986, pp. 212-15.
8. Robert Root-Bernstein, *Rethinking Aids — The Tragic Cost of Premature Consensus,* The Free Press, New York, 1993.
9. J. Ward *et al., New England Journal of Medicine,* vol. 321, 1989, pp. 947-52.
10. *Daily Telegraph,* 5 May 1993.
11. *Lancet,* vol. 345, 1995, p. 1242.
12. Simon Garfield, 'The Rise and Fall of AZT', *Independent on Sunday,* 2 May 1993.

13. W. Lenderking *et al., New England Journal of Medicine,* 17 March 1994, pp. 738—43.
14. 'Babies Treated with Contested Aids Drug', *Sunday Times,* 6 June 1993.
15. N. Mir and C. Costello, *Lancet,* 19 November 1988, pp. 1195-6.
16. J. M. McCune *et al., Science,* vol. 247, 1990, pp. 564—6.

Chapter 9: Science Fails the 'Aids Test'

1. A. Genesca *et al., Lancet,* vol. 2, 1989, pp. 1023-5.
2. R. J. Biggar *et al., Lancet,* vol. 2, 1985, pp. 520-23.
3. J. H. Jaffe *et al., New England Journal of Medicine,* vol. 314, 1986, pp. 1387-8.
4. D. M. Novick *et al., Alcoholism Clin. Exp. Research,* vol. 12, 1988, pp. 687-90.
5. C. Sterk, *Lancet,* vol. 1, 1988, pp. 1052-3.
6. T. A. Kion and G. W. Hoffman, *Science,* vol. 253, 1991, pp. 1138—40.
7. L. J. Conley and S. D. Holmberg, *New England Journal of Medicine,* vol. 326, 1992, p. 1499.
8. *Science,* vol. 263, 1994, p. 27.
9. P. Mortimer, *Lancet,* vol. 337, 1991, pp. 286-7.
10. P. Mortimer, *Med. Internal.,* vol. 56, 1989, pp. 2334—9.
11. G. Lundberg, *Journal of the American Medical Association,* vol. 260, 1988, pp. 674—9.E. P. Eleopulos *et al.,* 'HIV Antibody Testing: Autoreactivity and Other Associated Problems' (unpublished).
12. Edited by J. C. Petricciani *et al.,* and published by John Wiley & Sons on behalf of the WHO, 1987.
13. *Aids Testing,* ed. G. Schochetman and J. R. George, Springer-Verlag, New York, 1994.
14. O. Kashala *et al., Journal of Infectious Diseases,* vol. 169, February 1994, pp. 296-304.

Chapter 10: The Plague That Never Was

1. K. M. de Cock *et al., British Medical Journal,* 9 November 1991, pp. 1185-8.
2. C. F. Gilks, ibid., pp. 1189-90.
3. D. Serwadda and E. Katongole-Mbidde, *Lancet,* 7 April 1990, pp. 842-3.
4. F. Konotey-Ahulu, *What is Aids?,* Tetteh-A'Domeno Co., Watford, England, 1989.
5. Ranjit Kumar Chandra, *Science,* vol. 190, 1975, pp. 289-90.
6. W. T. Hughes *et al., Am. J. Dis. Child.,* vol. 128, 1974, pp. 44—52.

7. 'The Epidemic That's Wiping Out Africa', *Evening Standard,* 7 July 1992.

Chapter 11: Consternation at the Court of HIV

1. *Nature,* vol. 364, 8 July 1993, p. 96.
2. Richard Milton, *The Facts of Life,* Fourth Estate, 1992. Milton had also recently completed *Forbidden Science — Suppressed Research That Could Change Our Lives,* Fourth Estate, 1994.
3. *Nature,* vol. 368, 31 March 1994, p. 387.
4. *California Monthly,* September 1994, interview with Kary Mullis by Russell Schoch.
5. Lewis Wolpert, *The Unnatural Nature of Science,* Faber and Faber, 1992.
6. Jad Adams, *Aids: The HIV Myth,* Macmillan, 1989.
7. *Continuum,* published from 172 Foundling Court, Brunswick Centre, London WC1N 1QE, England.
8. Positively Healthy, PO Box 71, Richmond, Surrey TW9 3DJ, England.
9. HEAL Trust (London), 41c Ramsden Road, London SW12 8QX, England.
10. HEAL, PO Box 1103, New York 10024, USA.

Chapter 12: The Virus That Never Was

1. Jad Adams, *Reappraising Aids,* vol. 3, no. 9, September 1995.
2. *Physiological Chemistry and Physics and Medical NMR,* vol. 17, 1985, pp. 407-12.
3. *Cardiovascular Research,* vol. 23, 1989, pp. 662-5.
4. C. J. O'Hara *et al., Human Pathology,* vol. 19, 1988, pp. 545-9.
5. *Emerging Viruses,* ed. Stephen Morse, Oxford University Press, 1993.
6. S. Wain-Hobson, *Nature,* 12 January 1995, p. 102.
7. J. L. Marx, *Science,* vol. 241, 1988, pp. 1039-40.
8. H. Farzadegan *et al., Annals of Internal Medicine,* vol. 108, 1988, pp. 785-90; C. R. Horsburgh *et al., New England Journal of Medicine,* vol. 321, 1989, pp. 1678-80.
9. J. A. Mikowits *et al.,* vol. 1, abstracts, 1991 International Conference on Aids, Florence, Italy.
10. B. Hahn *et al., Nature,* vol. 312, 8 November 1984, pp. 166-9.
11. M. S. Horwitz *et al., Journal of Virology,* vol. 66, 1992, pp. 2170-79.
12. A. Shih *et al., Journal of Virology,* January 1989, pp. 64-75.

Chapter 13: A Better Fit

1. Peter Duesberg, *Inventing the Aids Virus,* Regnery Publishing, Washington, DC, 1996.
2. *Continuum,* vol. 3, no. 2, June/July 1995.
3. S. Darby *et al., Nature,* 7 September 1995, pp. 79-82.
4. *Blood,* vol. 73, 1989, pp. 2067-73.
5. For a full discussion of 'HIV' mythology in haemophiliacs, including 'as close a proof as one can get that what has been called HIV infection in haemophiliacs is not caused by an exogenous retrovirus', see Eleopulos *et al., Genetica,* vol. 95, 1995, pp. 25-50.
6. J. M. Jason *et al., Journal of the American Medical Association,* vol. 255, pp. 212-15.
7. J. Goedert *et al., Lancet,* vol. 344, 17 September 1994.
8. Randy Shilts, *And the Band Played On,* p. 272.
9. A. Hassig *et al., GanzheitsMedizin,* September 1994. Obtainable from Study Group Nutrition and Immunity, Elisabethenstrasse 51, CH-3014 Bern, Switzerland.
10. *WorldAids,* July 1993.
11. 'Aids in Thailand: An Appraisal of the Data Professing Proof of Heterosexual Transmission'; in press.
12. J. H. Jaffe *et al., New England Journal of Medicine,* vol. 314, 1986, pp. 1387-8.
13. C. Sterk, *Lancet,* vol. 1, 1988, pp. 1052-3.
14. A. Singhanetra-Renard, *Social Science and Medicine,* vol. 37, no. 9, pp. 1147-54.
15. A. Kalinkovich *et al., Lancet,* vol. 343, 11 June 1994, pp. 1506-7.
16. *Science,* vol. 270, 10 November 1995, pp. 899-900.

Chapter 14: Shedding The Illusions

1. Ruth Hubbard, *Exploding the Gene Myth,* Beacon Press, Boston, 1993.
2. Richard Strohman, 'Ancient Genomes, Wise Bodies, Unhealthy People: Limits of a Genetic Paradigm in Biology and Medicine', *Perspectives in Biology and Medicine,* vol. 37, no. 1, 1993.
3. B. Childs, 'Persistent Echoes of the Nature-Nurture Argument', *American Journal of Human Genetics,* vol. 29, 1970, pp. 1—13.
4. John Lauritsen, 'Truth Is Bustin' Out All Over', *New York Native,* 18 July, 1994.
5. *Spin,* vol. 10, no. 4, July 1994.

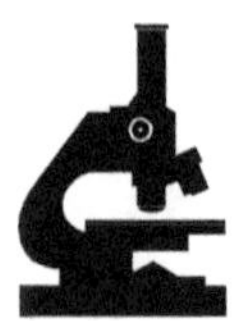

APPENDIX: SIX MISTAKES THAT CREATED AND SUSTAINED 'HIV'

What came to be called the Human Immunodeficiency Virus (HIV) was announced by the US Government as the 'probable cause' of Aids in 1984. A group of scientists in Perth, Western Australia, have challenged this theory throughout the years since.* They have faced relentless efforts to silence them and discredit their extraordinarily persistent and painstaking work.

The suppression has been so successful that most people do not even know of the existence of the group. If, even today, you go to a popular site like Wikipedia** to learn more about them, you will see them written off as 'Aids denialists', along with claims that their questioning of the HIV orthodoxy contributed to hundreds of thousands of premature deaths in South Africa. Their scientific arguments remain unaddressed.

Although mud-slinging does not advance understanding, history may well show us that it is the HIV/Aids protagonists who are truly in denial, because they find it so difficult to admit they could have been fooled into believing fervently in a non-existent virus. Why otherwise would they take every opportunity to abuse and belittle the work of a handful of scientists in a far-flung corner of the world?

It is also striking how passionately the white-dominated medical profession in South Africa has attacked any questioning of the HIV theory. It prefers to blame high death rates among black people on a mythical virus rather than the destructive economic and social legacy of 50 years of apartheid.

---

* See for example: The isolation of HIV: Has it really been achieved? *http://www.theperthgroup.com/CONTINUUM/PapadopolousReallyAchieved1996.pdf*

** https://en.wikipedia.org/wiki/The_Perth_Group#Influence

In 2017, the Perth scientists summarised their decades of research in a detailed, 80-page paper*. The work describes five mistakes which, they say, accompanied development of the HIV hypothesis by the first Aids researchers, and its premature acceptance by the scientific and medical communities.

A sixth mistake, which came later, helped to sustain the theory.

In essence, the group's critique asserts that:

- Groups at risk of the set of diseases that came to be known as Aids had in common repeated and heavy exposures to oxidising substances – reactive molecules that cause detrimental changes to all cells in the body, including immune cells.

- In the feverish atmosphere of fear and anxiety that arose when Aids first struck, biochemical signals arising from this disorder became misinterpreted as evidence for the presence of a deadly, new, sexually transmitted virus.

- Once the global alert was sounded over 'HIV', it became almost impossible for contrary views to be heard.

Even today, the group says, despite thousands of claims to the contrary, there is still no proof such a virus has been isolated and purified from the tissues of Aids patients – the procedure virologists use to prove a particular virus exists.

Calling for a review of the entire 'HIV/Aids' belief system, the Perth scientists express the concern that the true causes of Aids are not being adequately addressed, and that millions globally are being burdened with a false diagnosis of 'HIV' infection.

In addition, many people who have tested 'HIV'-positive, and even who are at risk of doing so, are being strongly advised to take drugs whose claimed benefits come at the cost of serious toxicities. Although the drugs are used to prevent and treat the immune decline said to cause the onset of diseases

---

* Papadopulos-Eleopulos, E *et al.* HIV – A virus like no other. *www.theperthgroup.com/HIV/TPGVirusLikeNoOther.pdf*

indicative of Aids, there is no proof such benefits are due to an 'anti-HIV' effect.

The group emailed their manuscript to seven leading scientific and medical journals, offering to prepare a concise version if the critique was thought 'worthy of being brought to the attention of the scientific community'. Three failed to reply, despite repeated requests. None took up the offer.

I too wrote to several senior biologists in the UK about the paper, asking for guidance on how to obtain an independent, authoritative assessment of the critique, in the hope of opening up the virus theory to detailed scientific inquiry. The arguments are complex in places, involving intricacies of molecular biology, and of course the implications are far-reaching. I received no replies.

At the heart of the group's challenge lies the work of the late Eleni Papadopulos-Eleopulos, a biophysicist at the Royal Perth Hospital, who in 1982 published in the *Journal of Theoretical Biology* a new theory about how the functioning of our body cells can go wrong. The essence was that the chemical process known as redox, in which cells take in, and give out, energy in order to do work, becomes unbalanced. When over-oxidised, their store of potential energy is depleted. The theory postulates that conditions such as cancer, cardiovascular diseases, ageing and blood clotting abnormalities involve such an imbalance.

In the course of developing this theory, Papadopulos-Eleopulos became aware of the pathological effects of many of the agents to which patients belonging to Aids risk groups were exposed – and that they shared the common property of being oxidising as well as carcinogenic agents. These included semen, especially when received anally; nitrite inhalants in common use among 'at risk' sections of the gay community at that time; recreational drugs; a wide range of infectious agents and the drugs used to treat them; and Factor VIII concentrates obtained from blood donors, given to people with the clotting disorder haemophilia.

By the end of 1984 the HIV theory was almost universally accepted as the cause of the collapse of the immune system seen in Aids. It triggered a global alert, with predictions that most sexually active people were at risk of becoming infected. The risk was said to be exacerbated because of a potentially long time lag between infection, and knowing one was infected because of the onset of an actual illness.

But the Perth scientists say the theory was questionable from the start, as it was already known that over-oxidation leads to the appearance of opportunistic infections seen in Aids. In their non-infectious theory of Aids, the primary causes are the biological effects of the oxidising agents to which individuals belonging to the risk groups are exposed. The theory also predicts that Aids can be prevented and treated by the use of antioxidants.

In the early 1980s Papadoulos-Eleopulos was joined by Valendar Turner, a consultant emergency physician at the Royal Perth Hospital and John Papadimitriou, Professor of Pathology at the University of Western Australia, and subsequently several other scientists.

For nearly four decades the group has critically analysed all aspects of the HIV theory, including the evidence said to prove the existence of a new virus, and the validity of diagnostic tests based on those claims.

Efforts to silence them have come especially from beneficiaries of the multi-billion-dollar HIV/Aids industry, including publishers of leading scientific and medical journals, as well as governments, lawyers and politicians who find it difficult to believe the global scientific and medical communities could have made such a mistake, and left it uncorrected for so long.

The following is the essence of the group's explanation of how the false and unproductive HIV/Aids paradigm came about.

MISTAKE ONE: The enzyme

The first mistake, which came at the earliest stage of laboratory research, concerns an enzyme whose role is crucial in defining the very nature of retroviruses, the virus family to which HIV is said to belong. Retroviruses carry their genetic endowment in the form of RNA rather than DNA. To replicate, they first need to copy their RNA into DNA. This is engineered by an enzyme known as reverse transcriptase (RT) which the HIV experts claim is carried inside the virus particles. The activity of this enzyme can be measured and when the HIV pioneers detected this phenomenon in laboratory cultures they chose to interpret it as proof for the presence of such a virus, despite it being known as early as 1973 that the enzyme is not specific to retroviruses.*

In a 1988 *Scientific American* article describing the history of the purported discovery of HIV, Robert Gallo and Luc Montagnier, the two scientists most identified with pioneering the theory, wrote: 'The specimen [tissue from the swollen lymph node of a gay man at risk of Aids] was minced, put into tissue culture and analysed for reverse transcriptase. After two weeks of culture, reverse-transcriptase activity was detected in the culture medium. A retrovirus was present.' This was despite Gallo having been among those who showed there could be RT activity in cells free of retroviruses, long before the alleged discovery of HIV.

Nearly a decade later, in a 1997 video interview Montagnier gave to the French investigative journalist Djamel Tahi, he still claimed RT activity 'is truly specific to retroviruses'. This belief was central to the case that he and his team were the first to discover HIV, a discovery for which in 2008 he and his co-worker Françoise Barré-Sinoussi received the Nobel Prize.

Yet it is now known that at least two fifths of the human genome is made up of retrotransposons, mobile genetic elements that can amplify themselves within cells by first being transcribed from DNA to RNA, and then reverse transcribed to DNA. RNA plays a major role in gene expression, and reverse transcriptase is ubiquitous within cells. Detection of RT activity does not mean the presence of a retrovirus. Furthermore, several 'non-HIV' microbes reverse transcribe, including some bacteria, and hepatitis B virus which infects many Aids patients.

More than 100 plant and animal viruses which reverse transcribe have also been identified.

MISTAKE TWO: The particle

The false assumption that the reverse transcriptase activity in cell cultures meant a retrovirus was present led to a second huge error in the construction of the HIV theory. This involved by-passing a vital step in virus identification:

* *http://theperthgroup.com/HIV/ReverseTranscriptasesFinal.pdf*

the separation of viral particles from cellular material. This step is known as purification. 'Viruses are particles,' the Perth scientists say. 'Without proof for the existence of particles there is no proof of the existence of a virus.'

It was not that the Montagnier and Gallo teams did not try. Both regularly attempted to purify particles from cultures of cells taken from Aids patients, or at risk of Aids, using a technique long-established in retrovirology known as sucrose density gradient ultracentrifugation. In this, a drop of the culture fluid is spun in a high-speed centrifuge containing a sucrose solution, whose concentration (and hence density) increases the further down the tube the material under investigation travels. Any retrovirus particles present gather at a characteristic density. The material at that density is harvested, and examined with an electron microscope (EM) in the hope of demonstrating the presence of particles.

Montagnier's group cultured cells from a 33-year-old homosexual man with swollen lymph nodes, who indicated that he had had more than 50 sexual partners a year and had travelled to many countries. He had a history of several episodes of gonorrhoea, and just three months previously had been treated for syphilis.

In the first of several cell culture experiments the group identified reverse transcriptase activity, which they interpreted as meaning a retrovirus was present. RT was also detected in their second experiment, where cells from their patient were co-cultured (mixed) with the cells of a healthy blood donor. Despite repeatedly looking, however, they failed to report particles in either of these experiments.

In the third experiment, Montagnier took lymphocyte cells from umbilical cord blood, obtained from two placentas, and cultured these with fluids from the second experiment from which all cells had been removed. The idea was to see whether a transmissible agent was present in the fluids. In this case a single micrograph of the (unpurified) cell culture did show a few particles resembling a retrovirus, which the group took to be 'HIV'. But umbilical cord cell cultures are known to produce such particles, independent of 'HIV' infection or indeed any viral infection whatsoever. No control experiment was done, to see whether the umbilical cord lymphocytes by themselves would produce a similar result.

Even if the particles did originate from the patient's swollen lymph nodes, and not from the umbilical cord cells, that would still not make them a retrovirus, let alone 'HIV'. In an extensive, blinded, 1988 electron microscope study from Harvard, 'HIV particles' were found in 18 out of 20 patients (90%) with enlarged lymph nodes attributed to Aids, and in 13 out of 15 patients (87%) with enlarged lymph nodes not attributed to Aids.

In other words, particles that simply look as if they might be retroviruses are non-specific. They can be detected in individuals with non-Aids-related illnesses; and also where no illness is present.

This is why it is so important to purify, in order to then be able to examine virus particles, precisely characterise their constituents, and prove they are infectious.

In her biography for the Nobel Prize announcement, Barré-Sinoussi gives the impression that purification was achieved when she states that 'it was important to visualise the retroviral particles, and Charles Dauguet [the team's electron microscopist]...provided the first images of the virus in February 1983. The isolation, amplification and characterisation of the virus rapidly ensued'.

However, when Djamel Tahi pressed Montagnier on this issue in a 1997 interview, asking 'Why do the EM photographs published by you come from the culture and not from the purification?', Montagnier replied: 'We saw some particles [in the "purified virus" material] but they did not have the morphology typical of retroviruses. They were very different.' Of Gallo's work, he said: 'I don't know if he really purified. I don't believe so.'

Dauguet later went further, telling Tahi: 'We have never seen virus particles in the purified virus. What we have seen all the time was cellular debris, no virus particles.'

This goes to the crux of the matter. Cellular debris means broken-down pieces of cells used in the cultures. Yet because of the RT activity, Montagnier was convinced he had found a retrovirus. This being the case, the patient from whom he believed the virus had come would have produced antibodies which would react with the virus proteins. When Montagnier incubated blood serum from the patient with what Dauguet called 'cellular debris', three proteins were identified as producing a reaction, and Montagnier concluded that one of these was 'specifically recognised' as viral.

But there was no scientific justification for this conclusion. It has been seen subsequently that many healthy humans have antibodies that react with this third protein, identified as p24 (a molecular weight of 24,000). It is also known that at least one non-viral, ubiquitous, normal cell component in the 'debris' is a protein with the same molecular weight. Yet it became the basis of Montagnier's case for having isolated a new virus; and for the subsequent Nobel Prize. Even today, the detection of this protein, p24, in blood or culture is taken to prove the presence of the virus, and described as 'virus isolation'.

In May 1984 Robert Gallo published four papers in *Science* with many similarities to the French group's experiments, though he tested samples from more patients, and used an immortal (cancer) cell line to obtain large amounts of proteins for diagnosis and research. His claims to have found the virus that was 'the probable cause of Aids' held no more validity than Montagnier's, however, because he too failed to observe, purify and characterise actual virus particles.

In 2003 the Perth group emailed Gallo asking if he was aware of Montagnier's admission that there were no electron microscope pictures of 'purified virus' from the original patient, and whether clinicians had cause for concern about the implication of Montagnier's answer. Had clinicians spent two decades diagnosing patients with a non-existent virus?

Gallo replied: 'Montagnier subsequently published pictures of purified HIV as, of course, we did in our first papers. You have no need of worry. The evidence is obvious and overwhelming.'

Gallo's reassurance has no basis in fact, the Perth scientists say. Not a single electron micrograph of purified 'HIV' was published by Gallo in 1984, or since. Neither has Montagnier published such pictures. Fourteen years later, European and US groups who tried to make good this deficiency were still unable to provide clear evidence of the existence of 'HIV'. Their electron microscope photographs showed that the density gradient material called 'purified HIV' since 1983 contained extensive cell debris – it was anything but pure, neither in regard to particles nor alleged HIV proteins.

MISTAKE THREE: The test

The 'HIV test' looks for a reaction between antibodies in a person's bloodstream with proteins (antigens) defined as coming from 'HIV'. But the 'HIV' antigens were identified as such not on the basis of being shown to belong to a specific virus, but on the basis that they reacted with antibodies in patients with Aids or at risk of Aids. Those patients were then diagnosed as being infected with 'HIV', with all the many consequences the diagnosis brings. This reasoning was entirely circular. It lies at the root of the erroneous 'HIV/Aids' construct which dominated public health concerns for decades.

Gallo, whose team developed and marketed the first test kits, stated in 2006 that 'no test in medicine is perfect, but done correctly and with a confirmatory second test, the HIV blood test developed in our laboratory comes close...HIV tests were highly accurate from the time they were developed in 1984 and have become much more accurate over time as the underlying technology has evolved. HIV tests are among the most accurate available in medical science.'

However, the principle behind the tests is just the same today as it was in 1984, and it remains just as false.

Remarkably, the problem was half-acknowledged by public health experts in the early years of Aids. Delegates at a 1986 World Health Organization (WHO) meeting in Geneva heard that the test kits were licensed to protect blood supplies and plasma donations, as they served as a broad screen for possible abnormalities in blood. Patients with Aids and at risk of Aids suffer a range of active infections and other blood abnormalities, some of which are transmissible. However, a lack of evidence that the antibody reactions were specific to 'HIV' meant that the kits should not be used to diagnose or screen for HIV as such, the experts were told.

People with severe immune deficiency, such as Aids patients and those at risk of Aids, have abnormally high levels of antibodies, any of which could react with the protein in the antibody test kits. Something more was needed to distinguish genuine 'HIV' infection or indeed determine if there were truly such a thing as 'genuine HIV infection', the meeting heard.

Subsequent research has repeatedly confirmed that many different conditions cause raised levels of these antibodies, putting a person at risk of being labelled 'HIV'-positive when in fact there is no such virus present. They include mycobacterial infections such as TB and leprosy, widespread among impoverished people, and the cause of millions of misdiagnosed 'Aids' cases in Africa.

Gay men leading 'fast track' sex lives with multiple partners, along with drug addicts, blood product recipients, and others whose immune systems are exposed to multiple challenges that put them at risk of Aids – including malnourished people in poor countries – are more likely to have raised levels of the antibodies looked for by the tests than the general population.

The 100 experts from 34 countries heard at the WHO meeting that a so-called 'confirmatory test', called western blot, relied on the same principle as the test kits it was supposed to be checking and so was also incapable of being used to diagnose HIV/Aids.

How, then, did the 'HIV' test take off as a diagnostic tool and 'HIV/Aids' become a global belief system? Despite all the cautions being sounded, a representative from the US Food and Drug Administration told the Geneva meeting that public health needs had caused usage to expand and 'it was simply not practical' to stop this.

In retrospect, it was like Pontius Pilate washing his hands before the crucifixion, although the atmosphere at the time was such as to make it immensely difficult for reason to prevail.

Soon afterwards, epidemiological studies showed a close association between testing 'HIV'-positive and risk of developing Aids. These studies were interpreted as providing proof of the viral theory. But the link was artificial, a consequence of the circular reasoning behind the way the test kits were constructed.

As the HIV/Aids paradigm won worldwide acceptance, increasingly complex procedures for trying to make a reliable diagnosis came into being. But the basic problem – not being able to validate any of these procedures against pure virus taken from patients – still remains.

MISTAKE FOUR: The genome

HIV's existence, and the viral theory of Aids, became the consensus view before data were accumulated on genetic sequences said to comprise the virus's genome. As described, public health experts set aside their reservations about the validity of the 'HIV' test because in the febrile atmosphere of the time they felt it was 'simply not practical' to stop the test from being used to diagnose Aids or risk of Aids.

As time went on, claims that a full-length genome had been sequenced seemed to offer reassurance that despite the failure to obtain virus particles, 'HIV' was a tangible reality.

Gallo's complex and ingenious work was the foundation for these claims and is still the best available proof for the existence of an 'HIV' genome. It fails close examination, however, for the same reason as the 'HIV' test: lack of actual virus particles from which to obtain the genome and to validate the assumptions made.

One fundamental flaw came to light through a two-year US National Institutes of Health Office of Scientific Integrity investigation into Gallo's laboratory practices, following an allegation of scientific misconduct. It found that a cell line which Gallo claimed to have infected with HIV had not been exposed to material from an individual Aids patient, but to culture fluids from first three and then ultimately from 10 patients. The inquiry, which found this to be 'of dubious scientific rigour' (one scientist called it 'really crazy'), was told by one of Gallo's co-workers that he had to pool the cultures because none 'individually was producing high concentrations of reverse transcriptase'. It was like getting 10 patients with suspected pneumonia all to spit in the same pot.

Gallo's team further claimed that the virus genome, the RNA, was obtained from purified virus particles. In fact, Gallo never published electron microscope pictures of the so-called 'purified virus' material. The RNA obtained was a type called messenger RNA (mRNA) that cells use as an intermediate between DNA and the synthesis of proteins. It had long been known that such cellular RNA bands in the centrifuge at the density considered characteristic of retroviruses.

When the RNA was reverse transcribed into DNA fragments of varying size, and those fragments were shown to bind to RNA obtained from 'infected' but not 'uninfected' cell lines, Gallo interpreted the fragments as the genome of a retrovirus. In further studies, he reproduced this 'genome' through molecular cloning techniques.

However, this was another example of circular thinking. The binding between DNA and RNA in the genetic sequences he was manipulating was to be expected, since the same material (what he was calling 'purified virus') was used both to obtain the 'HIV RNA' and to infect the cell cultures. Under such circumstances it would be impossible *not* to demonstrate DNA-RNA complementarities. Furthermore, since RNA of the type seen is not unique to retroviruses, he had no valid grounds for assuming the presence of a new viral agent. At no point did Gallo provide evidence to support the claim that 'virus particles were purified', nor even that they existed in the material with which he was working.

When Gallo did test Aids patients directly for the presence of the purported 'HIV' genome, he failed to find evidence for it.* In other words, contrary to the HIV theory of Aids, Gallo was not able to prove the existence of the HIV genome in Aids patients.**

Neither Gallo nor Montagnier, nor any other researcher from that day to this, has defined the 'HIV' genome by obtaining RNA from purified retroviral particles. After all these years, there is still no proof of the existence of the genome of a new virus, nor of the existence of the whole 'HIV' genome in even one Aids patient.

Tiny segments of the purported genome can be detected through the polymerase chain reaction (PCR) test, and are often wrongly taken as confirmation of an 'HIV' diagnosis, even though the segments vary to such an extent that the experts have to create 'consensus sequences' for the purpose of diagnosing infection. The variation can often be as high as 30-40 per cent. That compares with less than two per cent between the human and chimpanzee genome. Even 50 per cent variation is accepted by most

* *http://theperthgroup.com/HIV/TPGVirusLikeNoOther.pdf#page=39*

** *http://theperthgroup.com/CONTINUUM/PapadopolousReallyAchieved1996.pdf*

researchers without their questioning whether they are really working with a unique viral entity.

This huge variability is much more consistent with the sequences being newly generated RNA of abnormally stimulated cells than of a virus for which no researcher has ever published proof of purification. Whether the stimulus comes from chemical agents used on cells in the laboratory, the many biological and non-biological chemicals to which Aids patients or those at risk are exposed, or from the variety of infectious agents to which the Aids risk groups are repeatedly exposed, the common factor is the 'shock' to the cells and not the common presence of a mythical virus. This interpretation is supported by the finding of so-called 'HIV' sequences from tumour tissue in several types of cancer.

What this means is that an army of people around the world are doing tests for a virus never proved to exist using proteins and nucleic acids originating from normal cells, albeit abnormally stimulated. It is a tragedy blighting millions of lives.

MISTAKE FIVE: The STD

Along with rapid acceptance of the virus theory, the idea quickly caught on that Aids was a sexually transmitted disease with heterosexual as well as homosexual intercourse as the main route of transmission. Governments across the world launched health education campaigns warning that as the predicted pandemic spread, almost all sexually active people would become at risk.

Even after nearly 40 years, however, there is no microbiological proof of sexual transmission based on the isolation of 'HIV' from genital secretions of index cases followed by tracing and testing of sexual contacts. And except in the context of poor countries where many diseases of poverty have been renamed as 'Aids', the syndrome has remained confined to groups at risk because of lifestyle factors rather than because of exposure to a non-discriminatory STD.

Pioneers of the virus theory felt supported in their belief that Aids was an STD by the fact that many early studies documented a relationship between different types of sexual activity and the presence or appearance of 'HIV' antibodies, for which almost all Aids patients tested positive.

This association was real. But it came about because of the flawed way the test was developed, not because a new virus was present.

A positive test indicates elevated levels of antibodies induced by the many immune-stimulating agents to which those in the Aids risk groups have been exposed. Epidemiologists and others documented such exposures from day one.

This means that people who tested 'HIV'-positive should never have been given to understand that they were under a death sentence, as was the case for many years because of the 'lethal new virus' belief. If exposure to the true causes of 'HIV'-positivity is reduced or ended, the increased risk of ill-health may disappear unless the damage caused to the immune system is already irreversible.

This was seen particularly clearly in haemophiliacs. Early ways of treating their blood clotting disorder involved exposing them to concentrates made from blood donations from hundreds of thousands of people. Many tested positive as a result of this challenge from foreign protein. When genetic engineering made it possible to produce the clotting factor they were missing in a pure form, they showed signs of immune system recovery.

Similar results have been seen in drug addicts, another of the groups at risk of Aids. For example, the former head of the Australian national serology reference laboratory has published a study which showed that HIV-positive drug addicts lose their 'HIV' antibodies and revert to HIV-negative when they give up their habit. If, however, such individuals continue to be exposed to risk factors that caused them to test positive in the first place, they will face an increased risk of illness that has nothing to do with 'HIV'.

The Perth scientists say that one of the main true causes of both 'HIV'-positivity and Aids is exposure to anally deposited semen. They cite numerous studies in homosexual men that have shown that whereas a person exposed to frequent, unprotected, receptive anal sex is at high risk of testing positive, and subsequently developing Aids, no such risk is associated with the insertive (semen-donating) individual. In heterosexual studies the evidence is the same: the only sexual risk factor for acquiring a positive antibody test is passive anal intercourse.

For Aids to appear, they say, a high frequency of receptive anal intercourse over a long period is necessary. In contrast to vaginal intercourse, anally deposited semen is retained and absorbed. Whereas the rectum is lined only by a single layer of absorptive cells, the vagina has a multi-layered, skin-like protective lining.

Early acceptance of the virus hypothesis of Aids meant that the role of heavy exposure to semen in causing the condition remained largely overlooked and unexamined. Nevertheless, further evidence in support of this claim includes the fact that semen is one of the most potent biological oxidants, and there is theoretical and experimental evidence for it being both carcinogenic and immunosuppressive. In addition, rectal and colonic trauma accompanying passive anal intercourse – facilitating the absorption of semen – are proven risk factors. Volatile nitrite inhalants, widely used to facilitate gay sex in the early years of Aids, may also facilitate absorption of semen as well as being potent oxidising, immunosuppressive agents in their own right.

'The evidence shows that Aids is not a disease of sexual orientation but of sexual practices, passive anal intercourse in men and women', the Perth scientists say. 'It is not the sexual act *per se* but high frequencies of passive anal intercourse with ejaculation combined with drug use and trauma to the intestinal lining which facilitate system absorption of semen and other toxins.'

MISTAKE SIX: The drugs

Protagonists of the virus theory of Aids maintain that HIV was proven to be the cause in 1984, with publication of the original Gallo and Montagnier papers. Any remaining doubt, they say, was dispelled by the success of a 'cocktail' of drugs introduced in 1996 specifically to control 'HIV' replication. Known as HAART – Highly Active Antiretroviral Therapy – the drugs are said to have transformed HIV infection into 'a manageable chronic condition'.

The Perth scientists acknowledge that the drugs do help prevent the onset of familiar diseases which, in the presence of 'HIV' antibodies, have been defined as Aids. But they refute the claim that this confirms 'HIV' as the cause, on several grounds:

1. Regardless of their putative 'anti-HIV' effects, numerous studies demonstrate that the drugs are toxic to microbes causing some of the most common and severe Aids-defining diseases, including tuberculosis and fungal infections.

2. Changes in the definition of Aids created an illusion of a fast-growing epidemic, as more and more conditions of *decreasing* severity – and even no symptomatic illness at all – were brought under the umbrella diagnosis of 'HIV'/Aids. Between 1981 and 1984, the young homosexual men who were the first victims had essentially two lethal illnesses, an aggressive form of fungal pneumonia and a rare cancer called Kaposi's sarcoma. All had been leading fast-track lives with multiple sex partners and heavy drug use as part of the 'gay liberation' fight. In March 1985, the US Food and Drug Administration licensed the first commercial 'HIV' test for screening the blood supply, and in April 1987 a supposedly confirmatory test for diagnosing 'HIV' infection was introduced. With none of these tests actually capable of diagnosing the (imaginary) 'HIV', the authorities were able to make successive redefinitions of Aids in 1985, 1987 and again in 1993. These took the number of Aids-defining conditions to six, 23, and 26 respectively, including 'mild and moderate' diseases. The 1993 change brought a doubling of Aids diagnoses in the US and elsewhere, as it also required physicians to report HIV-positive individuals with a low T4 (immune cell) count as Aids cases, even in the absence of disease. Not surprisingly, these changes brought a rapid decrease in the death rate from Aids several years before HAART began to be introduced in 1996. Deaths fell significantly in 1995 and the introduction of HAART in 1996 made no obvious difference to the rate at which they kept falling in 1996-7.

3. Other factors that help explain a falling death rate before the introduction of HAART include behaviour change in homosexual men, who were first to recognise the relationship between the two original Aids diseases and intense sex-and-drugs activity. Those

> who had been most heavily exposed during the 1970s would have died during the 1980s. Also, an increase in federal funding in 1994 for Aids patients led to better prevention and treatment of opportunistic infections.

Finally, evidence from the outcome of hundreds of clinical trials of HAART, far from confirming the HIV theory of Aids, has instead disproven it 'beyond reasonable doubt', the scientists say.

HAART is believed to save lives by interrupting the replication cycle of 'HIV', reducing the purported 'viral load' (also known as 'HIV viraemia') in patients and thus reversing the decline in their immunity, thought to be indicated by a falling T4-cell count. According to the virus theory of Aids, these two measures are central to the disease process: HIV is held to be the cause and declining T4 cells the mechanism leading to Aids and death.

However, a 2008 review of data obtained from 178 randomised clinical trials of the drugs found that whereas most HAART therapies do appear to offer high levels of control over these two markers for assumed risk of Aids, the changes did not correlate with actual Aids cases and deaths.

Papadoulos-Eleopulos and her colleagues conclude: 'Even if you were to accept that HIV exists, these clinical trials show it has nothing to do with the deaths of millions of people from Aids. And since, to date, nobody has published proof that the "HIV" RNA, whose measurement is used to determine the "viral load", originates from a retroviral particle, the explanation that there is no virus must hold true. There is no "HIV" causing Aids because there is no HIV.'

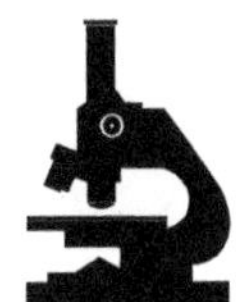

EPILOGUE

Oxford, January 2023

Two key differences, I feel, separate the HIV/Aids story from that of Covid.

One is that whereas Covid is caused by a highly infectious virus, Aids has never been proved to be an infectious disease, which is why it never spread as predicted. I hope the evidence to that effect cited in this book may finally pave the way to a rethink.

A second, related difference between the two is that whereas a novel 'vaccine', now shown to be not only dangerous but largely ineffective, was thrust upon us almost from the start of the Covid pandemic, 40 years of research have failed to find an equivalent for Aids.

That is because 'HIV' does not exist as a distinct viral entity. The political and social context in which a belief in HIV arose allowed it to take root and flourish, but to this day the mainstream scientific community has not even acknowledged, let alone answered, the work of other scientists who challenge the virus theory.

Hundreds of billions of dollars flowed into HIV/Aids research and treatment, much of it coming from US taxpayers. This windfall contributed to astonishing advances in molecular biology, giving scientists refined tools capable of manipulating the genes of both microbes and people. But these advances had the less happy result of setting in motion developments that led directly to the Covid crisis.

Defence experts became concerned that bioweapons of unprecedented lethality were now within reach. American and Chinese scientists, among others, collaborated with the aim of producing instant 'vaccine' antidotes to such agents. In the course of that research, they turned a bat virus into the microbe that causes Covid.

When this escaped from the laboratory in Wuhan, China, an industry specialising in global health security already had in place machinery to persuade governments and people worldwide to adopt mass immunisation as the main means to combat the virus. Pandemic planning exercises had included 'psy-op' rehearsals involving media manipulation and mass censorship. Transnational organisations such as the Davos-birthed Coalition on Epidemic Preparedness, with key players including the Gates Foundation and Wellcome Trust, swung into action, seeking billions more to counter future threats.

Just as with HIV/Aids, the science went badly off course. Data soon emerged showing the Covid virus to be much less harmful than statistical models had predicted. This, however, did not suit the fear-mongering narrative.

Wrongful use of the polymerase chain reaction test as a diagnostic tool created a mountain of false positive results – as had also happened with Aids. Deaths of very sick and elderly people were inappropriately reclassified as involving Covid, making the crisis look far worse than it really was.

Those scientists who persisted in challenging official doctrines were ruthlessly censored and often denigrated, discredited and intimidated by the medical establishment and mainstream media.

With Aids, challenges to the HIV theory were labelled homophobic. With Covid, questioning the official narrative was deemed disloyal. Facebook even removed factually correct posts that made people 'feel unsafe'.

When *Aids: The Failure of Contemporary Science* was published in 1996, I was convinced it would only be a matter of months before the edifice of illusion collapsed.

I could hardly have been more wrong. The closest we saw as a correction and apology was in June 2008, a quarter of a century after Aids was first identified, when the World Health Organisation admitted that the universal prevention strategy promoted by the major Aids organisations 'may have been misdirected': the threat of a global heterosexual pandemic had disappeared. Millions were still said to be dying in Africa, however, where as we have seen, misinterpretation of diseases of poverty has brought prolonged and far-reaching harm.

No official inquiry into the mishandling of Aids has ever been held. Most people have had no means of knowing that the 'Don't Die of Ignorance' propaganda campaigns to which a generation of young people were exposed have been discredited.

With Covid, the harm has been far greater. Many have now recognised the folly of scare tactics such as social distancing and mask mandates, the unnecessary disruption of children's development and schooling, the ill-treatment of old people forced to die alone, the crisis in health care, and the economic mayhem brought by lockdowns.

Perhaps the sheer scale of the damage will be enough this time to force a reckoning. One hopeful sign is that the advent of the internet has meant censorship could not be as near-total with Covid as it was with Aids.

As I write, however, the biggest disaster of all remains largely unaddressed: mass administration of an experimental vaccine which in many people, especially the young, is more of a threat to health than the virus itself. Millions of injuries and thousands of deaths have been reported globally in the wake of the jabs. Thanks to some outspoken doctors and scientists we now know much about the mechanisms of immediate harm, and as I write, unprecedented changes in the immune system following multiple jabs are being linked to increased vulnerability to infections and cancer.

Yet regulators, manufacturers, and rich medical funding agencies continue to insist the Covid jabs are 'safe and effective' and are even trying to persuade us that the same experimental mRNA technology can be used to tackle Aids.

David Bell, a public health physician and Brownstone Institute scholar, has observed that inventing truth can be more effective than bending it.

In a paper called *Global Health and the Art of Really Big Lies*, he writes of having had a boss whose fantasies, 'massive in scope and delivered with sincerity', went unchallenged. Over time, colleagues who raised questions learned that 'integrity was a poor career choice, whilst good team players supported false narratives.' In the same way, holding to the new dogma in public health 'enables a positive career path and financial security - as did siding with the Inquisition centuries ago.'

Error correction is supposed to be one of the strengths of science but in the case of both Aids and Covid, it has failed dismally. 'HIV/Aids' was and is the first Really Big Lie of our era, and it stands uncorrected to this day. While we continue to avoid facing up to such massive deceptions, further disasters must be expected.

The human intellect is a magnificent tool, capable of redirecting the course of history. Can it yet come to our rescue?

www.ingramcontent.com/pod-product-compliance
Lightning Source LLC
Chambersburg PA
CBHW082119210326
41599CB00031B/5809
* 9 7 8 1 9 1 5 3 3 8 5 0 1 *